Herbs for Health and Healing

by Kathi Keville
Director of the American Herb Association

with Peter Korn

Medical Reviewer: David Edelberg, M.D.,
Medical Director, American Holistic Centers

Rodale Press, Inc.
Emmaus, Pennsylvania

A FRIEDMAN GROUP BOOK

Copyright © 1996 by Kathi Keville
Illustrations copyright © 1996 by Roman Szolkowski
Photographs copyright © 1996 by Alison Miksch

Art Director: Lynne Yeamans
Cover Designer: Faith Hague
Illustrator: Roman Szolkowski
Cover Photographer: Alison Miksch

Printed in the United States of America on acid-free ∞,
recycled paper ♻

Library of Congress Cataloging-in-Publication Data
    Keville, Kathi.
        Herbs for health and healing / by Kathi Keville with Peter Korn.
            p. cm.
        Includes bibliographical references and index.
        ISBN 0–87596–293–9 hardcover
        ISBN 0–57954–045–7 paperback

    1. Herbs—Therapeutic use.   I. Korn, Peter. 1955– .   II. Title.
RM666.H33K47 1996
615'.321—dc20   96–10561

Distributed in the book trade by St. Martin's Press

6   8   10   9   7   hardcover

2   4   6   8   10   9   7   5   3   1   paperback

─── **OUR PURPOSE** ───

*"We inspire and enable people to improve
their lives and the world around them."*

DEDICATION

I dedicate this book to everyone who strolls down the path of natural healing. May it be lined with healing herbs and lead to health and happiness. I especially want to dedicate it to my family: my father, Jesse Keville, who shared with me his love of chemistry; my mother, Naomi Keville, who imparted her appreciation of art and nature; and my sister, Janna Buesch, who furthered my understanding of nutrition.

ACKNOWLEDGMENTS

A warm thank you to the herbalists who have given me suggestions and support: Steven Foster, David Hoffmann, Sara Smith, Rosemary Gladstar, Mindy Green and especially Christopher Hobbs, Beth Baugh and Bob Brucia, who also let me use their extensive herbal libraries. I also thank the many people who allowed me to share their herbal success stories in this book and to all my students—who have taught me how to share herbal knowledge. My sincere appreciation to my team of editors, Sharyn Rosart, Peter Korn and especially Ben Boyington. They all worked diligently to help make botanical chemistry, natural medicine and physiology easy to understand and to use.

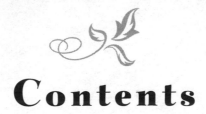

Contents

PART III: Living with Herbal Wisdom

Introduction

Opening Ourselves to Nature's Wisdom

Herbs have fascinated me for years. The first thing that captured my attention was the beauty of the plants, which I realized could fill my garden with color and texture. Using the first edition of Rodale's *Encyclopedia of Organic Gardening* as a guide, I planted dozens of herbs among my vegetables and flowers.

I soon realized that herbs offered a wide variety of wonderful flavors—the cooking possibilities, it seemed, were nearly endless. As I read more, I found that herbs could be used to improve my complexion and health and that their fragrances could even affect my emotions. As my interest grew, so did my herb garden—until I was cultivating more than 400 different species. Learning about these plants has become a lifelong passion.

When I first began studying herbalism in 1969, I never imagined that it would grow to be as popular as it is today. In time, my initial interest grew into a vocation—I am now a professional herbalist. I grow hundreds of herbs in my garden, I give seminars on herbs throughout the United States and I write articles on herbalism for national magazines and books for various publishers. Since I became a practitioner of this ancient art, I have watched enthusiasm about herbs swell. I have seen an increased response to my seminars on herbs. And my friends in the herb industry tell me that sales are soaring. Indeed, the entire Western world is taking a renewed interest in the age-old tradition of using herbal treatments for health and beauty.

Today, herbs are commonplace as ingredients in most cosmetics and gourmet foods, but the most impressive renaissance of herbalism is in the field of medicine. Once regarded as "alternative" medicine, herbalism is now recognized as a "complementary" approach to be used in conjunction with typical Western medical methods. Even after nearly three decades of working with herbs, I continue to be amazed by their effectiveness. Just yesterday, a friend called to say how excited she was that herbal formulas had healed a disorder she had been fighting for years. I have seen many remarkable cures effected by herbs, and I have chronicled some of them here. After you start using the recipes in this guide, I am sure that you will be able to tell some impressive herbal healing stories of your own!

In case the personal accounts in this book are not enough to convince you that herbs are effective, I have also cited evidence from numerous scientific studies. As you read about these studies, keep in mind that even the scientists who conduct them do not regard their results as conclusive, but as pieces of a puzzle that can help us understand how plants work. I have tried to cite only studies done on people or in laboratory test tubes, primarily because I find them more reliable than studies done on animals. The drug thalidomide, for instance, was shown to be safe for laboratory animals, but caused serious birth defects in the children of women who took the drug. Curiously enough, the problem was originally blamed on an herb. My other reason for avoiding studies done on animals is more controversial—I hate to see animals put through misery to prove the usefulness of an herb, especially one that herbalists have been using successfully for hundreds of years. (By citing animal studies, I would be condoning this practice.) Making helpless creatures suffer seems an odd way to improve our knowledge of healing and our ability to heal.

Before you start reading, remember this: Herbal therapy does not have to be mysterious or complicated. This book can help you treat many conditions that you would diagnose yourself anyway, and it will enable you to choose your

own medications at a drugstore without a prescription. For example, when you come down with a cold, you may buy a cough syrup to ease your cough and an antihistamine to clear sinus congestion. After reading this book, chances are you will be visiting a natural food store or your garden to get the herbal alternatives to the drugs you normally use. If you know nothing about medicinal herbs, do not worry. The remedies I recommend are totally safe—call them "over-the-counter" herbs, if you like.

As soon as I discovered how well herbs work, I threw out all my drugs and cosmetics and turned to nature's pharmacy and beauty salon instead. You may react the same way—or you may feel more comfortable working herbs into your medicine cabinet more gradually. Whatever your approach, think of herbalism in a new light—one different from standard medicine. Herbalism embraces the principles of holistic medicine. This means that most herbalists are not interested in simply replacing a drug with a handful of herb pills.

The holistic approach takes the whole person into consideration and listens to all complaints, no matter how minor or unrelated they may seem. As researchers have proven over and over, your emotions do affect your health. The best way to achieve deep and lasting healing—instead of just relieving your symptoms—is to treat the causes. This means that you will not keep coming down with one thing after another or experience recurring bouts of the same illness. Say you get an ulcer or a bladder infection. Once it is healed, what keeps you from getting another one? The aim of herbalists is not only to address the immediate problem, but to strengthen your system to prevent further attacks. They also want to uncover the reason for an ulcer or a particular infection occurring in the first place.

Another difference between herbalism and conventional medicine is that herbalists almost always recommend other complementary therapies, including acupuncture and massage, and lifestyle changes, particularly with regard to nutrition and exercise. There may be elements of your lifestyle that are detrimental to your health; no herbal formula can make up for a poor diet or a sedentary lifestyle. This approach means that you have to take more responsiblity for your own health, and it may require you to change your life in certain ways. In the long run, though, the hard work is well worth it. Again and again, I have seen holistic herbalism work wonders for people who have been suffering from all sorts of conditions that standard medicine has been unable to heal.

To help you choose the right herbs, this book is filled with general formulas using my favorite herbs. These are recipes that have, in my experience, proven beneficial to many people over the years. If I could, I would prefer to custom-design a formula for each of you that would address all your conditions in a more holistic way. As you become more familiar with herbs, you may want to alter my formulas to best suit your needs. It is also a good idea to get an herb book that lists herbs in alphabetical order, such as my *Herbs: An Illustrated Encyclopedia*, which lists 140 herbs. If you don't have the time to make your own remedies, you can buy commercial herb formulas in tinctures, teas and pills. Although these will not always include exactly the same herbs that I suggest, the information in this book will help you select the commercial remedies that are best for you. Be wary, however, of brochures produced by companies that sell specific products—you cannot always trust advertising.

If you are interested in the possibilities offered by herbalism and holistic health in general, this book can be your stepping-stone into natural healing. You will discover, as I have, that healing plants can bring more health and happiness into your life.

Part I

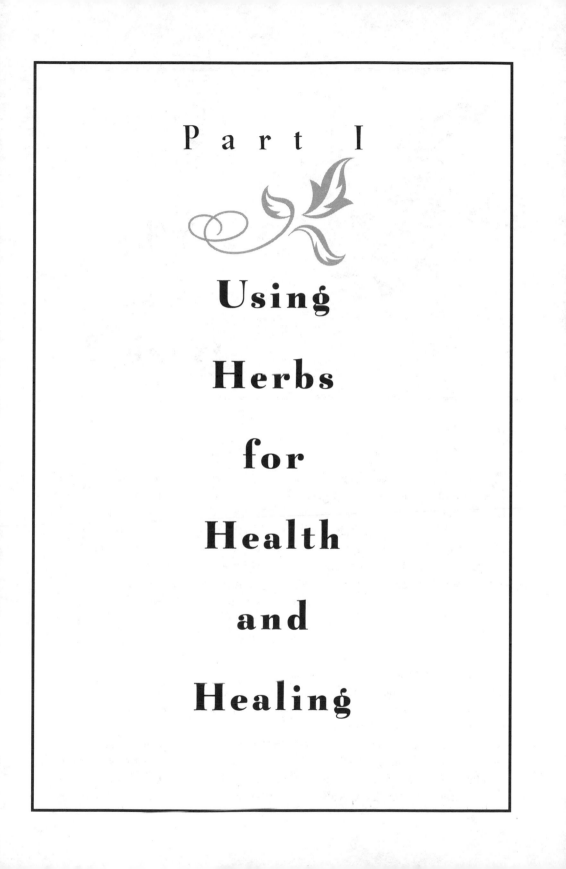

Using

Herbs

for

Health

and

Healing

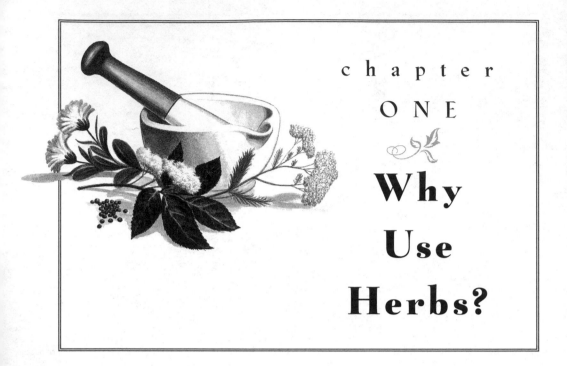

Nearly three decades ago, I began tending a culinary herb garden that slowly took over the area I had set aside for growing vegetables. Curiosity about using those herbs for purposes other than cooking soon sent me searching for information on practical uses for herbs—and eventually led me to a career as an herbalist.

Herbs were not as "in" then as they are now. Today, more and more people are rediscovering the art of healing with herbs. Some are undoubtedly attracted by herbalism's wholesome yet somewhat mysterious image. Others are simply looking for a more efficient, less dangerous alternative to conventional drugs.

Herbs *can* effectively treat many medical problems, but there is also a great deal herbs cannot do. We cannot always look to herbs as an alternative to medical science—especially in life-threatening situations. I do think, though, that we would all benefit if we filled our home medicine cabinets with herbal remedies. This book will teach you how to do just that. It will help if we lay down a few ground rules.

HEALING, NOT JUST RELIEVING

Herbal medicine works best when practiced holistically—that is, with an intent to heal the entire body and get at the sources of physical and emotional imbalance, instead of just treating the symptoms. For example, if you tend to get headaches, you can use herbs not only to ease the pain but also to eliminate the underlying condition causing the pain. This would eventually restore health and balance so that you no longer get headaches. That is real healing. To achieve this kind of result, a new look at health and healing is required. You must consider not only what you may be taking as medicine—both herbs and drugs— but your diet, your lifestyle, your mental attitude and the role that these factors play in keeping you healthy or contributing to disease.

Both traditional herbalists and modern herbal researchers believe that herbs, when properly used, encourage the body to heal itself. Herbal researcher Hildebert Wagner, Ph.D., of the Institute for Pharmaceutical Biology at the University of Munich specializes in studying herbs that improve immunity. He describes herbs as inherently health-promoting, rather than disease-killing: "With herbal remedies, it is not so much a case of totally blocking a reaction in the organism, as, for example, with cortisone or chemotherapy. Herbal preparations serve very often to regulate and stimulate the organism to promote self-healing tendencies."

The actions of many herbs can be compared to a tap on the shoulder, whereas the effects of drugs can be compared to a kick in the pants. In some cases, the body will take longer to heal itself with herbs than it would with quick-acting drugs, but the long-term result is much deeper healing. For many people, it's well worth the wait.

Herbalism also emphasizes preventive medicine—the point of many herbal treatments is to keep you from getting sick in the first place. We could all take a hint from the traditions of ancient China, where doctors were paid only when they kept their patients well.

NATURE'S THERAPY

Most medicinal herbs contain many natural compounds that play off one another, producing a wide variety of results. Even medical science does not always understand how the compounds work together, or even exactly what they all are. As botanist Walter Lewis, Ph.D., and microbiologist Memory Elvin-Lewis, Ph.D., put it in their book *Medical Botany*: "Nature is still mankind's greatest chemist, and many compounds that remain undiscovered in plants are beyond the imagination of even our best scientists."

Some herbs that regulate the body almost seem to have an inner intelligence, with the ability to perform many different functions, depending upon what the individual needs. For example, ginger can raise or lower blood pressure, depending on what needs to happen to bring an individual's blood pressure to a healthy level. And tonic herbs do more than clear up immediate, acute symptoms—they have the more general effect of renewing strength and vitality. Marshmallow, for instance, strengthens your digestive system and improves the functioning of your immune system while relieving your stomach distress.

Although 80 percent of pharmaceutical drugs are based on herbs, these drugs are generally based not on the whole herb but on one "active ingredient" derived from a plant. Modern medicine has become captivated by what it calls a "magic bullet"—a single substance that zeros in and destroys a germ or relieves a symptom. Whenever possible, the chemical structure of the active component found in an herb is duplicated in the laboratory and produced synthetically. This enables a drug company to produce formulas of consistent quality and strength and avoid the hassle and expense of collecting plants in the wild. (Not incidentally, it also enables them to patent the remedy and charge more money for it.)

These magic bullet drugs have several problems. First, they treat only specific problems. Well-known plant researcher and botanist James Duke, Ph.D., points out that "the solitary synthetic bullet offers no alternatives if the doctor has misdiagnosed the ailment or if one or more ailments require more than one compound." Herbs, on the other hand, can cover many bases at once.

Also, magic bullets don't give the body a chance to find its own solution. Dr. Duke theorizes that our bodies take fuller advantage than we realize of the complex chemistry in medicinal herbs. He believes that each herb contains hundreds of active compounds, many of which act "synergistically." That means that all these compounds somehow combine to produce a greater effect than each has alone, and that the body extracts the compounds it needs and discards the others. One possible reason that scientific studies sometimes fail to confirm an herb's traditional use in healing is that the studies often focus only on the isolated compound, not on the whole plant.

Years ago, researchers extracted an active compound called silymarin from the herb milk thistle and turned it into a pharmaceutical drug to treat liver damage. Only later did German scientists discover yet another compound in milk thistle—betaine hydrochloride—that may be equally important.

The popular immunity-enhancing herb echinacea has a similar story. For years, complex carbohydrates from echinacea were thought to be its sole active ingredient and were extracted to produce a drug. But then a team of German researchers headed by Dr. Wagner discovered that echinacea contains other compounds that enhance immunity.

In the case of the sedative herb valerian, medical researchers found that two compounds—valeric acid and essential oils—caused its calming effects, but for some time they remained unaware of still a third set of highly sedative compounds called valepotriates. And ginkgo, which is used to boost brain functions and circulation, has been found to be more effective when used in its whole form instead of its isolated active compounds.

SIDESTEPPING SIDE EFFECTS

Unfortunately, even when a potent magic bullet drug is right on the mark when it comes to resolving a certain problem, it often creates side effects—new problems. "Scarcely a month goes by without a drug being removed from the market because it is harmful," says Dr. Wagner. "This has helped to let the pendulum swing back and has brought a renewed consideration for our old treasures of experience with herbs."

The Food and Drug Administration (FDA), the governmental agency that regulates the sale of drugs in the United States, receives more than 10,000 reports of side effects from newly approved drugs every year, according to the Center for Drug Evaluation and research in Rockville, Maryland. This is especially sobering when you consider that about 25 percent of these side effects resulted in someone being hospitalized or dying. And that's only the tip of the iceberg. National surveys indicate that only about 5 percent of serious side effects from drugs are even reported to the center. The Environmental Protection Agency (EPA) says that 125,000 Americans die each year because they take their prescribed medicines incorrectly. In fact, some studies indicate that as many as half of all pharmaceuticals are not being taken correctly.

The herbs suggested in this book, however, produce few side effects, and many of them contain protective compounds that keep their potency in check. The herb meadowsweet, which contains natural aspirin (salicylic acid), is a perfect example. As you probably know, a big problem with taking chemical aspirin is that it can injure the stomach and even cause bleeding. Meadowsweet functions like aspirin to ease the pain and inflammation of

rheumatism and headaches, but it also contains astringent tannins and soothing mucilage, which researchers believe to be compounds that buffer salicylic acid's adverse side effects.

Dr. Duke speculates that the effectiveness of herbs and their less toxic effects on our bodies may be due to our long history of using medicinal plants. "We have adapted ways to be more responsive to herbs," he says. "In many cases your body, through evolution, has been exposed to these natural compounds. Perhaps it has evolved protective mechanisms against their negative effects while embracing their positive effects."

With so many reasons to use herbs, why are drugs so popular? An explanation would have to take into account doctors' medical training, the high cost of developing drugs, and patients' expectations about having their symptoms relieved. To understand this, we need to go back to 1935, when sulfa drugs, the first broad-spectrum antibiotics, revolutionized the medical world. Their success prompted heavy financial investments in pharmaceutical drug companies and rapid development of new drugs. Doctors and the public began to regard herbal medicine as old-fashioned.

BACK TO THE FUTURE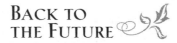

In an ideal medical system, herbalism would be viewed as a legitimate medical therapy, not as an outsider or "alternative" therapy. Recently, instruction in herbal therapy has been integrated into some medical curricula in Germany. So there is hope.

Unfortunately, in North America, medicine is extremely drug-oriented, and the American and Canadian Medical Associations have strong ties to pharmaceutical companies. It is no surprise that doctors, who are trained to use drugs, are hesitant to study herbs. Herbalist Michael Moore, author of *Medicinal Plants of the Pacific Northwest*, sums it up well: "I have known perfectly intelligent physicians whose sole regularly used reference manuals were the *Physician's Desk Reference* and *Goodman and Gillman,* both of which are drug manuals. Their patients have come to expect, and receive, prescriptions as their only therapy."

Obviously, doctors are not the only ones who consider drugs their first option for treatment. The pharmaceutical companies are also not likely to change the way they do business. They can easily spend anywhere from $50 million to $100 million, mostly for safety testing, when submitting a new drug application to the FDA for approval. These companies are willing to pay that much because a new drug can reap incredible profits for the firm that holds the patent rights. Herbs, however, are available to anyone with a garden, and they cannot be patented. Drug companies are understandably reluctant to invest in a product that their competitors can pick up after the research is done. The result is that few herbal remedies are manufactured commercially, and drug use (especially use of specific brands of drugs) is encouraged.

ENVIRONMENTAL AND ETHICAL CONCERNS

Another plus for herbal medicine is that it is environmentally sound. One person who has considered the relationship between environmental pollution and drugs is English herbalist David Hoffmann. Author of a number of herb books, including *The Holistic Herbal* and *Successful Stress Control,* Hoffmann's major issue when he ran for Parliament in England was global ecology. He focused on what happens when you regularly take a common drug used to treat stomach ulcers and gastritis: "You become very involved in an ecological cycle that involves all of the pollution produced in the factories that prepare the drug. It just happens that this process is a very messy one. In the process of healing our ulcers, we buy into killing fish, into environmental destruction, and we legitimize the destruction of laboratory animals. Is that healing? I suggest that it is not."

Hoffmann also points out that the pharmaceutical industry is one of the biggest practitioners of vivisection (operating on a living animal for research purposes). The research and development of new drugs generally involves killing thousands of laboratory animals. The resulting drugs are then tested on more animals before being declared safe for humans. "You can sip herbal tea without worrying that a rat or a guinea pig had to die to enable you to do so," he says.

Instead of contributing to destroying the environment, herbs bring us closer to it. Herbalist and acupuncturist Michael Tierra, author of *Planetary Herbology*, believes that herbs can make us more conscious of our place among all of Earth's living things: "The path of the herbalist is one that can offer a vital link to the natural and interaction with nature's wilds. It gives us a point of view by which we can see ourselves as being connected with the entire process of life."

Although herbalism in the United States and Canada is only beginning to recover its lost prestige, other countries have successfully combined it with conventional medicine. In China, for example, traditional medicine that includes herbs is fully integrated into the nation's health care system, and natural remedies are used in nearly half of the cases treated there. In fact, only about 15 percent of the world's population has access to Western-style health care services. Most people in developing nations still rely on herbal treatments.

The World Health Organization, the United Nations agency that monitors health and health problems around the world, considers traditional medicine well-suited for the Third World for several reasons. It is less expensive than Western medicine, it is usually effective for local health problems and it is already well-integrated into most Third World cultures. The first two of these reasons are arguments in favor of reintroducing herbalism into industrialized countries.

As public opinion begins to sway from complete faith in drugs, interest in herbs is increasing. Perhaps the day is not far off when the designations of traditional and modern medicine will have no significance, and all health care practitioners will feel comfortable working in a new system that incorporates both disciplines.

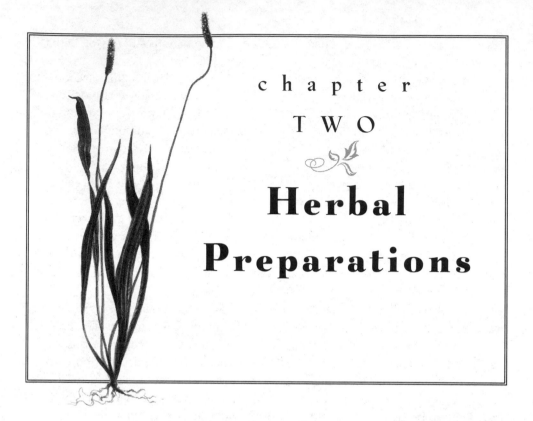

An herbalist's definition of an herb differs from that of a botanist. The botanist defines an herbaceous plant as one with a fleshy stem that dies back in the winter. The herbalist, however, considers all medicinal and cosmetic plants as herbs. This broad definition of herbs includes trees, shrubs, mushrooms, lichens and, of course, fruits and vegetables that have medicinal properties. In many of my recipes, you will find items that you consider food rather than herbs, such as apple juice or shiitake mushrooms.

There are countless different herbs and combinations of herbs that are used for health and healing. But even the most potent herb can become worthless if not properly prepared. Fortunately, there are only a few basic kinds of preparations that are used in treating illnesses and wounds herbally; these are the delivery systems for the healing powers of herbs.

These preparations transform dried or fresh herbs into something that can be taken internally, such as a tea or capsule, or applied externally, as in a skin salve or a massage oil. In many cases, more than one preparation is applicable for a specific treatment.

Some preparations, such as tinctures and body oils, can be made from either fresh or dried herbs. The best method for extracting an herb's properties varies from herb to herb. For example, Saint-John's-wort, oat berries and feverfew lose most of their properties when dried. A significant portion of the essential oils in fragrant herbs such as peppermint and chamomile is lost in even the most careful drying process. On the other hand, herbs that contain a great deal of water—comfrey and calendula flowers, for example—are sometimes best when used in dried form; otherwise, the final product will be too diluted.

Whenever one type of preparation is better than another to treat a specific condition, the reason is explained in that chapter. For example, if an aloe vera lotion is better for a burn than a salve is, you will find out why this is so.

Most of these preparations can be bought ready-made from natural food stores—either as individual herbs or in blends of several different herbs. If you feel ambitious enough to make your own concoctions, I have also provided a number of recipes. When deciding which preparation is the most suitable for you, consider availability, cost, convenience and, of course, effectiveness.

Many herbal recipes will use as their basic ingredient not herbs, but essential oils derived from herbs. These oils carry many medicinal properties of the herbs from which they are extracted. They are easy to use but are also highly concentrated, so they must be diluted and used moderately to prevent overdoses. As a result, they are mostly used externally, and appropriate cautions are given throughout this book. Do not confuse essential oils with vegetable oils such as olive oil, which are used as carrier oils in skin products.

Treatments are divided into internal preparations and external preparations, as the nature of the ailment generally determines the nature of the treatment.

PREPARATIONS FOR INTERNAL USE

The following preparations are designed to be taken internally. Included in the descriptions are definitions—for example, what makes a tincture a tincture?—basic directions and average doses.

GLYCERITES

Glycerites are syrupy liquids that provide an alcohol-free alternative to the more popular tincture (see page 12), in which an herb's properties are extracted using alcohol. A glycerite is created using glycerin in place of alcohol. Glycerin has a sweet taste, but does not affect blood sugar like honey, sugar and other sweets. In fact, a well-known nineteenth-century American herbalist, Edward E. Shook, N.D., preferred glycerites for most of his medicines.

One friend of mine preferred giving her baby glycerites instead of alcohol-laden tinctures. After discovering that her baby—and many others—turned up her nose at anything that even hinted of alcohol or vinegar, she started a business making herbal glycerites designed just for children.

There are two types of glycerin: One type, derived from animal fat, is a by-product of soap making; the other is derived from vegetable oil. Although soap itself is not edible, glycerin is. It is even used in some foods, such as frosting and baked goods, to hold ingredients together and keep them moist. Animal fat glycerin is sold in pharmacies. Vegetable glycerin can be ordered through natural food stores. A synthetic glycerin derived from petroleum is becoming increasingly popular.

An average glycerite dose is about 30 drops, a quarter teaspoon or half a dropperful (based on the one-ounce droppers used for most commercially available tinctures). This dosage should be diluted in water, tea or juice, as it may irritate the mouth otherwise. Glycerites are not as potent as tinctures and are more expensive than teas. Like tinctures, however, they are easy to carry and to make preparations from—for instance, a glycerite can be used to make instant tea. They also make a great base for syrups and they have a long shelf life.

PILLS

Tablets and capsules release their herbal contents in the stomach as they dissolve. They provide an easy way to down herbs, as long as you do not mind swallowing pills. They are slower-acting and generally less potent than tinctures, but like glycerites, they do not contain alcohol. They certainly offer a faster and more convenient method of treatment than tea—which has to be prepared—and they allow you to avoid tasting unpalatable herbs. They are more expensive than tea because you pay for the convenience of having the herb powdered, processed, bottled and marketed. For most users, the convenience outweighs the expense. Compact and easiest to carry of any herbal preparation, they are very handy in a traveling herbal first-aid kit. When carefully stored in a cool place, they last at least a year. Since capsules are a popular way to take herbs, you will find a large selection available at natural food stores and some pharmacies. (Powdered liquid

extracts, tinctures or freeze-dried herbs are sometimes put into capsules or tablets. Because they are so concentrated, they are usually mixed with a filler to give them more bulk.)

Capsules and tablets do have some disadvantages beyond cost. Many herbalists feel that the body better assimilates an herb that has been tasted. Bitters, for example, stimulate digestive juices when tasted. Indeed, what a surprise it must be when your stomach gets hit with a bitter herb such as goldenseal without any advance warning from the taste buds. Another potential problem is that the herbs used by some manufacturers may be of poor quality. Manufacturers get away with this because it can be difficult for the consumer to determine the quality of pills. One thing you can do as a responsible consumer is to examine the contents by opening a capsule or mashing a tablet with the back of a spoon. The herbs inside should still carry the color, fragrance and taste of the original plant.

If you want to fill your own capsules—either to save money or because you cannot find the herbal formula you want—you can buy empty capsules at natural food stores. I find this a tedious job, however. It involves powdering the herbs, scooping them into the capsule and packing them in with a chopstick or similar tool. You can speed the process along by using one of several types of capping machines sold through natural food stores.

The typical tablet or capsule is roughly comparable to half a cup of tea or one-sixth of an ounce of herb. Consult the product label for dosage.

SYRUPS

A syrup is a tincture, liquid extract, glycerite or sometimes a strong tea that is sweetened and thickened with sugar, honey, glycerin, molasses, rice syrup or fruit syrup. (*Caution:* Do not give honey to children under two years old, as it can hurt them; for more information on honey, see chapter 13.) Glycerin is often preferred since it will not ferment like honey. A syrup makes an ideal cough remedy because it coats and soothes the throat, but other remedies can also be taken as a syrup.

While syrups are tasty, easy to carry and long-lasting, the added sweeteners in them can pose a problem for people who have sugar "problems"—diabetes, hypoglycemia and the like. If you suffer from a disorder of this kind, avoid syrups. The other potential problem with syrups is that their herbal content is often low because of overdilution. The average dose of a syrup is one tablespoon.

TEA

Tea offers one of the simplest and least expensive ways to prepare herbs. In fact, a cup of tea usually costs only a few cents, and the typical dose is one teaspoon of herb per cup, one cup three or four times daily. Making tea can help you become familiar with the herbs as you feel, smell and taste them. Relaxing for a few minutes while you drink your medicine is a healthy way to remind yourself to slow down. Some remedies— for example, many fever-reducing teas and some diuretics—work only when taken as hot tea because the heat promotes sweating.

Tea has its advantages, but you may find you don't have time to make it every day. Of course, drinking tea sounds like a great idea until you brew up some foul-tasting herbs, then try to drink *that* a few times a day! Tea can also be a problem if it means having to lug a Thermos around with you. Refrigerated tea will keep for a couple of days.

There are several different methods of preparing tea.

Infusions are made by pouring hot water over herbs and steeping for five to ten minutes in a saucepan, teapot or cup. Flowers and leaves are the usual ingredients. Commercial herb teas that come in tea bags are cut extrafine to produce tea quickly, usually in five minutes. To retain heat-sensitive essential oils contained in the herbs, cover the pot or pan.

Decoctions are prepared by gently simmering the herbs in water for 15 to 30 minutes. The most common ingredients in decoctions are roots and bark. The Chinese prefer to simmer root and bark teas even longer. The high heat releases more properties from heavy barks and roots than steeping does. Keep the heat very low when simmering aromatic roots such as valerian, elecampane and angelica so that their essential oils aren't lost into the air. Some barks and roots can be brewed a second time.

Cold Infusions are made by soaking herbs in cold water for about eight hours. Because this method takes such a long time, it is generally reserved for delicate, fragrant herbs that lose their essential oils when heated.

Two modern versions of tea are increasingly finding their way to market. Flavor-enhanced tea has essential oils or flavorings, such as almond, mint, cinnamon or citrus, added to increase its flavor. Instant tea is made using herbs that have been quickly dried in a high-heat chamber. This removes their water but retains most of their properties and flavor, making the tea very concentrated. Instant tea is then added to a substance that dissolves easily, such as lactose or dextrin, to increase its bulk.

TINCTURES

Tinctures, also called herbal extracts, are a concentrated liquid form of herbal medicine. A tincture is easy to carry, easily assimilated and needs no refrigeration. It will keep for years, another important consideration for anyone with an on-the-go lifestyle. This concentrated form of herbs makes it easier to down strong-tasting herbs or take large doses. In fact, because a tincture is so concentrated, it is best to dilute it into an instant tea by adding it to water or juice; the average dose is about 30 drops, a quarter teaspoon or half a dropperful (based on the one-ounce droppers used for most commercially available tinctures). Certain tinctures are used externally, mostly as skin antiseptics. All tinctures take effect quite quickly.

The liquid medium of a tincture is alcohol. The alcohol draws important properties from the herb (or herbs), leaving behind the more inactive substances, such as starch or cellulose. It also extracts compounds that are not water-soluble. This means that a few herbs, such as goldenseal and black cohosh, and gums such as myrrh, are stronger when made into a tincture.

Making a tincture requires no heat, so essential oils are retained.

One ounce of tincture contains about 600 drops or six teaspoons, which equals 20 to 24 doses per bottle. Price-wise, that's about 35 to 40 cents a dose. This means that tinctures are more costly than tea, but most people don't mind paying for the convenience. When using the herbs suggested in this book, it is not necessary to use the exact number of drops; estimating is fine. (Remember, we are talking about very safe herbs, not drugstore pharmaceuticals.)

A tincture is much easier to get down than a strong-tasting tea. I find tinctures handy for dispensing herbs to children and animals, as well as to reluctant adults. For example, when my friend Don pulls out his tincture bottles, his nine-year-old daughter, Libby, holds her hand over her mouth saying, "Wait, wait! What is that?" If he says it is gold-enseal or some other "yucky-tasting" herb, she replies, "Wait, I need more water!" But she readily takes the tincture, even though she will reject medicinal tea or pills.

If you have religious, health or other objections to using alcohol, tinctures may not be for you. Otherwise, do not be concerned; many doctors consider a small amount of alcohol healthy and an aid to digestion. A typical four doses a day totals less than half a teaspoon of alcohol. Studies show that most people can handle 6 to 12 times that amount, unless they have liver problems. If you prefer, you can even eliminate much of the alcohol by dropping a dose of tincture into a cup of boiling water. The alcohol evaporates, leaving the medicine behind. Do this with only one dose at a time, since the tincture will spoil without alcohol to preserve it.

Do not confuse herbal tinctures with homeopathic remedies or flower essences, which are used differently. Although all three products are preserved with alcohol and sold in the same type of dropper bottle, homeopathic remedies and flower essences are so dilute that there is often no detectable trace of the original herbs in them. Remember that these products are not interchangeable; each has different effects.

There are a number of variations on the tincture theme, and this often makes it very confusing for the consumer. To make matters worse, these terms are used loosely and sometimes interchangeably. These definitions should help.

Concentrated Liquid Extract. This is a tincture that has had most of its water and alcohol removed, making it a thick, semisolid liquid that can be blended into pills or reconstituted with glycerin or alcohol into a liquid preparation. This is one way to make alcohol-free tinctures.

Double Extraction. This is a double-strength tincture that is made by making a regular tincture, straining out the herbs, then combining that tincture with a fresh batch of herbs to make a second tincture. Because twice as much time and twice as much work are required to make a double extraction, only a few herb companies bother with this method.

Standardized or Guaranteed Extract. This product, usually a tincture or pill, is guaranteed to contain a specified quantity of the herb's main active compound. Laboratory tests are used to determine the amount of an active ingredient in an herb. If that quantity is lower than guaranteed on the label, that herb is rejected and one that meets this requirement is used in its place. In a few cases, such as with the herb ephedra, a purified amount of the active ingredient is added to increase potency to the stated level. To achieve this, certain important compounds are isolated and others are often discarded. Some herbalists refuse to use herbs that have been altered in this way, but many laboratory scientists prefer them for their consistent strength.

USP Standardized. Until tinctures began to be replaced by synthetic drugs following World War I, they were commonly sold in pharmacies and were made according to proportions set down in the *U.S. Pharmacopoeia* (USP), the pharmacist's guidebook. Today, few herbal companies can afford pharmaceutical licenses, and herbs in general cannot legally be advertised or sold as specific medicines. Because manufacturing methods and herb qualities vary, products are often of different strengths, even when they come from the same company. These traditional USP standards are still used by some companies.

VINEGARS

Herbal vinegars are prepared like tinctures, but the herbs are infused into vinegar instead of into alcohol. Though vinegar does not draw out an herb's properties as well as alcohol, herbal vinegars offer the con-venience of a tincture without the alcohol. Because most herbal vinegars are designed for culinary use, they are not medicinal strength. Also, the selection is limited. An herbal vinegar is easy to take, provided you like the taste of vinegar, and it can be used surreptitiously in a meal as salad dressing or in any recipe calling for vinegar; the typical dose is one to two teaspoons. Herbal vinegar also makes a fine sore throat gargle. In addition, it can be used externally as a hair rinse, as a skin wash for fungal infections and in douches.

~ HERBS FOR DINNER

Food is certainly the most basic way to use herbs. In many cultures, including Chinese, medicinal herbs are incorporated into soups, stews and other foods. Herbal honeys—powdered herbs mixed with honey into a thick paste—are used as medicine in India and the Middle East. They make an instant drink and can be used as a spread. And while burdock is considered an herb in North America, the Japanese use it as a vegetable. On the other hand, North Americans eat parsley, which is considered medicine in most European cultures. Actually, nearly all the herbs and spices we use to season food have medicinal properties. Preparing herbs for use in cooking does take some time, but no longer than it takes you to make your meal—and as every serious cook knows, herbs make food taste better.

Caution: Vinegar eats away at tooth enamel, so be sure to rinse your mouth thoroughly after drinking it.

PREPARATIONS FOR EXTERNAL USE

The following preparations are designed to be used externally. Included in the descriptions are definitions—for instance, what is a compress?—as well as basic directions.

AROMATIC WATERS

Scented waters are used to treat many different skin problems, ranging from acne to burns. They can also be used for purely cosmetic purposes. Because the essential oils they contain are so dilute, aromatic waters can be applied directly to the skin and taken internally. They also come in handy for soaking herbal compresses to treat skin and complexion problems. But they are often expensive and hard to find.

BODY OILS

Body oils made from herbs or essential oils are suitable for massage, but can also be offered as an alternative to some internal remedies. I recall taking care of a child with a stomachache who refused every natural remedy from my well-stocked cupboards. He finally settled for a tummy rub with a body oil containing essential oils that aid digestion. Later, he claimed it was the best medicine anyone had ever given him and even asked for a bottle to take home!

If you add heat-supplying herbs or essential oils such as cinamon, cloves and cayenne to your body oil, it becomes a liniment suitable for rubbing into sore muscles. Body oil is also the basis for making facial creams and skin lotions. While herbal body oils are extremely versatile, they usually take longer to act than internal remedies.

COMPRESS

A compress is quick to assemble yet very effective for a variety of problems: headaches, bleeding, bruises, muscle cramps, sore throats and almost any time alternating hot and cold is needed to increase circulation. It is also used to bolster immunity and to increase lymph flow, especially when there is an internal infection or a growth, such as a fibroid. Making a compress is easy—soak a soft cloth in a strong herbal tea, diluted tincture or glycerite, essential oils or aromatic water, wring out the cloth, then fold it and lay it on the skin. A castor oil pack is a compress in which the cloth is soaked in warm castor oil (sometimes combined with essential oils). The soaked cloth is placed on the skin and covered with a hot water bottle to retain heat. The one inconvenience with a compress is that to use it you must either lie down or tie it in place.

HERBAL BATH

Besides providing a relaxing and luxurious way to take your medicine, a bath can combine herbs with other therapies, including aromatherapy—the use of fragrant herbs or essential oils—and hydrotherapy, which uses alternating hot and cold water treatments to stimulate circulation. Heat relaxes the muscles, and cold reduces swelling. When you

Making and Using a Compress

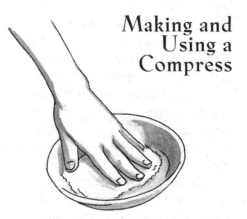

1. Soak a cloth in herbal tea, tincture or glycerite.

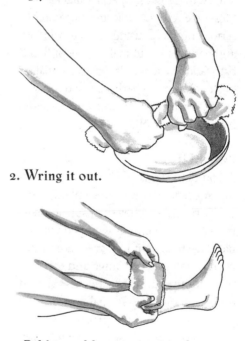

2. Wring it out.

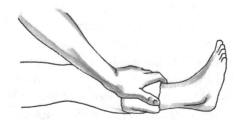

3. Fold it and lay it on injured area.

4. Hold or tie the compress in place.

consider that stress is the most common factor in promoting disease, an herbal bath may be one of the most important herbal treatments available! Baths are also useful in treating certain skin problems, and the steam that rises off a bath containing essential oils can be a treatment in itself for various breathing and circulation problems.

A variation on a full body bath is a foot or hand bath, popularized by the French herbalist Maurice Messegue and the French aromatherapist Marguerite Maury. In his book *Of People and Plants,* Messegue reports some amazing cures for serious problems using only herbal foot and hand baths. To make a foot or hand bath, add five to ten drops of essential oil or a cup of strong herb tea to a quart of water in a large basin, and stir well to distribute essential oils.

POULTICE

A poultice is made by pounding, blending or even chewing a fresh plant into a sticky paste, which is then spread on an injury and sometimes wrapped with a bandage to keep it in place. I admit that it may look a little strange and can be quite messy, but its effectiveness should outweigh any of your qualms.

My friend Gary, a carpenter, was accustomed to getting splinters while working in his wood shop, so he did not think much about a splinter in his leg last year—until he discovered that a nasty infection had developed. He tried an herbal salve, but it was no match for the infection. He spent weeks trying a variety of antibiotics, and the boils did heal, only to reappear persistently in different locations, sometimes opening into raw,

Making and Using a Poultice

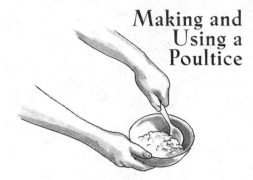

1. Use fresh herbs or mix moist clay with dried herbs to make a paste.

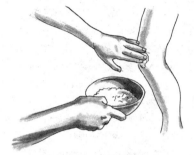

2. Spread paste on injured area.

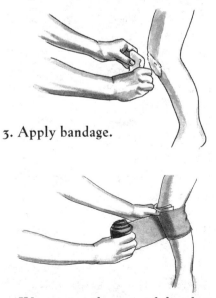

3. Apply bandage.

4. Wrap injured area with bandage to hold poultice in place.

painful sores. Gary decided to turn back to herbs, but with a different approach. He applied three poultices of fresh plantain and comfrey daily. It took a few weeks for his sores to heal completely, but he was finally free of the infection.

Another type of poultice is made from clay and/or dried, powdered herbs that are moistened into a paste using a tincture, strong herb tea or water. Sometimes, essential oils are added. Because this type of poultice comes in handy so often, I usually carry some with me for emergencies. Once, when I was attending an herb retreat, someone tapped me on the shoulder. "Quick," he said urgently. "A woman working in the dining room just got stung by a bee and she is allergic to them." When I reached the victim, another herbalist had already given her some echinacea and someone had run to her cabin for a prescription antidote. As I coated the swollen hand with my poultice, she said, "Oh, that feels so good!" I nodded, preoccupied in watching for signs of a reaction. Indeed, red lines were radiating from the sting and a deep red flush was creeping up her neck. Then, as quickly as they had appeared, both the red lines and the flush receded and disappeared. (For more information on this remedy, see "Bites, Stings and Splinters" on page 245. *Note*: Anyone suffering a severe allergic reaction *must* immediately see a doctor or take medicine prescribed for the allergy.)

SALVE

A salve is basically a thickened herbal oil. Olive oil, which is considered healing to skin, is the most common salve base, but other vegetable oils can also be used. To help a salve adhere to the skin, try adding beeswax.

Salves are used on almost all skin problems, including minor bruises and cuts, scrapes, rashes, eczema and swelling. Exceptions include any burn beyond a minor one (because of its oil base, a salve will hold the heat of a burn and cause more pain), the oozing stage of poison oak or poison ivy, and infected, open wounds. I once taught a weekend herb seminar attended by Juan, who clearly was paying little attention. He did, however, take home some herbal salve we made. Recalling that I had said it was a first-aid kit in itself, he took the salve to Mexico, where he encountered other travelers with all sorts of skin problems: foot blisters, chapped lips, scrapes and cuts, infected slivers, diaper rash, a rash from an unknown plant, bruises, hemorrhoids and sunburns. He doled out small amounts of salve, and as word spread through the village, the locals began requesting his *crema herbal* (see the Herbal Healing Salve on page 257). Juan returned home with an empty jar, and immediately called to sign up for next year's herb seminar, promising to pay attention this time! He learned more the second time, but to this day he claims that the herbal salve is the most important item in his first aid kit. Just about the only disadvantage of salves is that they can stain your clothes.

HOMEMADE MEDICINAL AND COSMETIC HERBAL PRODUCTS

If you are ambitious enough to make your own herbal products, these basic, generic recipes will guide you. The general uses to which these preparations can be put are discussed earlier in this chapter, where the different types of preparations are explained. To find the recipes suitable to treat a particular condition, look up the specific maladies you wish to treat in the other sections of this book. Your homemade products will cost a fraction of what the same preparations cost in the store, and you can avoid a lot of the unwanted extras, such as preservatives, stabilizers and colorants that are found in many products sold in natural food stores. Manufacturers, for instance, tend to use a lot of fixatives and preservatives, because they are concerned that someone might sue them for a spoiled product. However, many herbs and most essential oils contain their own natural preservatives, and beeswax is a great natural preservative.

You probably already have everything necessary to transform your kitchen into an herbal laboratory. In cooking up herbal formulas, be sure to use Pyrex measuring cups and pans made of stainless steel or some other nonreactive material. The proportions can change slightly according to the weight and absorbency of the herbs.

Tincture Formula

1 ounce dried or powdered herbs
5 ounces vodka
Chop herbs finely with a knife or in a blender, then place them in a clean glass jar; do not pack them tightly or the alcohol will not be able to saturate them. Cover herbs with just enough vodka so that they are completely submerged and can slosh around a little. (Vodka contains only alcohol and water. One hundred proof vodka is preferable, but 80 proof vodka will do: the former is 50% alcohol and 50% water; the latter is 40% alcohol and 60% water.) If there seems to be too much or not enough vodka, adjust the amounts as necessary. Put a tight lid on the jar and store for 2 weeks at room temperature. A dark shelf is fine, since tincture does not need light to process. Shake the contents once or twice a day to redistribute the herbs in the alcohol. If you are using powdered herbs, stir them with a spoon every day to keep them from clumping together. After 2 weeks, strain the herb pulp through a coffee filter or fine kitchen strainer. Stored in a cool place, a tincture can last 6 years or longer.

Glycerite Formula

1 ounce herbs
6 ounces glycerin
4 ounces distilled water
Chop herbs finely with a knife or in a blender. Place herbs in a clean glass jar; do not pack them too tightly. Combine glycerin and water; pour this mixture over herbs. Put a tight lid on the jar. Keep at room temperature. Shake the contents every day to redistribute the mixture. After 2 weeks, strain out the herb pulp through a coffee filter or fine kitchen strainer. Stored in a cool place out of direct sunlight, glycerite will last at least 2 years.

Herbal Vinegar Formula

1 ounce fresh or dried herbs
5 ounces vinegar (any kind)
Chop herbs finely with a knife or in a blender. Place herbs in a clean glass jar; do not pack them too tightly. Pour in just

enough vinegar to cover herbs (different herbs have different levels of absorbency, so you may need more or less vinegar than indicated above). Put a tight lid on the jar. Keep at room temperature. After 2 weeks, strain out the herb pulp through a coffee filter or kitchen strainer. Your herbal vinegars will last years.

Herbal Syrup

6 tablespoons herbs
1 pint water
4 ounces glycerin
1 ounce rice syrup or fruit syrup
    (or honey, for children over 2 years
    old) for sweetener

Bring herbs and water to a boil in a large uncovered saucepan. Remove from heat, cover and let steep for 30 minutes. Strain herbs from resulting tea. Return to heat, allow tea to simmer, then turn off heat. Measure out 1 cup of tea and stir in glycerin and sweetener while the mixture is still warm. Let cool. Stored in a refrigerator, this syrup will last for at least 6 months.

Herbal Pills

1½ teaspoons honey
1 tablespoon powdered herbs
Enough extra powdered herbs to roll pills

Warm honey in a saucepan and add powder bit by bit, stirring as you go. The consistency should resemble thick, sticky dough. Roll into small balls between the palms of your hands or on wax paper spread on a table. (Tack or otherwise hold down wax paper.) Let dry about 30 minutes, then roll in more powdered herbs so that the outside is not so sticky. This makes a soft pill that can last a year or more.

Body Oil

2 ounces dried herbs
1 pint vegetable oil

Chop herbs very fine, place in a container and pour in just enough vegetable oil to cover. (Use more or less oil as needed.) Stir to release trapped air bubbles. (Avoid using powdered herbs; they absorb oil like a sponge and clog the strainer. If powdered herbs are all you have, stir the powder every day to keep it from clumping together.) Heat herbs and oil for about 5 hours at about 80°F. You can use a double boiler on the stove top, or an oven, electric turkey cooker or slow cooker set on the lowest temperature. (If the setting on your appliance is not low enough, turn it on and off and monitor the temperature.) Or you can put the herb-oil mixture outside on a hot day; the temperature of the oil in the jar will be about 10 degrees cooler than the surrounding air. This will take 2 to 3 days, unless the air temperature is in the 90s. When done, strain out the herbs with a fine kitchen strainer, pressing out the oil with the back of a spoon. If any herb particles come through the strainer, re-strain the oil through a coffee filter. (These fine pieces will irritate skin when the oil is rubbed over it.) Stored in a cool place, herb oil will keep several months; stored in the refrigerator, it will keep even longer.

Body oil can be thickened by adding a natural thickener such as cocoa butter, lanolin or beeswax and then heating the mixture slightly. For every cup of vegetable oil, add ¼ teaspoon cocoa butter, ½ to 2 teaspoons liquid lanolin, or ½ ounce (by weight) beeswax. If the consistency is not exactly what you want, reheat the mixture and add more oil or thickener.

Body oils can also be made with fresh herbs, though this takes a little more care since these oils can easily spoil while you are preparing them. Herbs that contain a lot of water, such as comfrey, are better used in dried form, but some herbs, such as Saint-John's-wort, are far more potent when fresh. If you use fresh herbs, follow the same directions given above for making oils from dried herbs, but take extra care to make sure that they are completely submerged and all air bubbles are stirred out. Because fresh herbs contain a certain amount of water, you may have some water in the bottom of the container when you are done preparing this formula. If so, discard it after you pour the oil off the top, even if it means throwing away the last bit of oil.

Body Oil with Essential Oils

4 ounces vegetable oil
1/2 teaspoon (50 drops) essential oil
~ Combine ingredients and it's done!

Healing Salve

1 cup Body Oil (see page 19)
3/4 ounce beeswax (by weight)
8 drops essential oil (optional)
~ Combine Body Oil and beeswax, and heat mixture just enough to melt the wax. Add essential oil, if using it. Stir, then pour into widemouthed jars. Let cool. Stored at room temperature, this salve will keep for 6 months. If you have difficulty finding beeswax, check the telephone book for a bee supply or crafts store or beekeeper, and ask for pure beeswax.

Herbal Compress

5 drops essential oil
Small bowl of water
Soft cloth
~ Add essential oil to water. Soak cloth in water and wring out. Fold cloth and apply to afflicted area.

Skin-Healing Poultice

1 handful herbs
4 ounces water
~ Blend ingredients in blender into a thick slurry. Spread on wound, holding the poultice in place by wrapping gauze around it. Leave poultice on wound for 20 minutes to 1 hour. To store for future emergencies, freeze the poultice in ice-cube trays. Keep cubes in a plastic bag or freezer container. When you need a poultice, thaw out a cube in a pan.

CHOOSING THE BEST HERBAL PRODUCTS

Herbal preparations are only as good as the herbs themselves. Unless you are fortunate enough to have your own herb garden where you can be assured of quality, you should purchase your herbs from a reputable store or mail-order business.

As with any plant, a number of factors can influence the potency of herbs, including growing conditions, harvesting method, drying and storage processes, even the time of year and time of day when the herbs were harvested. Don't underestimate freshness—the moment an herb is picked, enzymes released in the plant begin to break down its active compounds. Light, heat and air all

(continued on page 24)

🙠 HERBAL PREPARATIONS: QUICK REFERENCE

PREPARATIONS TAKEN INTERNALLY

Description	Advantages	Possible Disadvantages
Food	Easy to take.	Small, often diluted doses of medicinal properties; preparation time; limited to foods and herbs that taste good.
Glycerite: Herbs extracted into glycerin. An average dose is about a quarter teaspoon or half a dropperful. Dilute in water, tea or juice or it may irritate the mouth.	Quick and easy to carry, makes instant tea, sweet-tasting, easy method for taking strong-tasting herbs, does not contain alcohol, long shelf life, good base for syrup.	Not as potent as tincture, relatively expensive, small selection.
Pills (Tablets and Capsules): Powdered herbs enclosed in gelatin or vegetable-based capsules or pressed into tablets with sticky binders. The typical capsule is "00" size, roughly comparable to half a cup of tea or one-sixth of an ounce of herb. Consult the product label for dosage.	Fast, convenient, easy to carry, wide selection, no unpleasant taste, no alcohol.	More expensive than tea, can't taste bitters (which play an important role in healing), uneven quality, short storage life.
Syrup: Sweetened and thickened tea, tincture or glycerin. An average dose is one tablespoon.	Sweet taste, easy to take, transportable, makes strong-tasting herbs palatable, no alcohol, coats sore throat, lasts a year.	Herbs can be overdiluted; added sweeteners can pose problems for those who suffer from diabetes, hypoglycemia and other sugar "problems"; potential to ferment; very small selection.

(continued)

HERBAL PREPARATIONS: QUICK REFERENCE—CONTINUED

PREPARATIONS TAKEN INTERNALLY—CONTINUED

Description	Advantages	Possible Disadvantages
Tea: Herbs extracted into water; sold chopped in bulk or in tea bags. Typical dose is one teaspoon of herb for every cup of water, one cup of tea three or four times a day.	Inexpensive, relaxing to drink, very wide selection.	Strong taste with some herbs, does not keep long, does not extract all properties of some herbs, bulky to carry.
Tincture (also called herbal extract): Herbs extracted into alcohol and water. An average dose is about a quarter teaspoon, or half a dropperful. This equals about one cup of tea. Certain tinctures are used externally, mostly as skin antiseptics (the alcohol itself is antiseptic).	Concentrated medicine, quick and easy to take even with strong-tasting herbs, makes instant tea, easily carried, pulls out most medicinal properties, quick effect on body, can take larger doses, keeps for years, good antiseptic base, wide selection.	Contains alcohol, strong alcohol taste, expensive.
Vinegar: Herbs extracted into vinegar. Dosages vary with application, but one or two teaspoons is typical.	Ideal against fungal infections and as a gargle, easy to carry, preferable for some strong-tasting herbs, no alcohol, lasts for years.	Can harm tooth enamel if not rinsed off, strong vinegar taste, not as potent as tincture, very small selection.

PREPARATIONS USED EXTERNALLY

Description	Advantages	Possible Disadvantages
Aromatic Waters: These fragrant waters are either by-products of distilling essential oils (called hydrosols), or essential oils combined with water.	Easy and pleasant to use, already diluted.	Expensive, difficult to find.

Description	Advantages	Possible Disadvantages
Bath: Herbs (quarter-cup), herb tea (four cups) or essential oils (a few drops) added to bath water.	Inexpensive, provides steam treatment and relaxation, can be used for hot or cold therapy to aid circulation.	Takes time and, of course, you need a bathtub.
Body Oil: Herbs extracted into vegetable oil, often olive or sesame oil. A shortcut is to add essential oils to vegetable oil. Depending upon which herbs and essential oils are used, it can be a massage oil, hot liniment, facial cream or skin lotion. These more sophisticated preparations are explained later in this book in their appropriate categories.	Beneficial to skin and complexion, can be applied directly on a skin affliction, adheres well to skin, holds in heat, can be combined with relaxing massage, quick preparation when essential oils are on hand, the base for many herbal remedies.	Must be rubbed into skin, oily, takes longer to act than internal herbal treatments, can stain clothes.
Compress: Cloth soaked in herbal water.	Quick, easy, inexpensive, very versatile; can be combined with hot or cold treatment; provides method to apply tincture, glycerite, essential oils or herb wash externally.	Must be held or tied to skin.
Poultice: Fresh, mashed herbs.	Very effective, especially for infection; no added cost.	Messy, requires fresh herbs, takes time to prepare.
Salve: Herbal oil thickened with beeswax to make it adhere to skin.	Beneficial to skin and complexion, can be applied directly on a skin affliction, adheres well to skin, versatile.	Holds in heat of burn, can stain clothes.

increase oxidation, which causes herbs to deteriorate.

Store herbs in airtight containers, preferably glass, away from heat and direct sunlight. Herbs in large pieces will keep longer than those that are finely cut or powdered. Plan on keeping leaves and flowers for at least two years, roots and barks for three years. Since there is no exact cutoff date, use an herb's color, taste and aroma as guides to tell you how much potency remains. Even after it is dried, an herb should retain its taste and color, and a fragrant plant should still have its characteristic aroma. For example, if dried chamomile looks brown instead of yellow or if you cannot detect much of peppermint's characteristic fragrance, these herbs are probably no good.

The savvy consumer needs to be open-minded to new, improved methods of extracting and preparing herbs, but wary of sales pitches that promote one product over another. One of the best ways to sort through this marketing confusion is to educate yourself and to seek out a store with knowledgeable clerks. Herbs are wondrous healers, but be realistic about their abilities. Take a hard look at products that sound too good to be true. Do not trust product literature as fact. As with other commodities, herbal advertising sometimes stretches the truth, uses tricky wording or tells only part of the story. Most herb companies claim that their products and processing techniques are the very best. They probably believe this, but that doesn't mean it's true.

Part II

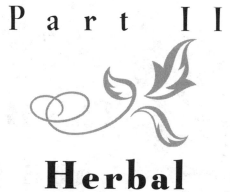

Herbal

Medicine

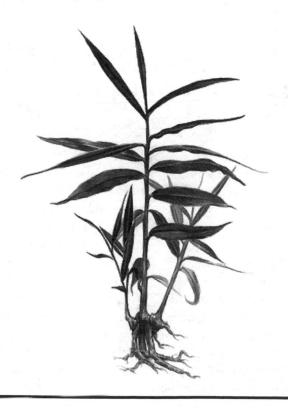

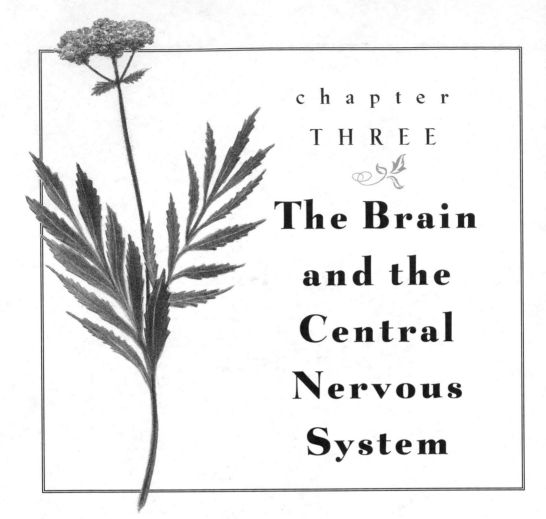

chapter THREE

The Brain and the Central Nervous System

The brain is perhaps the body's greatest mystery. It is enormously complex and it controls so much—yet we know so little about it. Despite years of research, we also know precious little about medicines used to treat the brain and nervous system—mostly, we can only observe the effects of such drugs as aspirin and Prozac and wonder how they work. Similarly, herbs for the brain and nervous system are shrouded in mystery.

The brain is only part of the central nervous system, which also includes the spinal cord and the peripheral nerves. This system is responsible for conveying information from the outside world to you and relaying messages from one part of your body to another. This is a big job, which is done mostly by chemicals called neurotransmitters, or "nerve transmitters." These transmitters carry messages to nerve cells called neurons and help these messages jump their signals from cell to cell across narrow gaps called synapses. Your brain's cerebral cortex alone—the part of the brain that is responsible for coordinating higher nervous activity—contains about 50 billion of these nerve cells.

There are many different types of neurotransmitters. If you end up with too much or not enough of a particular transmitter, the chemistry of your brain can be disrupted, and this will affect not only your mental functioning but also your emotional balance—indeed, your entire body may be affected. For example, one particular neurotransmitter, serotonin, is important because it promotes sleep, lowers pain sensitivity, hinders aggression and acts as an antidepressant. All sorts of problems, ranging from prolonged stress to inflammatory bowel diseases, can alter the levels of accessible neurotransmitters.

The central nervous system controls many functions, so problems with it can lead to a number of different conditions, including headaches, depression and pain. Fortunately, herbs, and even aromatherapy, can hasten healing in many central nervous system conditions. While natural treatments do not take the place of professional counseling or medical treatments in overcoming addictions or serious depression, they certainly can be good allies.

The herbs mentioned in this section come from all over the world. Although some of these plants have unusual names, all of them are available in natural food stores. You will find them sold separately or in combinations designed to help various nervous system disorders. Also, be sure to check out chapter sixteen, where I discuss aromatherapy techniques and cover the specific fragrances used to treat depression, anxiety, insomnia and stress.

ADDICTION

Addiction and recovery, once taboo subjects in our society, have become common topics of discussion during the nineties—it is hard to imagine a party or social gathering where at least one person doesn't have a story to tell. Nevertheless, the causes of addiction are just beginning to be understood.

While an emotional crisis or problem can lead people to drink alcohol, smoke cigarettes or use other drugs, many researchers believe that a chemical imbalance in the brain is actually responsible for addiction. What makes substances such as cocaine, heroin, alcohol and nicotine so attractive are the pleasurable sensations they create. After a few rounds of artificial stimulation, the brain responds only to the drug instead of to pleasurable events in life. In most cases, the more often you take the drug, the more you need to take to feel pleasure. This leads to addiction—an intense craving and even physical need for the drug. If addicts cannot get the drug, they can become nervous, anxious and even desperate.

Breaking an addiction is hard work. Cigarette smokers, for instance, often quit, start again, quit, start again—they are caught in a vicious cycle. In the words of the great Mark Twain: "To cease smoking is the easiest thing. I ought to know. I've done it thousands of times."

Besides creating an unending cycle of addiction, drugs can cause the addict a variety of other physical problems. For example, smoking damages the lungs and promotes lung cancer, and drinking destroys brain cells and can ruin your liver. Nicotine and caffeine also stimulate the production of too much cortisone and adrenaline, often triggering anxiety, panic attacks, depression, nervousness and heart palpitations. In some people who have psychiatric problems, caffeine can promote the intensity of mental illness.

Since addiction and depression often go hand in hand, if you have a problem with addiction and are seeking answers here, be sure to read "Depression" on page 30 and "Anxiety" on page 31 as well.

Also read the section in this book that covers herbs to treat a liver damaged by alcohol (pages 114 and 118).

While herbs do make a difference, by themselves they usually offer little help for someone dealing with an addiction. Most recovering addicts find that they also need to make lifestyle changes that bring new meaning to their lives. Regularly doing any aerobic exercise— even walking three times a week for 20 minutes—can change brain chemistry enough to help fight addiction or depression.

Take Sue and Marjorie, friends of mine who are both admitted alcoholics. Sue had tried everything imaginable, however briefly, to overcome her addiction—except herbs. She told Marjorie that she considered them her last hope. Unfortunately, she devised a treatment that consisted only of herbs, and as is often the case with alcoholism, the herbs just weren't enough by themselves. So Marjorie decided it was time to take another route and focus on several methods at once. She had already tried all the

standard methods (quitting "cold turkey," joining 12-step programs and so on), but had never backed these methods with an herbal program. She tried, unsuccessfully, to persuade Sue to do the same. I was not surprised to hear later that Sue was drinking again. Marjorie, however, has stayed sober—with the help of herbs.

Here's the lowdown on the herbs that often prove helpful. Capsules of gamma linoleic acid (GLA) from evening primrose, borage or currant seed oils are among the best herbal aids for controlling alcoholism. Brian Leonard, Ph.D., who studies evening primrose at the University College in Galway, Ireland, believes that supplements of this herb not only help recovering alcoholics to stay sober, but also slow down the damage that alcohol is known to cause to brain cells.

According to the latest research, the relaxant herb valerian may also slow brain cell damage that results from excessive alcohol consumption. Herbalists in Europe use valerian—in tea, tincture or pill form—to help people overcome and lessen alcohol withdrawal symptoms. In Brazil, passionflower is preferred.

In the nineteenth century, Eclectic doctors who used several natural treatments, including herbs, found that another sedative, skullcap, could be used to reduce anxiety and nervousness resulting from emotional or physical exhaustion. Herbalists today use it as one ingredient in formulas for addiction. The key to the addiction-fighting effects of valerian, passionflower and possibly skullcap may lie in the adjustments these

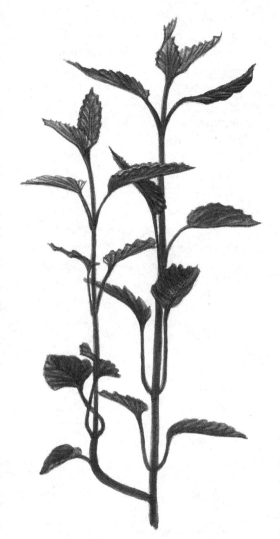

Skullcap, one of nature's "brain herbs," was once a well-known treatment for rabies.

herbs make in brain chemistry by changing the levels of neurotransmitters. Another secret to their success could be their roles as bitter digestive aids. Eclectic physicians of the early nineteenth century recommended bitters to overcome drunkenness. They were especially fond of a formula that included the extremely bitter quassia and gentian, which they found diminished the desire for alcohol. (Bitters are also good for getting rid of a hangover—bartenders recommend Angostura bitters, which have gentian as the main ingredient.)

For centuries, Asian herbalists have suggested kudzu to reduce alcoholism and drunkenness. This perennial vine from Japan, which was introduced to the southeastern United States around 1876, has made itself so much at home that it has taken over acres of land. Preliminary studies on experimental animals conducted at the National Academy of Science have gotten positive results, but so far no studies have been conducted on people. There are plans to investigate kudzu's effects on people. It should make southerners happy to know that there may be a practical use for this highly invasive weed.

The Chinese also use shizandra to enhance both mental and physical balance. It has been successfully used for over a decade to treat mental disorders related to alcoholism.

Turning away from alcohol addiction, let us consider smoking. Oatmeal is probably one of the last things you would think of to help in overcoming an addiction, but modern herbalists report that fresh oats are indeed useful, especially during nicotine withdrawal. (Practitioners of Ayurvedic medicine have been recommending it for at least a thousand years to treat opium addiction.) A 1971 study on this herb showed that a tincture made from fresh oats can indeed help people stop smoking.

In a 1994 study, researchers tried an Ayurvedic remedy on people who had recently quit smoking—they had them sniff the essential oil of black pepper (you can also just sniff raw peppercorns—if they don't make you sneeze). This treatment alleviated the anxiety and other symptoms that usually accompany nicotine withdrawal.

Withdrawal Tincture

½ teaspoon each tinctures of valerian rhizome and skullcap leaves

1 teaspoon tincture (or glycerite) of fresh oat berries

½ teaspoon each tinctures of Saint-John's-wort leaves and passionflower

❧ Combine ingredients. Take 2 to 5 dropperfuls a day. If you are a recovering alcoholic, use a glycerite instead of a tincture, which is alcohol-based. (If you are not sure what a glycerite is, see "Glycerites" on page 9.)

DEPRESSION

Been feeling down in the dumps for a while? You might be suffering from depression—North America's most common psychological complaint. While mood swings are a normal part of life, chronic depression is a serious disorder that limits the quality of life and suppresses the immune systems of more than 30 million Americans.

Statistics show that depression has been on a steady rise in North America since the early twentieth century. So is anxiety, a closely related disorder associated with nervousness and fear, which can bring on sudden hyperventilation, a pounding heart and feelings of suffoca-

tion, often at the most inappropriate times. It may be little consolation, but if you are depressed or anxious, you are in good company: The romantic poets Shelley, Keats and Byron, as well as the American novelist Ernest Hemingway are among the many legendary artists thought to have suffered from major mood disorders.

Fortunately, herbal antidepressants do exist. In fact, I know quite a few people who have successfully lowered or gone off their antidepressant drugs—sometimes after taking them for years—and now use herbs instead. Most of these folks find that they need to continue taking at least a minimal maintenance dose of the chemical antidepressants, but they are happy to have switched almost completely to a more natural alternative. Keep in mind, though, that antidepressant herbs are not as fast-acting or powerful as their pharmaceutical counterparts. Moreover, do not switch to herbal treatments for serious emotional disorders without consulting a professional health care practitioner, preferably one with whom you have a close working relationship.

Because depression is quite often a symptom of some other condition, you should attempt to eliminate its source instead of just looking for a quick fix from a drug or an herb. Michael F. Breslos, M.D., a psychiatrist at the University of Arizona, found that even a single cup of caffeine-laden coffee or cola produces anxiety attacks in susceptible individuals, and ten cups can cause almost anyone to have an attack.

Allergies to food and other substances, as well as low blood sugar levels (hypoglycemia), can also make you feel low. Some prescription drugs are notorious for causing depression, especially when used in combination with certain other medicines—if you are taking any prescription medicines, ask your doctor about bad combinations or read up on the side effects of your medications in the *Physician's Desk Reference* at the library.

Many commonly prescribed antidepressants work by keeping the neurotransmitter serotonin circulating in the brain. If you are at all familiar with antidepressant drugs, you have probably already heard of tricyclic drugs, MAO (monoamine oxidase) inhibitors and serotonin uptake reinhibitors such as Prozac. What you may not have heard is that Siberian ginseng, licorice and Saint-John's-wort also increase the availability of serotonin in the brain. In clinical studies, Siberian ginseng has repeatedly proved helpful for people who are depressed or have other serious emotional problems. According to a 1980 study, licorice is more effective than one of the commonly prescribed MAO inhibitors.

In a series of studies that were presented in 1992 at the Fourth International Congress on Phytotherapy in Munich, Germany, Saint-John's-wort helped well over half of those who were mildly to moderately depressed. In less than a month of taking this herb, the depression and accompanying disturbed sleep and fatigue experienced by participants in these studies generally improved.

In a 1984 study conducted in Germany, depressed women were given a tincture of Saint-John's-wort. These women's symptoms, including anxiety,

anorexia, lack of interest in life and psychomotor problems, all changed for the better. They even had fewer feelings of being worthless.

Research on Saint-John's-wort was also conducted in Russia—the herb was combined with psychotherapy to treat alcoholics suffering from depression. One of the major advantages of Saint-John's-wort is that, unlike many antidepressant drugs, it does not impair your attention, concentration or reaction time.

Antidepressant Tincture

1 teaspoon tincture of Saint-John's-wort leaf

½ teaspoon tinctures of licorice root, ginseng root, lemon balm leaf and ashwaganda leaf (if available)

Combine ingredients (if you do not or cannot drink alcohol, buy glycerites instead of tinctures). Take 1 dropperful 3 times a day.

ANXIETY

Anxiety, which is also very common, often accompanies depression. It is characterized by a feeling of impending disaster and an inability to deal with the pressures of everyday life. If your anxiety is stress-related, try taking ginseng or the Ayurvedic herb ashwaganda. In a study conducted in 1982, nurses who switched from a day to a night shift were tested to see how efficient they were and how they reacted psychologically as they struggled to adjust to their new routine. Some of them were given ginseng to help them maintain emotional balance; another group was not given anything. Those who took ginseng felt less moody and were much more steady emotionally than those who did not take the herb. In a 1990 study, ashwaganda, also known as Indian ginseng, was given to people who had been diagnosed with anxiety disorders. Ashwaganda treatments improved the mental condition of most participants in only three months.

If you visit a Chinese herbalist complaining of anxiety, expect a recommendation of herbs with the unusual names of zizyphi seed and ligustrum. Ligustrum is one of the herbs commonly used to support the adrenal glands when a person is under stress. Studies conducted in China showed that these herbs are successful anti-anxiety agents. In the same studies, both herbs proved even more potent when combined with licorice and the Chinese herbs poria and bunge root. This ancient Chinese combination is known as *Suanzaorentang*. A 1986 study showed that this treatment is almost as effective as the anti-anxiety drug diazepam (known commercially as Valium) in dealing with anxiety, weakness, irritability and insomnia. When taken three times a day, the herbal combination, unlike the drug, improved psychomotor skills and produced no side effects. In another 1986 study done in Europe, this same combination helped people whose anxiety attacks were so severe that they often experienced heart palpitations, chest pains and shortness of breath.

In Polynesia, we find that a drink made of the root of kava has traditionally been used to lift the spirits. Throughout the South Seas, kava ceremonies are held to celebrate important events. Even when taken out of the party atmosphere and into a scientist's laboratory, kava still

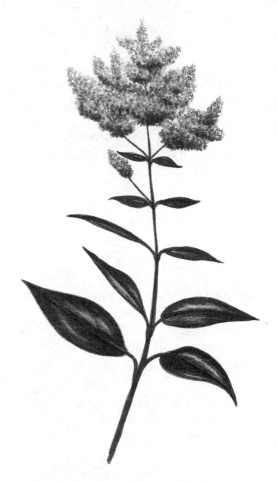

Ligustrum is a main ingredient in the Chinese anti-anxiety formula *Suanzaorentang*.

makes people feel relaxed and friendly. In one of several clinical studies, kava helped more than 50 people reduce both depression and high anxiety levels—a difference was noticed after only one week. And in a study conducted in Germany in which kava was given to women suffering from anxiety, depression and other symptoms associated with menopause, the symptoms were relieved, and the women reported an increased sense of well-being.

According to German researchers who measured the brain waves of people subject to anxiety, kava has been as effective in treating some forms of anxiety as the powerful tranquilizers known as benzodiazepines. And unlike this drug and others used for similar purposes, kava does not dampen alertness or lead to addiction. In fact, it improves alertness, vigilance and memory. Kava is available in tincture and pill form at natural food stores, usually as part of a formula with other herbs used to treat the nervous system.

Valerian has also been compared with various prescription drugs. It is no wonder, considering that this herb affects the same nerve receptors as benzodiazepines. The most popular of these tranquilizers is Valium, which doctors have long prescribed to relieve symptoms of anxiety. The drug is also used to lessen the anxiety, agitation and tremors that occur during alcohol withdrawal. (If you have heard the popular rumor that Valium was derived from valerian, you should know that it's not true—this myth probably arose because their names are so similar.)

Physicians in Germany commonly prescribe valerian in place of Valium or Xanax (another very common anti-anxiety drug) for mild and even moderate cases of anxiety. Some recommend fairly large doses—up to two teaspoons of the tincture at least twice a day. I know several people who have needed to take this much for the first few weeks after they stopped taking their antidepressant drugs. For most people, a dosage of this size creates no problems, but for a few it leads to upset stomachs or headaches. If you are taking Valium, Xanax or related drugs on the advice of a physician, do *not* discontinue them without your doctor's approval. No prescription drug should be discontinued before the prescribed stop date without consulting a doctor.

The results of one study conducted in 1993 showed that valerian and hops are calming to the central nervous system. When volunteers took this combination, several measurements showed that they experienced less depression and anxiety. In fact, the herbs worked faster than if the subjects had been given prescription drugs—hops and valerian worked in only two weeks, as opposed to the six weeks required for drugs. The herbs also caused far fewer side effects. You should know, though, that if you are used to strong prescription sedatives, herbs such as valerian seem to have a harder time taking effect.

Finally, folklore is filled with stories of herbs being used to improve mood. Around A.D. 1000, the Persian herbalist Avicenna recommended lemon balm "to make the heart merry." In Europe, this herb was sipped in cordials.

Motherwort—recognized today as a heart herb that also increases blood circulation in the brain—was recommended by the seventeenth-century herbalist Nicholas Culpeper to prevent melancholy. In modern times, it has been studied in Germany, where it is recognized as a mild sedative effective for treating anxiety and sleep disorders.

Modern herbalists find that both lemon balm and motherwort help alleviate depression, especially when combined with other antidepressant herbs. And aromatherapists commonly use the scent of lemon balm to treat depression.

One final remedy that I would suggest for relieving depression and anxiety is capsules of GLA, which is found in evening primrose, borage and black currant seed oils. In studies done at the London Children's Hyperactive Clinic in England, evening primrose oil was shown to reduce depression and nightmares in children.

HEADACHES

More than 45 million Americans have headaches severe enough to send them to a doctor, according to the National Headache Foundation in Chicago. If you suffer from recurring headaches, it is important that you see your doctor. Recurring headaches can be symptoms or indications of serious disorders such as tumors, meningitis, blood poisoning or infection in or near the brain.

The majority of headaches, however, are tension headaches, which tighten up muscles in your head. They are triggered by stress, illness, bright lights, food sensitivities or even changes in the weather. Next time you experience this type of headache, remember that it can be eased with relaxation techniques, gentle massage of the back of the neck and sedative herbs. In fact, a good way to deal with most headaches is to reduce the stress in your life.

Hangover, hunger, migraine, cluster and "ice cream" headaches (brought on by sudden cold, such as eating ice cream too quickly) are examples of circulation

or vascular headaches. They are helped by taking herbs that promote relaxation, along with those that dilate blood vessels in the head.

In some cases, long-term use of typical commercial headache relievers—codeine, acetaminophen, meperidine (Demerol), ibuprofen and even aspirin—makes your headaches more frequent, more severe or both. When the New England Center for Headache in Greenwich, Connecticut, took people who experience chronic headaches off their daily dose of five or six painkillers, a surprising two-thirds of them were having fewer headaches by the end of the month. After two months, four-fifths of these people were experiencing even less pain than when they were taking the pills. And the immediate side effects of the drugs—digestive problems, drowsiness and dizziness—are nothing to shrug off.

If these statistics alone are not enough to persuade you to turn to herbs the next time a headache strikes, consider the long-term effects of the typical painkillers. The results of a 1994 scientific survey suggest that there might be a direct correlation between the habitual use of acetaminophen—at least one tablet a day for a year or more—and the development of kidney failure. The survey also indicated that people who take large quantities of other pain relievers, such as ibuprofen, naproxen and indomethacin, may increase their chance of kidney failure eightfold. The majority of painkillers also cause stress on the liver, especially in high or repeated doses. This is because they are detoxified in the liver.

Want some natural alternatives to ease your aching head? Try drinking a ginger tea. Numerous clinical studies have shown that this herb can be used to relieve headaches. Researchers believe it does so by relaxing the blood vessels in the head and diminishing swelling in the brain. It also activates natural opiates in the brain that relieve pain, and it reduces prostaglandins, which are responsible for causing inflammation.

Other traditional headache teas are made with chamomile, lemon balm and linden (the flowers of the lime tree), which is is far more popular in Europe than in North America. In *The British Herb Pharmacopoeia,* linden is listed as a sedative for treating nervous tension and headaches. Researchers suspect that this herb heals migraines (and other vascular headaches) by improving blood circulation.

For other ways to ease tension headaches, see the information on natural aspirins and muscle relaxants in "Pain: Inflammation" on page 44. You should also consider using herbs known to reduce stress (see "Stress" on page 52)—these may take care of your stress headaches.

In a 1994 study on headaches, the essential oils of peppermint and eucalyptus relaxed both mind and muscles. When these herbs were diluted in alcohol, then sponged on the foreheads of study participants, both greatly reduced sensitivity to headaches. My own favorite headache herb is lavender. A tincture of lavender called Palsy Drops was recognized as an effective herbal treatment in the *British Pharmacopoeia* for more than 200 years. Until the

1940s, physicians used this tincture to relieve muscle spasms, nervousness and headaches.

The essential oils of any of these herbs—peppermint, eucalyptus and lavender—can also be used to make an excellent compress to place on your forehead whenever a headache hits. Most headaches respond best to a cold compress, but you may find that a warm or hot compress, or alternating cold and hot compresses, works even better. My rule of thumb is to do whatever feels best to relieve the pain. If you are using a compress on someone else, simply ask which the individual prefers. I find that placing a second compress on the back of the neck is especially helpful. When you are on the run and do not have time for compresses, dab a small drop of lavender, eucalyptus or peppermint essential oil on each temple.

Bathing can also be helpful, although some people cannot tolerate a hot bath—it only makes their heads pound more. But if you are one of those people for whom bathing does help, add a few drops of a relaxing essential oil (you can use lavender or see chapter 16 for other aromatherapy options) to your bath water.

One interesting technique that short-circuits a vascular headache, such as a migraine, is to regulate circulation by raising the temperature of the hands by 15 degrees. Simply place your hands in hot (but not too hot) water and add a couple drops of lavender, eucalyptus or peppermint essential oil to the water to increase its effect.

In one 1993 study on cluster headaches, a cream made from capsaicin—

the compound that makes cayenne and chili peppers hot—was shown to provide some relief. After two weeks of regularly rubbing this cream onto their temples, the people who participated in this study said that the capsaicin cream made a difference. One-quarter of the people who used it had far fewer headaches than the group using plain cream, and those who tended to get cluster headaches benefited the most. As you might expect, there were a few complaints about burning and runny noses! However, for most people, having the sniffles was far better than having a blinding headache. A study conducted in 1965 showed that capsaicin works by blocking a neurotransmitter called substance P (for pain)—it simply stops pain impulses from registering in the brain. For full blocking effect, capsaicin must be applied four or five times a day for four weeks.

Migraines are a particularly nasty and increasingly common type of headache. When you have a migraine, the pain, which often lasts all day, is usually felt on only one side of the head. It may also be accompanied by nausea, distortion in vision and a peculiar visual sensation, called an aura, that precedes the headache with flashes of light, tunnel vision and/or blind spots. These headaches seem to occur when arteries in the brain constrict, then suddenly relax. No one knows why, but twice as many women experience migraines as men, most often before or during menstruation.

In 1990 I read an article in a scientific journal about a woman who treated her migraines with ginger. When the migraine aura first started, she stirred 500 to 600 milligrams of powdered ginger into a glass of water and drank it down. Only 30 minutes later, her pain subsided. She took ginger again that day, and for several more days, to ward off future attacks. Encouraged by her success, she began adding fresh, uncooked ginger to her meals and found that she was having far fewer attacks. I know people who suffer frequent migraines who will not leave the house without carrying a little crystallized candy ginger or a piece of raw ginger root in their pockets. One friend told me that even cooked ginger seems to do the trick for her.

As you will read again and again in this book, ginkgo is wonderful for improving blood circulation—for this reason, it is a great choice for a remedy to treat circulation headaches. French scientists have done many studies on ginkgo. Several of these showed that treatments made using this herb were effective for reducing vascular headaches (migraines, cluster headaches, hangovers). In at least one of these studies, ginkgo reduced headaches in 80 percent of the people who took it, most of whom were experiencing migraines on a regular basis. People who participated in the study said that they had tried just about everything they could think of to get rid of their headaches, but nothing worked until they discovered ginkgo. The researchers responsible for this study concluded that ginkgo should be considered one of the most effective remedies for migraines. Ginkgo is also the remedy of choice to treat dizziness and tinnitus, or ringing in the ear, which are often associated with headaches.

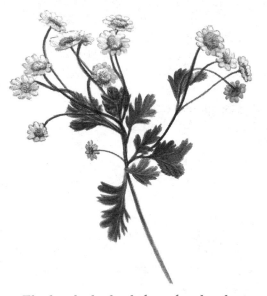

The headache herb feverfew has long been used as an aromatic to ward off diseases and repel insects.

Feverfew is also a good choice for the treatment of migraines and other vascular headaches. In his 1772 *Family Herbal*, John Hill stated, "In the worst headache, this herb exceeds whatever else is known." The City of London Migraine Clinic in England found that almost 75 percent of those with migraines who took feverfew had fewer, or at least less severe, headaches. In a study done at the Department of Medicine and Haematology at City Hospital in Nottingham, England, people who experience many headaches ate fresh feverfew leaves for three months and stopped using their usual headache drugs for at least the last month. The result was less severe headaches and fewer symptoms such as nausea and vomiting. The team that ate feverfew discovered an unexpected side effect as well—an increased sense of well-being.

When I first read about this study, I realized that the renowned sixteenth-century herbalist John Gerard may have been on to something when he suggested feverfew "for them that are giddy in the head . . . melancholic, sad, [or] pensive." Although feverfew has been studied for years, the exact way in which it works remains a mystery. Researchers have said that one way the herb appears to reduce migraines is by inhibiting the release of serotonin in the brain. It may also decrease swelling in the brain by reducing the amounts of prostaglandins, histamines and other substances that cause inflammation, according to Denis Awang, Ph.D., former director of the Natural Products Section of Canada's Department of Health and Welfare. The fresh leaves of feverfew are more potent than the dried, so when you buy a tincture or freeze-dried capsule, make sure that the product was made with fresh leaves (this should be clearly marked on the label).

Remember, though, an ounce of prevention is worth a pound of cure. If you suffer from migraines, you should follow the suggestion of the National Headache Foundation to avoid certain foods known to trigger migraines: ripened cheese (Cheddar, Gruyère, Brie and Camembert, among others), onions, pickles, cured meats, avocados, fresh bread, red wine, sour cream, nuts, chocolate, coffee, tea, cola and alcohol. (This list makes a cocktail party sound like a certain invitation to a migraine!) In an experiment at a Texas neurology clinic, over 25 percent of people who get migraines improved when these foods were removed from their diet.

ie Tincture
*...oon each tinctures of feverfew
leaves, ginkgo leaves, valerian
rhizome, ginger rhizome and
peppermint leaves*
🍂 Combine ingredients. Take a dropperful as needed, up to 8 times a day.

Lavender Headache Compress
*5 drops lavender essential oil
1 cup cold water*
🍂 Add essential oil to water and swish
a soft cloth in it. Wring out the cloth, lie
down and close your eyes. Place the
cloth over your forehead and eyes. Use
throughout the day, as often as you can.

INSOMNIA

My friend Amber struggled with a
chronic stress–related illness for years.
Insomnia was just one of her symptoms.
In fact, she had so many symptoms that
were similar to those resulting from
chronic insomnia that her physician
could not tell which were due to the illness and which resulted from lack of
sleep. He prescribed a strong barbiturate
so that she could sleep and so that her
life would be more manageable. In time,
Amber got better and was finally able to
get a job, but she still had trouble sleeping without the drugs. She would lie
awake for hours, and when she did doze
off, her sleep would be filled with bizarre
dreams. In the end, she always awoke to
find that she was more tired than when
she had gone to bed. Amber was sleepy
and easily distracted at work, and her
husband complained about her short
temper.

On the recommendation of a clerk at
a health food store, Amber tried a combination of all the best-known herbal sedatives, including valerian, skullcap, hops,
passionflower and chamomile. She felt
more relaxed in the evenings, but she
still could not sleep. Desperate to save
her job and perhaps her marriage, not to
mention her sanity, she turned back to
the barbiturates—and had to take a
double dose to fall asleep. They worked,
but she was groggy for hours the next
morning and felt off balance all day. She
tried her best to hide it, but could not
avoid embarrassing moments at work,
like the time she veered into the copy
machine. The same day, she collided
with another employee, and her file of
papers went flying. Amber's boss probably thought she was hitting the bottle.
And Amber feared she might become
addicted to her pills as she gradually
began upping the dose. Amber bravely
decided to give herbs another try.

This time, she sought the advice
of an herbalist who explained that the
health food store clerk had indeed been
on the right track. However, the 30
drops of tincture before bedtime that the
clerk recommended was barely enough
to begin addressing her problem. Amber
started taking Saint-John's-wort, Siberian ginseng, skullcap and lots of valerian
a few times a day, then an extra-large
dose an hour before bedtime. It was not
an easy transition going from drugs to
herbs, but she felt it was worth it in the
long run. Slowly, the herbs began to
work their magic, and for the first time
in years, she felt like she had a normal
life again. And yes, both her marriage
and job survived.

Have you, like Amber, ever stayed up all night counting sheep? If so, you may be able to imagine how lack of sleep diminishes the quality of life for the 20 million to 50 million people with chronic insomnia in the United States. It is important to get plenty of sleep to keep your nervous system operating smoothly.

While stress, worry or simply drinking coffee or eating just before bedtime can occasionally keep you from nodding off, chronic insomnia is another matter. It contributes to headaches, dizziness and mental confusion and eventually leads to emotional instability. Insomnia is actually a symptom of various disorders, not a disease in itself. If you suffer from more than the occasional sleepless night, you should get checked for thyroid and estrogen imbalances, low blood sugar, chronic heart and lung conditions, chronic pain and other disorders that can cause sleeplessness. You should also improve your sleeping environment: Make sure that your bed, pillow and room temperature are comfortable and that your bedroom is dark and quiet. Don't use your bed for anything except sleeping and sex—no reading or needle-work!—and wait until you're sleepy before going to bed. Relaxing music, a good stretching regimen, a hot bath, a massage and deep, rhythmic breathing also help induce sleep. So do sedative herbs, which in the long run are far better for you than drugs that promote sleep.

Sleeping pills certainly provide temporary relief, but long-term use of them may have side effects such as liver damage, high blood pressure and suppressed immunity. Besides, you can all too become dependent on them. For most people who take sleeping pills regularly, it takes only two to three weeks before they need to up the dose. And when they try to discontinue the pills, withdrawal often becomes a problem—and sleeplessness, agitation and fogginess often lead these troubled folks to reach for the pills again.

But who really needs sleeping pills anyway? Especially when natural alternatives abound. When the Nestlé Research Center in Switzerland decided to conduct laboratory tests on sleep inducers recommended in herbal lore, catnip, chamomile, lettuce, orange flower, poppy seeds, rosemary, almonds and especially valerian got high scores. And in a 1989 study, almost half of the people with insomnia who took valerian had a perfect night's sleep and almost everyone else found that their sleep improved to some degree. According to the results of several other studies, including one conducted in Germany in 1993, valerian helps you fall asleep more quickly, especially if you are elderly or a habitually poor sleeper. And once you do fall asleep, the deep sleep stages that are so important to a restful night are deepened. The results of another study conducted in Germany showed that a combination of valerian and lemon balm sent even the worst sleepers off to dreamland as effectively as the drugs commonly prescribed for sleep.

Valerian has been compared to various prescription drugs. One compound found in this herb depresses the central nervous system so well that the effect is similar to that of the sedative barbiturate

...d valerian does this ...ny dizziness, blurred ...s or poor physical per-...ncentration the next ...rs and barbiturates so often do. It does not even affect your dream recall or the ability to awaken refreshed in the morning. People in one study reported that they even felt much better the next day.

Another herb that is good for treating insomnia is catnip. For some reason, though, catnip has never been as popular as valerian, even though the two contain similar components that encourage sleep. Nevertheless, it did have its heyday. The English have long enjoyed their afternoon tea, and in pre-Elizabethan times, the beverage of choice was a relaxing cup of catnip tea. Times have changed, however, and now a stimulating cup of imported black tea is preferred. But catnip remains one of the favorite herb teas for sending children off to sleep.

Studies conducted in the late 1970s confirmed that catnip is indeed a potent sleep-inducer for humans. Like valerian, catnip calms you without disrupting performance the next day. And it is a plant that you can easily grow yourself. In fact, if you are lucky enough to have your own herb garden, you might already have catnip in it. Just be sure to protect it from your cats. Catnip and valerian both have the opposite effect on cats and rats as on people—they act as stimulants. According to legend, the Pied Piper's secret to ridding the village of Hamelin of rats was not his music, but the valerian he had tucked in his pockets!

Plenty of research has been done on chamomile's ability to relieve pain and insomnia. In a study conducted in 1973, almost all the people who drank chamomile tea instead of taking their regular pain medication fell into a deep sleep within ten minutes. The Germans call chamomile *alles zutraut,* or "capable of anything"—chamomile is so versatile that I sometimes think it can indeed do anything.

Passionflower has been a popular sleep inducer since the days of the Aztecs and the Incas, and it is still widely used in Brazil to treat insomnia, anxiety and nervousness. Combined with valerian, this herb makes one of the most popular sleeping aids in Europe, where you can find it sold in almost every drugstore. Passionflower is particularly helpful when tight muscles or an overactive mind disturb your sleep. Research from the Escola Paulista de Medicina in Brazil in the early 1990s showed that passionflower depresses the central nervous system.

If you are having trouble falling asleep at night or if you wake up too early in the morning and cannot doze off again, try Saint-John's-wort to help regulate disturbed sleep patterns. Like passionflower, it adjusts brain chemistry, helping to increase the availability of the neurotransmitter serotonin, which is responsible for promoting sleep and relaxation, as we know. When taken over a period of many weeks or even months, both of these herbs help people who suffer from chronic insomnia.

In India, gotu kola is taken to overcome insomnia and make one calm for yoga practice and meditation.

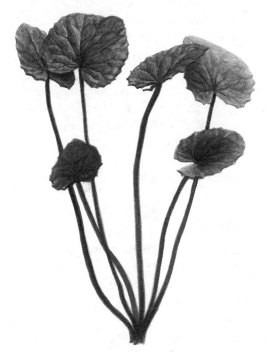

Despite its name, the sedative herb gotu kola is not related to the kola nut—a caffeine-based herbal stimulant.

Besides other sedative compounds, gotu kola contains an abundance of the "anti-stress" B vitamins.

Suanzaorentang, a Chinese formula used to treat depression, also improves sleep. It contains licorice, zizyphi seed, ligustrum, poria and bunge root. In a study conducted in 1985, people with insomnia who took this formula 30 minutes before bedtime found that they slept much better. Symptoms resulting from lack of sleep also improved significantly: People reported far fewer heart palpitations and stiff necks, less nervousness and less lower back pain. In general, they also felt an improved sense of well-being. Even after discontinuing the formula, the individuals involved in the study continued to sleep well for a week before returning to their former disrupted sleep patterns.

Hops is another important sleep-promoting herb with a unique way of working. It acts directly on the central nervous system, and takes effect in 20 to 40 minutes when taken as a tea or tincture or in pills. In studies conducted in Germany on people who have trouble sleeping, those who were given a combination of valerian and hops reported that they experienced a much sounder sleep. These favorable reports were confirmed by researchers who observed the participants in this study and measured their brain waves as they slept.

Even sniffing hops helps you doze off. Throughout much of Europe, bed pillows have for centuries been stuffed with dried hops for just that reason. Unlike most herbs, hops actually gets better with age—exposure to air increases its sedative effect.

Hops Sleep Pillow
2 pieces of fabric about 8 inches square
¼ cup hops strobiles
⅛ cup chamomile flowers
⅛ cup lavender flowers (optional)
🌿 Sew pieces of fabric together around the edge to form the pillow, leaving enough room to insert a tablespoon. Turn the pillow inside out so that the stitching is inside. Combine herbs and spoon them into the pillow. Sew up the opening. Lay the hops pillow under your regular sleeping pillow. If you are feeling creative, you can make the pillow any shape or size—just make more of this recipe to fill it. The hops should last about a year.

a Formula

*on each tinctures of valerian
___me, hops strobiles, passion-
flower and chamomile flowers*

🌿 Combine ingredients. These herbs can also be made into a tea, although most people prefer the tincture because the tea doesn't taste very good. Also, valerian is more effective as a tincture since some of its components are not water soluble.

MEMORY

Until recently, accounts of herbs improving intelligence and memory were regarded as whimsies of folklore. Now we know better. Scientists are learning that herbs *can* help us think better. Researchers are also dispelling a few myths about memory loss and aging. Medical experts know that in older people, being run-down or tired can lead to confusion. And increased anxiety can contribute to problems by cluttering up memory channels. The primary cause of age-related memory problems, however, is arteriosclerosis (see page 62), which slows the flow of blood to the brain. And this is a problem because the brain requires 20 percent of the total oxygen carried in the blood to function properly.

While it is true that you normally forget more things as you grow older, only about 10 percent of North Americans over 65 suffer from true senility or memory-loss disorders such as Alzheimer's disease. The good news, according to Stanford University psychiatrist Jerome Yesavage, M.D., is that most memory loss resulting solely from age

can be prevented. A study funded by the National Institute on Aging in which a group of people were charted for 28 years found that many showed no intellectual decline at all, even after they were well into their seventies. The researchers who conducted the study concluded that people turning 65 today are mentally sharper than those of previous generations, thanks to better nutrition and education.

This means that the odds are high that your mind will remain sharp as you grow older. And there are quite a few herbs to help ensure that it does. Clinical studies have shown that the four Gs—ginkgo, ginseng, Siberian ginseng and gotu kola—enhance mental abilities, including concentration, aptitude, behavior, alertness and even intelligence. And this seems especially true if you have experienced a decline in any of these.

In one study, proofreaders and radio telegraph workers, both of whom have stressful jobs that require close attention to detail, made fewer errors—only half as many as those who didn't take the herb—and had a quicker reaction time when they took Siberian ginseng or ginseng while working under pressure. They also managed to increase their reading speed and concentration.

In a Russian study in which people with senility or mental disorders due to atherosclerosis were given Siberian ginseng for one to three months, most participants experienced an improved memory and, as an added benefit, even felt stronger and more self-confident. In the ancient Chinese herbal known as the *Pents'ao,* ginseng is recommended for "benefiting the understanding."

In India, gotu kola has long been used as a brain tonic. There the herb is called *brahmi,* which is translated as "the highest order."

The best-known herb for improving memory is ginkgo. In dozens of studies done in Germany and France during the last decade, ginkgo helped elderly people feel more alert, attentive and sociable and less moody, generally after one or two months of taking it. It also improved their reaction time. One way ginkgo does this is by boosting the brain's ability to use oxygen.

Several scientific teams researching ginkgo in the mid-1990s found that this herb improves mental and even behavioral performance in the elderly better than a very popular drug for senility. And the herb produced no side effects and was not habit-forming. Ginkgo is good for long-term effects, but it is also fast-acting. When women took it only one hour before being given a battery of psychological and physiological tests, every woman improved her performance. In this 1984 study, researchers concluded that ginkgo has "a specific effect on the memory process."

I have even begun bringing a bottle of ginkgo to share with my students at the start of daylong herb classes. I pass around some more at the lunch break. Usually at least half the students say they can really tell the difference. And they tell me they feel even more alert when I combine it with some Siberian ginseng and ginseng. Over the years, quite a few of my students have attended college. They have relied on ginkgo, sometimes in combination with the other "brain herbs" (ginseng, Siberian ginseng and gotu kola), to help them get through. They dose up especially heavily with a dropperful or two of the tincture about an hour before an exam. All of these students, especially the older ones who are going back to school a second time, say that the herbs seem to help them think faster and more clearly.

Currently, research is under way to see if herbs might be used to help reverse or at least stop the progress of Alzheimer's disease, an increasingly common degenerative disorder in which memory and related aspects of cognition deteriorate over time. One of the herbs that researchers are most interested in is ginkgo. Another is the Chinese herb club moss, which is used in traditional Chinese medicine to promote circulation. In Alzheimer's disease, neurons are destroyed because of a defect in a neurotransmitter called acetylcholine. Chemist Alan Kozikowski, Ph.D., from the University of Pittsburgh, found that a derivative of club moss reduces the breakdown of acetylcholine. He found that the effect of this herb is three times stronger than that of drugs typically prescribed for Alzheimer's. It is hoped that herbs may offer part of the solution to this terrible disease.

Memory Tincture

1 teaspoon each tinctures of ginkgo leaves and Siberian ginseng root

½ teaspoon each tinctures of ginseng root and gotu kola leaves

🍂 Combine ingredients. Take half a dropperful a few times a day. Take extra tincture an hour or so before an exam or an important office meeting, or at any time you need extra focus.

Pain: Inflammation

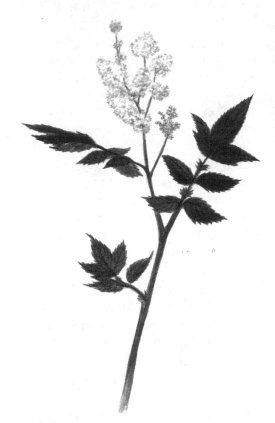

Pain occurs when the sensitive nerve endings in your body become irritated. This commonly happens when tissue swells — say, from a bruise, tensing of muscles or an overabundance of agents produced by your body in response to allergies, stress or a hormonal imbalance — and presses on the surrounding nerves. It also happens when your nerves are damaged from injury or strained from overuse. Whatever the cause, pain is your body's way of telling you that something is wrong. It is important to get to the root of what is causing the pain, but also to make yourself comfortable in the meantime. Chronic pain alone can cause a chain reaction in the body that can be quite detrimental: Pain leads to long-term stress, possibly to depression, then to greater sensitivity to pain and thus to more pain.

Herbs known to reduce inflammation can also help stop your pain. Herbs are also advantageous because they do not have the long list of dangerous side effects that result from long-term use of steroids and other anti-inflammatory drugs. As Lawrence J. Leventhal, M.D., pointed out in a 1993 article, many drug treatments for rheumatoid arthritis "are associated with adverse effects...that can often be as difficult to manage as the disease itself."

Most of the herbs suggested for problems such as arthritis do little to fight the disorder itself, but they do reduce the pain, and if you suffer from arthritis, you know that is a big step. You must have patience — it can take anywhere from a week to a couple of months for you to notice any

The word *aspirin* comes from "spirea," an ancient name for the natural pain reliever meadowsweet.

improvement, but the results can be dramatic. Sometimes the herbs help increase mobility of arthritic joints. In the most serious cases, herbs have at least enabled people with arthritis to reduce the amount of steroid drugs they were taking.

The best-known commercial pain reliever is aspirin. But did you know that there are natural aspirins like willow bark and meadowsweet? The magic ingredient in these herbs is salicin, which converts in the stomach to salicylic acid, a compound you have probably heard about in aspirin commercials on television.

Salicylic acid was first synthesized by chemists in the mid-nineteenth century. It was hoped that this new purified form would not irritate the stomach as natural aspirins did, but the new drug turned out to be even more irritating, and it was terribly bitter. Then the slightly less irritating acetylsalicylic acid was developed. Reflecting its herbal heritage, this new compound was called "aspirin," from "spirea," the old name for meadowsweet (not the ornamental spirea bush).

No one heard much about aspirin until Felix Hoffman, an employee at the Frederick Bayer drug company, became concerned about his father's problem with rheumatoid arthritis. He began thumbing through old medical journals, discovered aspirin and thought his dad might as well give it a try. Thanks to Hoffman and his investigations, the Bayer company started selling aspirin tablets as an over-the-counter drug in 1899. Today, aspirin is the most widely sold painkiller and anti-inflammatory in the world. Unlike its herbal counterparts, this purified, synthetic form is so potent that medical researchers say that if it were introduced today, instead of in the more lenient nineteenth century, the Food and Drug Administration, the federal agency that oversees the sales and dispersement of drugs in the United States, would demand that it be sold by prescription only.

Herbalists use willow bark or meadowsweet to fight many of the same symptoms for which you might pop an aspirin. Two cups of tea or 1 to 2 dropperfuls of willow bark or meadowsweet tincture usually does the trick. Ironically, it turns out that these natural aspirins are far less irritating to your stomach than the synthetic drug. This is especially true of meadowsweet, which herbalists even recommend to treat the pain of stomach ulcers. The results of numerous European studies indicate that meadowsweet protects the stomach from ulcers and other irritations, something that the Eclectic physicians knew a century ago.

Both natural and synthetic aspirins decrease pain by reducing the levels of pain-producing prostaglandins, hormonelike chemicals that are manufactured in the body. Prostaglandins serve many important functions, but for various reasons the body sometimes makes too much of them. Medical researchers believe that high levels of these chemicals are a typical cause of menstrual cramps and that they play a role in both migraine headaches and various types of arthritis.

Although feverfew contains different compounds than the other natural aspirins, it also stops inflammation and the resulting pain by reducing prostaglandin levels, according to several studies conducted in the United States—and it often works even better than aspirin. I have not found this to be consistently true for everyone. The best way to figure out the most potent pain reliever for you is to do a little experimenting—try the different herbs I've mentioned to see which works best.

Another herb that reduces pain by lowering prostaglandin levels is ginger, which has long been used in India to treat inflammation and pain. When Indian researchers investigated their culture's ancient claims for ginger, they discovered that it did indeed relieve pain. In a 1992 study in which ginger was given to people who suffered from muscle pain, all of the participants showed at least some improvement. In the same study, the ginger treatment provided substantial relief for over 75 percent of those who had painful rheumatoid arthritis or osteoarthritis. And best of all, no one experienced side effects, not even the people who continued to take it for more than two years. The recommended dose is 500 to 1,000 milligrams a day, although doses that are double and even triple that bring quicker and better relief. And ginger actually does double-duty—in addition to relieving pain, it also brings more blood to the injured, inflamed area.

The enzyme bromelain, from the stem of the pineapple, is also effective in inhibiting prostaglandins. In an extensive five-year study of more than 200 people experiencing inflammation as a result of surgery, traumatic injuries and wounds, 75 percent of the study participants had good to excellent improvement with bromelain—a much higher rate than that afforded by drugs. Most of the people in this study were discharged from the hospital in only eight days—half the usual amount of time. They also experienced no side effects. The results of several other studies showed that this enzyme also reduces inflammation resulting from arthritis or sports injuries. Bromelain is currently being used for pain relief in a number of U.S. hospitals.

In China, herbalists use bupleurum, ginseng and licorice to reduce or relieve pain resulting from inflammation. All three of these herbs stimulate the pituitary and adrenal glands to increase natural production of adrenal hormones such as cortisone that reduce the inflammation and consequent pain caused by conditions such as arthritis. And while prescription drugs such as prednisone produce adverse side effects, these herbs have quite the opposite effect—the drugs eventually shrink the size of your adrenal glands, impairing their function, but bupleurum and ginseng reduce adrenal shrinkage. According to the results of a 1984 study, when bupleurum is taken in conjunction with the prescription drugs, compounds in the herb even repair the damage already done by the drugs.

Some of the side effects that can come with taking cortisone are depression, thymus atrophy, high cholesterol and decreased levels of the neurotransmitter serotonin and the pituitary hormone ACTH. Studies have shown that licorice prevents all of these and also stops the liver from breaking down and deactivating your body's natural cortisone too quickly. Licorice also appears to enhance the action of bupleurum. Of course, it took Western researchers a while to catch on to licorice's versatility. At first, they were investigating how a licorice-based cream reduced the pain and swelling of skin inflammation problems such as eczema. Finally, they realized it might also have potential to help people with arthritis when taken internally. Sure enough, licorice proved very effective.

Licorice and ginseng offer another benefit to people with rheumatoid arthritis—they enhance the immune system. So do several other herbs used successfully to treat arthritis. Dr. Lawrence Leventhal, who was mentioned at the beginning of this section, is interested in the use of gamma linoleic acid (GLA), which is found in evening primrose, borage and black currant oils, to reduce inflammation, boost immunity and help maintain cell membranes in painful inflammatory disorders such as rheumatoid arthritis. In his study of people who suffer from this condition, GLA significantly improved the symptoms of joint tenderness and swelling in those who took it daily for six months.

Cat's claw, an herb that grows in South America and is described on page 105, not only enhances the functioning of the immune system, but also has been found to reduce inflammation. This herb is also used to treat rheumatoid arthritis—researchers have discovered that cat's claw contains anti-arthritic compounds.

You may be surprised to find that the famous immune enhancer echinacea also serves as an anti-inflammatory. The same compound—hyaluronic acid— that protects cells from germ and viral invasion also lubricates your joints. Unfortunately, rheumatoid arthritis breaks down this acid. Echinacea is an excellent herb to use for most inflammatory disorders for another reason: Many of them, including rheumatoid arthritis, are linked with immune system problems.

Guggul, a resin from a relative of the myrrh tree, has long been used by practitioners of Ayurvedic medicine to fight pain resulting from inflammation. The results of one study showed that people experienced significant relief from their arthritic pain after three months of

using a traditional Indian combination of guggul, turmeric, withania and the mineral zinc. One of the compounds responsible for the efficacy of this treatment is curcumin, the active compound in turmeric, the spice that makes curry powder yellow.

In fact, curcumin has been shown to be as effective as cortisone and phenylbutazone in decreasing inflammation. In one study with men who had surgery-related hernia, this compound reduced tenderness much more than the drug or a placebo. Like cayenne, curcumin contains pain relievers that stop the neurotransmitter substance P from sending its pain signals to the brain. It also works in several ways to decrease inflammation—by reducing prostaglandin activity. Researchers also believe that curcumin increases cortisone's anti-inflammatory action by making the body more sensitive to this hormone. So the next time you sit down to a curry dinner, consider that you are doing far more for your body than simply giving it a flavorful meal.

Other plants or plant compounds that have been compared to the anti-inflammatory drug phenylbutazone— but without the drug's long-term adverse effects—are Chinese skullcap, devil's claw and the compound lapachol from the South American herb pau d'arco. The Department of Antibiotics at the Federal University of Pernambuco in Recife, Brazil, has used this compound to develop an anti-inflammatory for use on the skin.

Research on Chinese skullcap conducted in China and Russia has validated theories about its sedative action and ability to stabilize nerve-related heart problems. This herb, which is related to European skullcap, has also been favorably compared to anti-inflammatory drugs such as aspirin and ibu-profen. As is true of most pain re-lievers, the reasons for the effectiveness of Chinese skullcap are not well under-stood. One thing we do know, however, is that it produces no side effects.

The curiously named devil's claw is so called because of the shape of its large fruit, which resembles a clawlike hand. In Europe, physicians give devil's claw as an injection, and it is also available as a tea and an external ointment for pain from inflammation. In southern Africa, this herb also has a long history of use for arthritis, rheumatic diseases, lower back pain and other inflammatory disorders.

Another important herb is yucca. In one study, people with arthritis were di-vided into two groups: One group was given an extract derived from yucca; the other was given a placebo. Almost three times as many of those who took the yucca reported reduced swelling, pain and stiffness as those who took the placebo. Some of these people felt better in a matter of days; for others it took weeks and for some it took over three months. While other scientific investiga-tions into the effects of yucca on people show little action, herbalists have reported success in using it. This may be because the longest of these studies lasted only three weeks, and long-term use of the herb is generally necessary be-fore any improvement is apparent. This proved true in a two-month study in France in which people with various types of arthritis took 1½ grams of yucca a day. About nine out of ten participants reported that the intensity of their pain decreased.

In this section, I have not men-tioned external treatments for inflamma-tion problems. For advice on liniments and muscle-relaxing oils that reduce swelling, see "Sprains and Strains" on page 266. In addition, herbs that increase circulation, such as prickly ash, ginkgo, hawthorn and gotu kola, can help increase the blood supply to an in-flamed area, thus speeding the healing process.

Inflammation Pain Tincture

½ teaspoon each tinctures of bupleurum
     root, ginseng root, licorice root,
     echinacea root, yucca root and
     turmeric (if available)

🌿 Combine ingredients. Take half a dropperful a few times a day or as needed. For long-term use, consult an herbalist.

PAIN: NERVE AND MUSCLE

Any time you experience nerve damage or injury, you can count on it being pretty unpleasant. Neuralgia is the term doctors use to describe nerve pain— the sharp, often tingling pain that runs along a nerve and can sometimes create an uncomfortable dullness or numbing sensation. Nerve pain can be caused by pressure on the nerve—say, from a rup-tured spinal disk—or by a simple injury such as a sprain. One common example of neuralgia is sciatica, a condition that involves pain running down the back of your leg, along the sciatic nerve.

Neuralgia can also result from repeated use of a particular nerve or muscle group. An example of this is the infamous carpal tunnel syndrome, in which a nerve in your wrist becomes compressed, causing great pain in the wrist and hand. This syndrome is fairly common in office clerks, writers and others who spend most of each day typing, and in carpenters who spend their days pounding nails. You can also develop compressed nerves by continuously leaning on your elbow or crossing your legs all the time.

Degeneration of the nerve fibers themselves, which is most common in elderly people, also leads to constant pain. And certain diseases, such as herpes and the closely related shingles, cause painful skin eruptions that break out along the nerves. The herbal treatments I suggest for nerve pain can be used to treat these disorders as well as to relieve the symptoms of nerve degeneration resulting from diabetes and nervous system disorders such as multiple sclerosis (MS), in which the protective sheath that surrounds the nerves is partially destroyed. While there is no known cure for either of these disorders, I have certainly seen herbs improve the quality of life of people who suffer from them.

None of the available herbs offers the significant pain relief given by prescription drugs. (Granted, there are some pretty strong painkillers derived from plants, such as morphine from opium poppies, but these are available only by prescription.) Unlike heavy-duty prescription drugs, however, the herbs men-

tioned here help heal your ner tem instead of only suppressin, And they don't dull the senses and a not addictive, as are many of today's popular prescription painkillers.

There are actually many herbs that can help relieve pain, and not all of them work the same way. Saint-John's-wort and vervain are nervous system relaxants that help you recover when your nerves are damaged, inflamed or strained.

Vervain is a bushy plant that has been used medicinally for thousands of years, but has fallen from favor in modern times. Still, some herbalists swear by its aspirin-like effects in relieving minor pain and reducing inflammation. Vervain is also considered a nerve tonic, especially when used constantly over several weeks—it improves the general action of the nerves and makes the system healthier. (It is also rumored to be a mild antidepressant, which may be one reason it used to be called "simpler's joy.") I find it works best when mixed with other nerve tonics.

Every spring, the hills around my home are covered with two excellent nervous system toners: California poppy and oats. Both of these herbs are available as ingredients in formulas and occasionally as individual tinctures.

All of these nervous system herbs help relieve pain. They can be useful in treating pain brought on by sciatica, herpes, shingles and carpal tunnel syndrome. These herbs can be taken internally as tinctures or pills. Saint-John's-wort can be used externally along with essential oils that reduce inflammation, such as chamomile, marjoram and lavender.

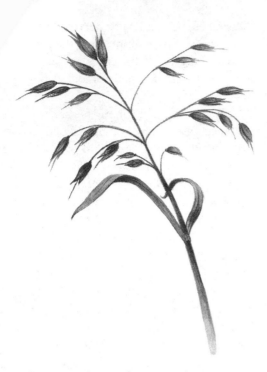

Oats aren't just for breakfast anymore—they're also a great treatment for nerve pain.

I know firsthand the benefits of such herbs. A few years ago, while writing my herb encyclopedia, I began experiencing nerve problems in my shoulders, arms and wrists. Sometimes problems like this creep up on you slowly when you are busy, and it takes something fairly dramatic to make you realize how dire things have become. For me, that day came when my wrists hurt so badly that I was unable to turn the doorknob to get into my house. It was obvious that something had to be done, and quickly.

I had given up my massage practice and my pastime of playing the recorder because of the pain. In fact, I could barely finish typing the encyclopedia. The next thing I knew, I was wearing

wrist braces, even at the wedding of my friends David and Diana. I did several things to cure myself and spare myself from impending surgery (which is not always successful). At David and Diana's wedding reception, I got a gentle lecture from David, who is also an herbalist, about practicing what I preach. The next day, I adopted an aggressive natural healing program that began with a visit to an excellent osteopath (whom I met at the wedding!) and a not-so-gentle lecture about the importance of herbs and exercise and reducing my stress level over deadlines. Then I started getting regular massages with relaxing aromatherapy oils and using herbs inside and out. I took the Nerve Pain Tincture (see page 51) with an extra dose of Saint-John's-wort. I also slathered liberal amounts of Saint-John's Strain and Sprain Oil (see page 268) on my wrists throughout the day. It paid off, although it took months before I was back to normal. As I sit here typing these words, I am thankful for the herbs—and the people—that allow me to be pain-free today without surgery.

While I am on the subject, I must also tell you about my friend Mary, since her story is slightly different. She came over to my house one day to pick up some facial cream I had made for her. As we walked back to the car, I could not help noticing that she was having difficulty walking. When I asked her what was wrong, she told me that she had sharp pains in her leg and hip and that these pains had been worsening for months. Now it was to the point where she could not even sit comfortably at the sewing machine to make her quilts or go out for walks. "You know how much I like to take walks," she said. "I cannot even make it up the hill to the top of our driveway anymore." She said that she felt like she was 90 instead of a spry mid-fifties. Guessing that Mary might have some nerve trauma that could benefit from herbal treatments, I sent her home with a tincture that I had made using Saint-John's-wort combined with the muscle relaxants valerian, hops, passionflower, chamomile and catnip.

Over the next few weeks, I received a series of phone calls from Mary, each one more excited, as her hip and leg got better every day. In one call, she gleefully announced, "Guess what? My headaches have also disappeared!" And in another, "Now I have no more PMS!"

The herbs ended up fixing all sorts of nerve-related problems that Mary had stoically never mentioned, at least until they were gone. That was years ago, but Mary has not stopped talking about her herbal success. Her enthusiasm is so strong that she has adopted herbalism as part of her life, and she and her husband, son, daughter, grandson and niece have all benefited from taking herbs for a number of different problems.

That this kind of pain relief is possible with herbs has not gone entirely unnoticed by the drug companies. The compound capsaicin, from cayenne, has been used as the basis for a number of over-the-counter creams for external use on painful skin problems such as diabetic neuropathy (nerve damage), facial neuralgia, psoriasis and post-surgical pain. A 1991 study showed that capsaicin also reduced pain and tenderness in people with osteoarthritis and rheuma-

toid arthritis. Capsaicin is used experimentally in some U.S. hospitals to reduce pain after a breast or limb has been removed. Clinical trials have shown that about 75 percent of the people with the painful condition called shingles experience substantial pain relief when they apply a capsaicin cream. For most people, this required applying the cream about four times a day for a month. A burning sensation is reported only occasionally, and becomes less of a problem the more the cream is used.

Herbs have also proved helpful in treating muscle spasms. Valerian, skullcap and cramp bark sedate the nervous system and also stop tight muscles from going into spasm. Other helpful agents include the same compounds that color berries and grapes red and deep purple. These compounds also calm and sedate the nervous system. You can get these substances, called anthocyanidins, by eating plenty of the fruit or buying the fruit-derived extracts in capsules sold in natural food stores.

In one study, a grape extract was found to reduce pain, nerve sensitivity, prickly skin and leg cramps at night— this is because of the anthocyanidins it contains.

Nerve Pain Tincture

1 teaspoon each tinctures of Saint-John's-
wort flowering tops, skullcap leaves,
fresh oats and licorice root
½ dropperful each tinctures of ginger
rhizome and vervain leaves
Combine ingredients. Take 1 dropperful every half hour, as needed during an emergency. To relieve chronic pain, take 2 to 4 dropperfuls a day

Stress

If you look beyond the symptoms of many physical ailments to the core problem, you will find stress. Even when it is not the cause, stress often aggravates a condition. Stress has such a powerful effect because of what it does to the body. When you sense danger, your body floods with adrenaline and other hormones, and nervous system reactions are heightened: Your heart pumps faster, blood rushes to your face, your eyes dilate and your muscles are primed to move—all in the matter of a few seconds. Your body even begins to sweat as a means of keeping cool during the crisis. Once vital for survival, these ancient responses are no longer always appropriate.

While you were born with reflexes that are more appropriate for a hunter or warrior, you don't really get to use them as nature intended. Instead, in these modern times your adrenal alarm goes off for much different reasons—you get caught in a traffic jam, your boss gets angry, your computer crashes, your washing machine overflows, a family squabble erupts. Responsible for pumping out adrenaline in response to stress, excitement or anxiety, your adrenal glands are controlled by your nervous system and they respond quickly to your emotions. After a while, constant stress overworks these glands and they become exhausted. The consequences of this can be far-reaching, since there is hardly a system in your body that is not influenced either directly or indirectly by adrenal activity. When your adrenal glands are exhausted, you and your body just do not respond to life the same way. You get sluggish and seem to be tired all the time. You may develop anemia and your blood sugar levels and blood pressure may be low, which will make you feel even more exhausted. Other typical symptoms include weight loss, digestive problems, skin discoloration and feeling overly emotional.

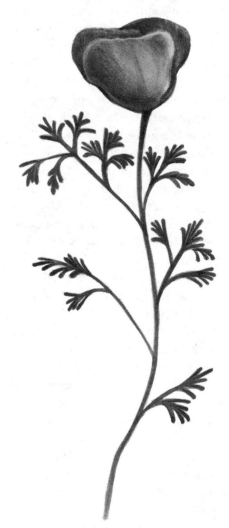

The beautiful California poppy is also an effective nervous system sedative.

Researchers say that stress itself is not the villain—what matters is how we deal with it. Those lucky individuals who are able to handle stress creatively are far better off than those who carry the woes of the world on their shoulders. For those who cannot handle it, years of stress eventually take their toll, perhaps leading to heart disease, ulcers, allergies or mental confusion. People who have a tendency to be hostile find extra amounts of adrenaline pumped out every time they get upset. And once the crisis passes, they have more difficulty calming down. As a result, researchers say, these people are more prone to high blood pressure and heart attacks.

If stress is a way of life for you, stay as far away as you can from recreational drugs, coffee and tobacco. For many people, sugar can also be problematic. Make sure that you are getting a sufficient supply of the "antistress" B vitamins. Also consider nervous system sedatives such as valerian, skullcap, chamomile and California poppy to help keep you calm and to repair damage that may already have been done.

The versatile herb valerian calms people who are agitated, but stimulates those who feel fatigued, according to one Italian study. During World War II, the British used valerian tincture to treat nerves shattered during bombing raids on London. (To get the full picture of just what valerian can do, read *Valerian: The Relaxing and Sleep Herb,* by Christopher Hobbs.)

A survey conducted in 1985 showed that passionflower is the most popular herbal sedative in Great Britain. It is also

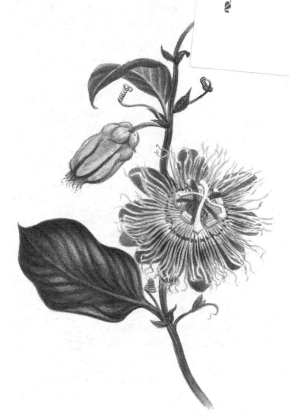

In the seventeenth century, passionflower came to be seen as a symbol of the Crucifixion: the five petals and five sepals are the ten faithful apostles (not including Judas or Peter); the corona is Christ's crown of thorns; the five stamens are His wounds; and the leaves are the hands of His persecutors.

well-liked in Romania, where there is even a sedative chewing gum made from passionflower to help ward off the nervous jitters and encourage relaxation. A German government commission designated the use of passionflower for "nervous unrest." One of the compounds it contains was originally called astelepathine, after "telepathic," because it made people mildly euphoric and more contemplative.

Ginseng and Siberian ginseng can help you handle stress by sedating or stimulating your central nervous system, according to your body's needs. Studies conducted in China showed that ginseng also increases your brain's utilization of amino acids, which is important because when you are under stress, your body uses more protein than usual. (Proteins are composed of amino acids.)

Another Chinese herb, shizandra, also has a regulating effect on the central nervous system. Studies show that this herb quickens responses and makes people more alert while actually stimulating the nervous system. A 1983 study conducted in China showed that shizandra relieves headaches, insomnia and dizziness and calms a racing heart. It has also been reported to control anger and aggression.

Since stress takes a big toll on your adrenal glands, consider using herbs such as licorice, bupleurum and ligustrum to support those glands. In China, all three of these herbs are commonly prescribed for people operating under a lot of stress. In China, in fact, herbal treatments are regularly incorporated with conventional methods. One report from that country details the herbal treatment of a woman suffering adrenal deficiency from extreme stress. She had undergone a lot of emotional stress in her life and had just had a very hard pregnancy and labor. Instead of following the usual medical method—cortisone and ACTH, a pituitary hormone that stimulates the adrenal glands—her doctor gave her licorice to promote corti-

sone production and ginseng, which researchers believe stimulates ACTH. The combination worked. The signs of adrenal exhaustion disappeared: She had more energy, she gained weight and her blood pressure returned to normal. The researchers attributed this success mostly to the licorice. Remember, though, that licorice should be used with care—it can raise blood pressure in sensitive individuals.

In Polynesia, kava tea is used to induce relaxation, restful sleep and a sense of mild euphoria. Even though it occurred about 20 years ago, I will never forget the complete sense of relaxation I experienced after a Fijian kava ceremony. I was in the middle of a very hectic trip, but the world seemed to stop after I drank some kava. Soon I was all smiles and so pleasantly relaxed that I actually fell asleep as soon as I got back to my hotel room.

It is often said that preparing kava fresh, the way it was done in that ceremony, makes it much more potent. Kava is available in natural food stores as a tincture or pills alone or in combination with other relaxing herbs, although I have to admit that I have never quite duplicated that experience by using kava in these forms. This herb is perfectly safe unless used in quantities you would never think of using—heavy kava users in the South Seas and Australia develop a scaly skin condition that remains until they cut down their dosage.

Strictly speaking, kava is not a true sedative. Instead, it is a muscle relaxant that reduces convulsions; one of its compounds stops muscles spasms up to ten times more effectively than a common anticonvulsant drug. Because of this, it is used to treat nervous tension, muscle spasms and tension headaches caused by a tight neck, as well as insomnia resulting from stress or tight muscles. I have found that kava lives up to its reputation of promoting peace and harmony among people. This is a pretty amazing feat for an herb, but I have experienced similar reactions after taking it and am convinced that all the world's leaders should sit down to cups of kava before their meetings.

Cool-Out Tincture

1 teaspoon each tinctures of valerian rhizome, licorice root, Siberian ginseng root, kava root and California poppy plant (if available)
🍂 Combine ingredients. Take as needed during emergencies, up to 1 teaspoon per hour. Otherwise, take ½ or 1 dropperful a day as a general relaxing aid. I find that tinctures of valerian

and skullcap made from the fresh root are stronger than those made from the dried root.

If the tincture doesn't work or if you're a person who enjoys hot baths, combining herbs with heat is one way to combine two stress-relieving methods. Simply add herbs or essential oils to warm compresses or baths. There is evidence that at least 20 minutes of heat in a sauna or hot tub or half an hour of deep massage changes brain chemistry for the better. If you have your own hot tub and you find that the heat relieves your stress, add a few drops of essential oil the next time you get in and see if that does not increase the relaxing effect. An aromatherapy massage is another ideal way to deal with stress. Some of the most relaxing essential oils to try include lavender, chamomile, sandalwood, orange, petitgrain and ylang-ylang.

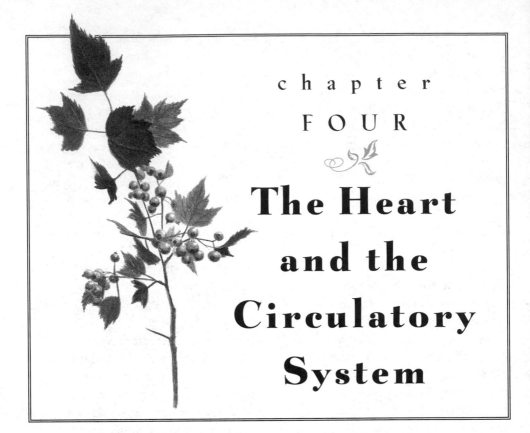

chapter

FOUR

The Heart
and the
Circulatory
System

Next time you find yourself philosophizing about the nature of progress, stop and consider cardiac disease, which is generally considered a twentieth-century ailment—and for good reason. Cardiac disease afflicts mainly people who live in Western, industrialized nations. It kills nearly one million Americans a year and is the leading cause of death in the United States. Scientists who study the history of disease believe that heart disease was rare among our earliest human ancestors.

The heart can be likened to an engine that drives the body. It uses a vast network of blood vessels to pump blood to every cell in your body. As you probably know, blood is responsible for transporting important life-giving commodities such as oxygen, nutrients, chemical messengers and infection fighters to your cells. It also carts away unneeded debris, such as carbon dioxide, urea and lactic acid, to your kidneys for disposal. Together the heart and blood vessels are called the cardiovascular system.

How have we managed to create a modern-day plague on the most basic of our bodily systems? Medical science points an accusing finger at a diet rich in fat, salt and too many processed foods, among other risk factors. People are taking this knowledge to heart, and dietary changes alone have dramatically reduced deaths from heart disease in the United States.

Stress and lack of exercise are also commonly named as factors contributing to heart disease. In addition, the American Medical Association warns that cigarette smoking increases your chance of dying from heart or artery disease by up to 300 percent! This is because nicotine constricts arteries and the carbon monoxide in tobacco smoke reduces the amount of oxygen in the blood.

Nothing can completely offset the effects of an unhealthy modern lifestyle, but in addition to eating healthily, exercising and not smoking, the use of humble herbs can reduce your risk of heart disease. Treating a heart condition is certainly more drastic than soothing a simple sore throat or headache, and a doctor's advice is required. That said, herbs do offer some of the best support for a healthy heart, especially when combined with exercise and a well-balanced diet. No, I do not suggest that you toss your heart medication into the trash and head for the garden, but herbs can help keep many heart and circulation problems from getting worse and can even prevent some of them from developing at all.

If your doctor has prescribed any type of heart medication, do not take it upon yourself to add herbal remedies to your regimen without consulting your doctor. Combining herbs with drugs can be tricky business, and the results can be disastrous. For example, hawthorn, a popular herbal heart tonic, can make you more sensitive to the potent prescription heart medication digitalis (which, by the way, is derived from the poisonous herb foxglove), slowing your heart's rate and increasing the force of its contractions. If you cannot find a doctor who is knowledgeable about herbs, your safest bet is to use the advice in this section only to treat minor disorders that have not yet developed into full-blown disease or to use my suggestions to help avoid heart problems in the first place.

ANGINA AND IRREGULAR HEARTBEAT

Your heart and blood system's first responsibility is to send oxygen-filled blood to the cells in your body. If your heartbeat is weak or irregular, or your arteries are laden with cholesterol deposits or stiffened from atherosclerosis, blood flow is diminished. The resulting lack of oxygen can leave you feeling dizzy and disoriented, and can turn your hands and feet numb. Even worse, it can lead to heart disorders such as angina pectoris and its painful chest constrictions.

The most reliable herb to help maintain your heart and blood flow is hawthorn. Herbalists around the world have used the bright red berries of this attractive tree for centuries, but scientists have recently discovered that the flowers contain equally important medicinal compounds, so most modern herbalists use both.

(continued on page 60)

☙ FIT FOR LIFE

Physical fitness has become a way of life for millions of North Americans, as they bounce, run, flex and prance their way to better health, bigger muscles and a fit physique. Vigorous yet prudent exercise combined with sensible eating habits is their route to a healthy, strong, muscular body.

Some fitness addicts feel that exercise and diet aren't enough to produce the body shape they want, and they turn to steroids—mostly testosterone—to bulk up muscles. Besides being unsportsmanlike and banned in professional athletics, steroids have plenty of nasty side effects: They raise blood pressure, increase nervous tension and cause headaches, nosebleeds and skin and digestive problems. They also lead to aggressive behavior, a diminished sex drive and eventually, sterility, a seeming contradiction until you consider that nature never intended a body to have that much of any one hormone. In short, steroids are dangerous, and experimenting with them is foolish. But there are alternative herbal methods for boosting training or general endurance and energy levels.

I can think of many men and women whose physical stamina has benefited from taking herbs: Dave, a bodybuilder; Maria, a swimming coach; and Greg, a competitive bicyclist. And I know people who take these herbs because they do hard physical labor for a living, such as construction, road maintenance, or farming. All of these forms of physical activity have at least one thing in common: They require lots of physical stamina. Impressive musculature is simply not enough.

Three herbs—Siberian ginseng, ginseng and shizandra—are all-stars when it comes to athletics. Studies from the Soviet Academy of Sciences have shown that these herbs improve mental efficiency, endurance, muscle strength, stamina and the general health of the cardiovascular system. These herbs also provide muscles with more energy by helping your body process carbohydrates. They help overtaxed muscles recover more quickly—an important concern not only for the professional athlete but for anyone just trying to stay in shape. The two types of ginseng also encourage muscle gain and the transportation of oxygen to muscles, thus preventing cramping, stiffness, panting and a racing pulse. In one study from the former Soviet Union, Siberian ginseng was also shown to increase the storage of energy in the muscles by almost one-third!

Millions of Russians—both men and women—greet each morning with a cup of Siberian ginseng tea. So do Russia's Olympic-bound athletes and their cosmonauts, who find it helps them withstand environmental and physiological changes. Russian cyclists who took Siberian ginseng during a Lesgraft Institute of Physical Culture and Sports event captured six of ten first-place awards in a ten-kilometer (six-mile) race. When given Siberian ginseng before training, Olympic sprinters, high jumpers, decathletes and marathoners had better endurance and performed better than a group that didn't take the herb. If Olympic athletes who already undergo maximum training can see these kind of results, imagine how it can help you with a workout twice a week or just keeping up with a grueling day at the office.

Ginseng has a very long history as a medicinal plant. Studies on this herb were being conducted in China more than two thousand years ago. In one such experiment, two people—one with a piece of ginseng in his mouth and the other without—ran five li (a bit under two miles). If the individual chewing ginseng did not feel tired or out of breath at the end of this run, the root was considered genuine.

Other cultures have relied on their own discoveries—ginseng is not the only herb known for its energizing abilities. The Nanai people of Japan hunt for a whole day after eating only a handful of shizandra berries.

Several other herbs have also gotten good marks for helping improve performance. Licorice apparently increases energy storage in the muscles. Licorice also gently stimulates the adrenals. (Remember, though, that licorice can sometimes increase blood pressure in people who already have high blood pressure.) Saw palmetto may help build up muscles. This herb was once prescribed for frail people or those who were weak from long-term sicknesses to make them stronger. The active ingredients are found in the fruits of this scrubby palm that grows in Florida and southern California.

For many men and women, the benefits of these herbs to muscles and the cardiovascular system may not be immediately apparent, but they do add up. Studies show that ginseng's antifatigue properties, for example, are much more pronounced after it has been taken for at least two months.

Stamina Formula

1 teaspoon tincture of Siberian ginseng root
½ teaspoon each tinctures of shizandra berries, ginseng root, saw palmetto berries and licorice root

Combine ingredients. Take half a dropperful twice a day, or as needed to increase stamina.

A popular medicine in Europe, hawthorn is an important ingredient in more than 36 pharmaceutical heart preparations in Germany alone. This is really not surprising, since German researchers have been studying it for more than 25 years, and their government approves its use to treat mild heart conditions.

European doctors often prescribe hawthorn as a tonic at the earliest warnings of heart or circulation problems, yet most North American doctors are unfamiliar with it. This is too bad, since hawthorn provides some of the same benefits as digitalis—without the harmful, accumulative side effects, such as an increased risk of irregular heartbeat and toxicity—and can often be used for mild heart conditions.

This wonderful herb increases blood flow through the heart by dilating the muscles that surround major blood vessels—something very important in the treatment of angina. Hawthorn decreases an accelerated heart rate, reduces spasms caused by angina and other heart problems and allows your heart to function effectively even when it is not receiving enough oxygen.

We can travel around the world and find other herbs to ease a troubled heart. Egyptian researchers have found that chicory slows a rapid heartbeat. Research conducted in Germany showed that compounds in the roots have a weak digitalis-like effect, but in doses that are low enough to make it safe for anyone to use. To take advantage of the benefits provided by these compounds, you can eat the roots in a dried or roasted form. Several commercial coffee substitutes contain roasted chicory, and there is also a recipe

for making your own tea (see page 66). In France and Italy, the roots not only are prepared as a drink, but also are considered an edible vegetable.

I have occasionally seen chicory greens sold in grocery stores as Whitlood chicory or Belgian endive, but if you are interested in eating the roots as a fresh vegetable, you may have to buy the seeds from a nursery catalog and grow your own plant (or buy a full-grown plant from your local nursery). Chicory is popular with gardeners because the roots of the plant can be replanted in a box in the cellar or garage at the end of the growing season, and the roots and greens can be harvested all through the winter.

In the 1980s, medical researchers examined several herbs traditionally used in China to treat heart-related problems. They learned that ginkgo and reishi, like hawthorn, improve blood flow to the heart, soothe chest pains, lessen the heart's demand for

For a healthy heart—try the "mushroom of immortality," the medicinal reishi mushroom.

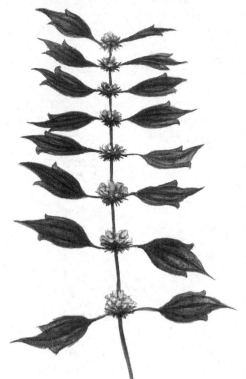

Motherwort's stout stems are tinged with red or violet, and in the summer it's covered with small white, pink or red flowers.

oxygen and reduce shortness of breath. Researchers have favorably compared ginkgo to metroprolol and diliazem, two drugs that are commonly used to reduce heart palpitations and lower blood pressure. According to Chinese researchers, reishi, which is actually a medicinal mushroom, steadies an irregular heartbeat. This is probably one of the reasons the Chinese call it the "mushroom of immortality" and sixteenth-century Ming dynasty texts say it "mends the heart."

The popular Chinese herb astragalus helps the heart develop a more regular rhythm. It also reduces damage to heart cells. Chinese physicians even use astragalus to destroy *Coxsackievirus B,* which infects the heart and causes an irregular heartbeat. This condition is becoming more of a problem in China, and astragalus is the only known treatment. Even though astragalus is a Chinese herb, it has become popular in North America—many natural food stores sell it along with their other bulk herbs.

Wu-han Medical College and other hospitals in China use a special type of ginseng (*Panax notoginseng*) called pseudo, or sanchi, ginseng to relieve angina spasms and pain. It is a little harder to find than regular ginseng, and equally expensive, but for many people, the price is worth it. In studies done at the college, it helped relieve symptoms in almost half of the people who took it. According to tradition, sanchi ginseng, which is similar to ginseng in its chemical makeup and effects, normalizes heart rate, blood pressure and circulation and helps to prevent fatigue and relieve stress.

All these Chinese herbs are sold in North America individually and in herbal formulas for the heart.

Another heart-healing herb that has found fame for hundreds of years—both in the East and in the West—is motherwort. Motherwort's botanical name, *cardiaca*, actually means "heart" in Latin. One study done in China showed that this herb slows a rapid heartbeat and generally improves the heart's activity. As a nervous system sedative, it also reduces the anxiety, stress or nervous tension that so often go along with heart problems.

While we are on the subject of stress-related heart problems, the sedative valerian is often helpful when used in addition to motherwort.

In the tropics, we find an unlikely candidate to treat various heart and circulation problems—pineapple. Herbalists and researchers look upon pineapple as more of an herb than a food. More than 400 papers, mostly from Germany, have been written on the medical uses of bromelain enzymes extracted from the pineapple stem. In a study from the early 1970s, people with angina who were given a daily dose of bromelain saw their symptoms disappear in 4 to 90 days, depending upon the seriousness of their condition. Their heart problems returned only after they stopped taking the enzyme.

You might also turn to traditional Indian Ayurvedic medicine to help your heart. The efficiency of a blend called *abana* to reduce the frequency and severity of angina attacks and improve heart function was reported in 1990. The herbs in this formula have long been used as heart tonics and are now establishing a reputation for themselves in the United States as well.

You may see yet another interesting plant making herbal headlines in the future. This is night-blooming cerus— a cactus called "pain in the heart" by Shoshone Indians who lived in the deserts of the southwestern United States and northern Mexico. It was once a favorite of both Eclectic and regular doctors, who made a tincture of it to treat angina, heart spasms, heart pains and shortness of breath. (Eclectic physicians were nineteenth-century doctors who used several natural treatments, including herbs.)

Heart Ease Tincture
1 teaspoon tincture of hawthorn berry
½ teaspoon each tinctures of motherwort leaves, ginkgo leaves, chicory root and reishi mushroom

~ Combine ingredients. Take half a dropperful a few times a day on a regular basis. Similar proportions can also be used to make a tea from these herbs. Even though astragalus is a Chinese herb, it has become so popular that many natural food stores now sell it with their other bulk herbs.

ARTERIOSCLEROSIS

Arteriosclerosis, commonly called "hardening of the arteries," actually defines several different related disorders. These disorders are marked by thickening of the arteries, loss of elasticity and hardening of the artery walls as calcium and plaque (resulting from high fat and cholesterol intake) are deposited. These deposits narrow the artery, thus interfering with the normal flow of blood through the vessel. This makes the heart work harder, which can cause a heart attack or lead to blood clots in the artery, which in turn can lead to a heart attack or stroke. Plaque buildup on artery walls occurs naturally as we age, but the process is accelerated by smoking, alcohol consumption, a high-fat diet, caffeine and lack of exercise. Stress is another risk factor. Heredity and some diseases, particularly diabetes, also contribute. All this points to the importance of maintaining a healthy diet and lifestyle, which will certainly help you avoid this dangerous disorder.

Arteriosclerosis can happen to any artery, but is most serious in those vessels that channel blood to the heart and brain. When vessels to the heart narrow, not only is blood flow to the entire body diminished, but a lot of stress is placed on your heart to work harder as it tries to pump blood through the narrowing passages. Symptoms include leg cramps while walking, changes in skin temperature and color, an altered pulse, headaches, dizziness and memory defects. The problem is that symptoms often do not arise until the problem has progressed to a dangerous phase. In fact, more deaths occur in the United States from arterial and degenerative heart disease than from heart attacks.

Dozens of studies have shown that garlic—a lot of it—keeps arteries healthy by thinning the blood and lowering cholesterol. Typically, the people in these studies took the equivalent of one to four cloves for every 35 pounds of body weight daily. I know that's a lot of garlic, but I've eaten that much for a day or two at a time—to knock out a cold—and still managed to keep most of my friends.

Since arteriosclerosis is worsened by high cholesterol levels, which contribute to the formation of dangerous blood clots, you should consider using the herbs recommended in "Cholesterol Reduction" and "Blood Clots" on this page and page 67, respectively. For example, compounds called anthocyanidins, which give foods such as bilberries, blueberries, grapes, hawthorn berries and cherries their bright coloring, reduce your chances of developing arteriosclerosis by slowing down both cholesterol buildup and the blood's tendency to clot. Anthocyanidins also stop a destructive enzyme from attacking the elastic fibers that support the arteries. You get some anthocyanidins when you eat deep red and blue fruits. They are also sold in pill form.

CHOLESTEROL REDUCTION

Cholesterol is on the minds, as well as the plates, of many people these days. In 1984 the results of the Coronary Primary Prevention Trial, a ten-year study on cholesterol involving about 4,000 men, were released. These results showed that lowering blood cholesterol from elevated levels will reduce the risk of heart disease. After that, the anticholesterol bandwagon started rolling.

But even public enemy number one has a good side. Our bodies produce their own cholesterol to make adrenal and sex hormones. You should expect to find *some* cholesterol in your blood, since that is how it is transported in your body. Problems develop when cholesterol begins collecting on your artery walls. This can begin happening as early as your twenties, but it may be many years before you start noticing any problems. Eventually, cholesterol contributes to arteriosclerosis and the formation of blood clots, which can lead to a heart attack or stroke. And a diminished flow of blood to the brain contributes to senility, depression and memory loss.

For simplicity's sake, I am using the term "cholesterol" in a generic sense. When I talk about lowering cholesterol, it is the LDL (low-density lipoproteins) —the "bad guy" cholesterol—that I am talking about, not the HDL (high-density lipoproteins), the "good guy" cholesterol. There are drugs that lower LDL levels, but these drugs can cause vomiting, headaches, liver damage, internal bleeding and vitamin deficiencies. Why experience side effects like these when a better way to keep cholesterol down to a heart-healthy level is to take herbs and cut fats from your diet? Numerous scientific reports show us that herbs can lower cholesterol almost as much as prescription drugs—about 16 percent.

If North American diets are responsible for our cholesterol problems, at least we can take heart in the knowledge that some of the best cholesterol fighters are found right in our kitchens. Onion, garlic, cayenne, rosemary, turmeric, fenugreek and ginger—add any of these herbs to your meals or take them as pills, teas or tinctures. When participants in a 1991 study were put on an experimental diet that included three ounces of fenugreek seed powder a day for 20 days, their LDL levels fell by about a third, while the HDL levels remained the same. Several other studies on fenugreek showed similar reductions.

Turmeric helps to prevent high cholesterol before it even gets into your bloodstream by interfering with its absorption in the intestine. Studies from India, where turmeric is a popular spice, show that it also improves the body's ability to break down and eliminate cholesterol.

If you are a connoisseur of south Indian–style curry, you may already know about brindal berry. This small yellow fruit is advertised in the United States mostly as a treatment for weight loss—one of its traditional Ayurvedic

uses—but modern studies show that it also lowers cholesterol.

Garlic lovers will be happy to learn that there is less heart disease in areas of the world where people eat lots of the "stinking rose," as some affectionately call it. When researcher Arun Bordia, Ph.D., was working in Udaipur, India, he could not help noticing the near absence of heart disease despite the locals' habit of dousing their vegetables in butter. He also observed that vast quantities of garlic were consumed regularly and decided to find out if that could be the secret to the low frequency of heart disease. Sure enough, even when he had volunteers eat butter, their cholesterol levels fell, providing they ate garlic along with it! Take away the garlic, and their cholesterol levels jumped.

Three onions (which are in the same family as garlic and share many of its healing properties) or five cloves of garlic a week are recommended, but if you find that even this much garlic puts too big a crimp in your social life, smaller amounts are also beneficial—or you can take garlic capsules instead. Liquid garlic tested at Loma Linda University in California noticeably reduced blood cholesterol. The German Association of General Practitioners found that dried garlic also reduced cholesterol levels.

Other herbs that keep cholesterol in line may seem even more like food than medicinal plants. In one German study, participants who were given compounds extracted from artichoke showed a consistent reduction in cholesterol levels, with an average decrease of 20 percent. So far, studies on eggplant have been done only on animals, but these preliminary studies indicate that it too may lower cholesterol levels. It's no wonder that India's ancient Ayurvedic medicine considered this vegetable a heart tonic.

The Ayurvedic herb guggul can also be used to slow cholesterol buildup. In studies conducted in India, more than 100 people who took guggul saw their cholesterol go down almost as much as it did in people taking the cholesterol-lowering drug clofibrate. Both the herb and the drug began taking effect about three to four weeks after the people started taking them, but only guggul increased HDL (the good cholesterol) in more than half of the people. A derivative of this relative of myrrh is generally used instead of the raw herb, which sometimes has side effects like skin rashes and diarrhea when used in doses large enough to have a medicinal effect. This derivative of guggul is most commonly available in pill form.

In China, we find that Chinese skullcap, ginseng and sanqi ginseng also keep cholesterol low. Even more impressive are two mushrooms used in China—shiitake and reishi. In various Chinese studies, these mushrooms have dramatically knocked high cholesterol levels down. Chinese skullcap and ginseng are available as bulk herbs, but you will probably need to get sanqi ginseng and reishi in pill form.

Lowering cholesterol can be that easy—just eat. During my class on making dried herbal wreaths, a student asked if any of the herbs we were using were medicinal. I said they were and spoke some about the medicinal effects of garlic. That was all the prompting Joyce needed to tell us her husband's story.

When George's physician told him that he was concerned about his high cholesterol reading, Joyce decided to take the situation into her own hands. "Well, I don't know much about medicine," she told us, "or herbs for that matter, but I read about the side effects of those drugs and knew there had to be a better answer. So, I did what I do know how to do best; I started cooking. George—he did what he knows how to do best; he ate everything I put in front of him. We started the day with garlic omelettes, and ate garlic pasta for lunch and anything you can imagine." It worked. George's cholesterol is still not as low as it should be, but they are not through with garlic, either. Joyce is still cooking up a storm, and she also discovered that they could buy garlic capsules.

Another thing George could try is a special type of fatty acid called omega-3, which some researchers believe reduces blood cholesterol. For a long time, the only known source was fish—until Artemis P. Simopoulos, Ph.D., former chairwoman of the National Institute of Health, cut up some purslane one night for her dinner. She had learned to cook this plant in her native Greece, but only now noticed how similar its slippery leaves were to fish oil. The next day, she brought some purslane into her lab for testing, and sure enough, she learned that it contains omega-3. It also has large amounts of vitamin E, probably the most important vitamin for the heart and circulation. Since then, small amounts of omega-3 have been found in flaxseed, soy beans, wheat and oat germs, radish seeds, rapeseed (canola) oil and nuts, especially walnuts.

Fiber is also important, as the proper amount of fiber in your diet keeps your liver healthy, and a healthy liver means that fats will be broken down properly—which is absolutely necessary for a healthy cholesterol level. One teaspoon of psyllium seeds (an herbal laxative sold in any drugstore) soaked in a cup of water, three bran muffins a day (be sure to buy the low-fat kind—most commercial muffins are unhealthy because they're loaded with fat) or a few servings a day of carrots, cabbage, apples, grapefruit, pinto or navy beans or agar will do the trick. You will probably find that herbalists will recommend all of these, since they generally find that the line between medicinal herbs and foods is a thin one. Even the natural fungicide in grape skins increases good cholesterol and lowers the bad. This fungicide is found in wine, but it has to be good wine—cheap, processed wines and those made from grapes treated with pesticides do not have this fungicide.

Remember, though, that dietary habits are not the only lifestyle issues implicated in cholesterol problems. Some of the African Masai of the former Tanganyika and some Jews in Yemen thrived on fat-laden, high-cholesterol diets, but never got heart disease until they emigrated to other countries and adopted a Western lifestyle. Researchers from San Antonio's School of Aerospace Medicine in Texas conducted a series of studies to determine whether stress might be a factor in elevating cholesterol. They found that cholesterol increases after only one hour of either emotional or physical stress, such as overexposure to cold. Worse, they found that if you stay stressed for a few hours, your cholesterol can remain high for more than a week. They even sent some lucky people to Hawaii to relax...and eat two eggs a day. In every case, their high cholesterol levels dropped and stayed low, until they returned home. Studies conducted at Stanford Research Center and Mount Zion Hospital in San Francisco showed that cholesterol also increases in medical students before exams and in accountants around tax time every year.

Of course, you do not have to move to a remote area of the world to keep cholesterol—and stress—under control. You can simply use the herbal treatments suggested in "Stress" on page 52. Two of your best choices are the sedative herbs valerian and motherwort, which also reduce high blood pressure. Since the cholesterol that you eat is processed in the liver, you might also consider taking herbs to keep your liver healthy. Herbs such as milk thistle can help keep your liver happy and your cholesterol low.

Low-Cholesterol Tea
*1 teaspoon each roasted chicory root and
    lime flowers*
*½ teaspoon each fenugreek seeds and
    ginger rhizome*
1 quart water
❧ Combine ingredients in a pan and bring to a simmer. Cover and steep for about 20 minutes. Strain herbs. Drink 1 or 2 cups a day. The formula can also be made into a tincture using the same proportions. If you prefer a tincture, take ½ to 1 dropperful a day.

BLOOD CLOTS

Blood clots are life-saving when they heal a wound, but turn life threatening when they create a blockage in a blood vessel. When this happens, your heart beats harder and harder trying to push the blood past the obstruction—the result can be a heart attack as the heart overexerts itself or a stroke if the blockage prevents the flow of blood to the brain. The accumulation of cholesterol in blood vessels is a serious risk factor for developing clots. All blood clots, especially in the legs, should be examined by a doctor. There is always a chance that clots in the leg will break away and travel to your lung, where they can produce a pulmonary embolism. (While strokes and heart attacks can also be caused by blood clots, only clots in the deep veins cause these body traumas.) If you have a minor clot in your leg, see "Varicose Veins and Hemorrhoids" on page 72.

It follows that treatments that reduce cholesterol also reduce your chances of developing blood clots. French scientists investigating herbs for the circulatory system have found that hawthorn, motherwort, ginkgo, bilberry, evening primrose oil and guggul, a relative of myrrh, are some of the best herbs for reducing the risk of blood clots. In addition, the enzyme bromelain from pineapple and the flavonoids known as anthocyanidins, which come from bilberry and other dark fruits, not only keep blood clots from forming, but also break down plaques of cholesterol that have already formed inside the arteries. Bromelain, evening primrose oil and anthocyanidins are usually available only

as pills, but you can buy the other herbs in a variety of forms. You can also get anthocyanidins into your system by taking pills that contain bilberry or other herbs that are high in these compounds. These pills are available in most natural food stores.

You might be surprised how many anticlotting herbs you already have in your kitchen: garlic, onion, cayenne, lemongrass, turmeric and ginger. If you are thinking that this sounds like a recipe for curry, that's because it is. Studies reported in 1977 showed that garlic breaks down fibrin—the substance that blood clots are made of—and thus stops clots from forming. A 1992 study showed that garlic works even better to reduce blood clots when heated slightly; when you cook with garlic, you get a small medicinal dose. Onions have the same effect, and along with motherwort, they also stop the blood's tendency to clot—even right after eating a fatty meal.

One study conducted in the early 1980s found that ginger prevented blood clots from forming even better than garlic or onions. And in another study, turmeric was found to be so effective that the authors who reported it in a 1986 article in a German medical journal regarded it as the treatment of choice for anyone prone to developing blood clots.

Doctors recommend an aspirin a day to reduce your chance of blood clots and strokes. The aspirin helps by thinning your blood. Perhaps someday they will instead recommend the mo-er mushroom, also known as black tree fungus. For centuries, the Chinese have claimed that this fungus increases longevity, but no one knew that it stopped blood from clotting. That is, not until a medical researcher happened to eat them one evening at a Szechuan restaurant, then gave himself a routine blood test the next day. When he saw the results, he was amazed at how much his blood had thinned. He correctly guessed that it was something he ate! It turns out that mo-er prevents blood cells from clotting. You can find mo-er in any Chinese grocery or in Chinese herb formulas, but don't over-do it. The mushroom is safe in average doses, but it works so well at thinning your blood that it can make your nose bleed if you take huge quantities of it!

Physicians in at least one cardiology clinic in Israel are recommending ginger instead of aspirin to all the patients in their clinic. (Aspirin is frequently used to prevent blood clots.) They suggest a half-teaspoon of powdered ginger a day to prevent clotting. Why? Because ginger inhibits the same blood-clotting compounds inhibited by aspirin—prostaglandins and thromboxane—without any of aspirin's notorious side effects. This interesting ability of ginger was discovered in the same way that the healing powers of the mo-er mushroom were discovered: A researcher at Cornell Medical School conducted a routine blood test on himself one day in 1979 and found that his blood was not clump-ing as it had been. By process of elimina-tion, he determined that it might be because of his favorite marmalade, which contained lots of ginger. A few tests confirmed his suspicions. Since then, researcher K.C. Srivastava, Ph.D., has conducted several studies on ginger's anticlotting action. In one of these, he found that eating 5 grams of ginger daily

for a week counteracted the detrimental blood-clotting effects of 100 grams of butter.

Blood Vessel Tonic

2 teaspoons hawthorn flowers
1 teaspoon each motherwort leaves and
   ginkgo leaves
½ teaspoon ginger rhizome
Hot water (enough to cover herbs)
❧ Cover herbs with hot water and let steep for 5 minutes. Strain and drink. The same proportions can be used to make a tincture.

Blood Pressure

Blood pressure is the pressure exerted by the blood on the walls of blood vessels as it is pumped through them. Numerous factors contribute to blood pressure levels—the most important thing for you to know is how to maintain a healthy blood pressure so that blood flows efficiently throughout the body. And while high blood pressure is prevalent in our society—and its dangers are relatively well-known—the less common low blood pressure can also present problems. But fear not—there are numerous herbs that can be used to help regulate your blood pressure.

HIGH BLOOD PRESSURE

Here's the most telling fact about high blood pressure, a quintessentially mod-ern disease—in remote regions of the world, there is almost no incidence of high blood pressure. It is not until peo-ple emigrate to more "civilized" areas that their blood pressure tends to increase. It may be that the change in their diet or the increased stress of a technological society is to blame, or it may be a combination of both.

Exactly why certain people get high blood pressure is not clear, except for the relatively few cases that obviously result from another disease. What we do know is that this condition, if it is not controlled, increases your chances of dying from a stroke or heart attack.

You are more prone to high blood pressure if you have problems with your kidneys, adrenal glands or blood vessels, eat lots of salt, are overweight or do not exercise regularly. The jury is still out on the long-term effects of caffeine on high blood pressure, but it is well documented that nicotine contributes to it. Stress also plays a big role—have you ever heard that just being nervous about a visit to the doctor can make your blood pressure jump? Actually, stress and nicotine work in a similar fashion. They both increase the release of adrenaline, which in turn raises blood pressure.

High blood pressure is nothing to fool around with—you should have your blood pressure checked regularly by a doctor, who will tell you what your reading means. Doctors in North America generally prescribe pharmaceutical drugs to treat high blood pressure. In Europe and Asia, where herbalism is generally more accepted than in the United States, physicians often prescribe herbs before turning to drugs.

If your blood pressure is only borderline high, like my neighbor Frederick's, you might try herbs and see if they work for you. I will admit that Freder

ick's doctor considered him one difficult patient—he kept asking about remedies called *Baldrian* and *Weissdorn* that he remembered from his native Germany. His doctor insisted that these drugs were not available in the United States and that it was unlikely that they had no side effects, as Frederick stubbornly claimed. So Frederick left the office without a prescription and called his brother in Germany. He discovered that his brother's doctor had indeed prescribed these remedies for his high blood pressure, but they were not drugs—they were the herbs known as valerian and hawthorn in English. Frederick easily found them in the local natural food store and wasted no time in starting an herbal and dietary program.

A month later, when Frederick went back to his doctor, his blood pressure was indeed lower. As stubborn as ever, he convinced his skeptical doctor to give the herbs a chance. After all, a respectable heart doctor had prescribed them to his brother in Germany. To help keep his blood pressure low, Frederick decided to take more time to relax, and he went back to Germany. He had some great stories to tell, but when the subject of American medicine came up, he always added, "Mein Gott, they do know a lot, but they still have a lot to learn about God's simple gifts of healing: the herbs."

Another way to maintain healthy blood pressure is to make your diet more herbal. Just adding garlic to a meal can keep your blood pressure lower for an entire day. In a 1987 study, the average blood pressure of volunteers dropped significantly when they took a daily dose of garlic oil—the equivalent of one-third of an ounce of fresh garlic—over a four-week period. When onion oil was given to people who had high blood pressure, their blood pressure also fell. As an added benefit, their cholesterol was also reduced.

There are also other dietary changes that can help you. If you drink coffee or black tea and also suffer from high blood pressure, consider switching to green tea. The Japanese neurologist Yoshikazu Sato, M.D., has found that green tea lowers high blood pressure. He believes that this may be why Japanese women who drink green tea experience only half as many deaths from stroke as those who don't, even though their diet contains large quantities of salt. The popularity of green tea in Japan may be one reason why the Japanese have less incidence of high blood pressure and heart disease than North Americans do.

Another way the Japanese are getting heart benefits is from all the kelp they eat. If you visit Japan, you can't help noticing that this plant appears in almost every meal—they even make noodles out of kelp! Japanese researchers, who are highly interested in kelp's health benefits, have done many studies on how kelp and other seaweeds keep blood pressure down. The results of these studies have been reported in various Japanese medical journals. One way to eat your way to a healthy blood pressure is to use powdered kelp and garlic as seasoning in place of salt. Although kelp contains some salt from the ocean waters it lives in, this is only a "sprinkling" compared to straight salt. The transition is simple. Dump the salt out of your saltshaker and replace it with one of the many salt substitutes sold in grocery stores that contain various herbs, including powdered kelp. You will also find recipes for using kelp in chapter 18. Kelp pills are sold along with other herbal supplements in natural food stores.

Since high blood pressure so often goes hand in hand with tension, the herbal sedatives valerian, skullcap, lemon balm, linden and motherwort hold promise. These herbs reduce stress and muscle tension and may also prove helpful in lowering blood pressure. There is some scientific evidence to support this, especially from studies on motherwort conducted by Italian and Chinese researchers.

Sedative aromas have also been shown to reduce blood pressure temporarily. See chapter sixteen to learn how blood pressure can be lowered simply by sniffing a cinnamon-apple blend or orange blossom essential oil (also called neroli). Even sniffing an orange will provide a similar effect, though to a lesser degree. Next time you feel your blood pressure rising, try biting into a fragrant apple or peeling an orange! Also try sniffing rose geranium oil to keep your blood pressure steady. All these scents can also be used in a relaxing, blood pressure–lowering massage or bath oil.

High Blood Pressure Tea

1 quart boiling water
1 teaspoon each hawthorn berries and
   flowers, ginger rhizome, valerian
   root and motherwort leaves
✎ Pour boiling water over the herbs and steep for 20 minutes. Strain herbs. Drink at least 2 cups a day. You can also

make these herbs into a tincture using the same proportions, or you can look for commercial tinctures with similar herbs in them.

Blood Pressure–Lowering Massage Oil
12 drops each orange and geranium
*   essential oils*
2 drops cinnamon essential oil
4 ounces vegetable oil
❧ Combine ingredients. Use as a massage oil or add a teaspoon to your bath, and stir well to disperse it before getting in the tub.

LOW BLOOD PRESSURE
You have probably heard people complain about their blood pressure being too high, but how about the reverse problem? While it is not too common, many people do suffer from symptoms caused by low blood pressure. If you have low blood pressure, you know that sometimes so little blood reaches your brain that simply getting out of a chair may be all it takes to make the room start swimming around you. But it is not just dizziness that results from low blood pressure—fatigue can also be a problem. And what are the causes? Low blood pressure can be caused by infections, fever and anemia, as well as more serious conditions, such as excessive bleeding and certain types of debilitating diseases.

If you have a relatively minor case of chronic low blood pressure—your doctor will tell you whether or not it is serious—that is not the result of an emergency situation, European physi-

cians have an answer for you. Rosemary infused in white wine is a centuries-old European treatment for poor circulation, low blood pressure and the headaches brought on by these conditions. Even today, German pharmacists sell a rosemary ointment that is designed to be rubbed over the heart to increase blood pressure. You can make your own version of this ointment by infusing rosemary leaves in a vegetable oil and using the infusion as a massage oil. For instructions on how to make this herbal oil, see Rosemary Heart Oil on page 72.

Herbalists have found that some of the same herbs that raise blood pressure also help lower it. Because of their complex chemistry, hawthorn, ginger, Siberian ginseng and ginseng apparently "normalize" blood pressure, adjusting it according to your body's needs. Studies have shown that a single compound in ginger can both raise and lower blood pressure. A study conducted in Great Britain in 1984 showed that ginseng works the same way. When given to people experiencing low blood pressure, shock and an irregular heartbeat, it helps increase blood pressure and seems to strengthen heart contractions.

Siberian ginseng has a similar story. As shown in studies conducted through the Soviet Academy of Sciences in the 1960s and 1970s, this herb elevates blood pressure only in persons whose blood pressure is low. The researchers who organized these studies observed that Siberian ginseng regulated blood pressure by tightening the walls of arteries. Both ginsengs have been proven to provide a much needed mental and physical boost in people who have low blood pressure.

Another potential blood pressure balancer is rose geranium. This herb is used in experimental outpatient clinics for the elderly in Azerbaijan. Doctors there write prescriptions for their patients to sit and sniff this fragrant plant twice a day. Just inhaling the scent of rose geranium is said to adjust blood pressure—either to raise or lower it—depending upon what the person needs. The Azerbaijani doctors use the actual plant, which is commonly sold in nurseries, but you can also buy the essential oil, which is usually sold as geranium. To take advantage of this essential oil's powers, add a few drops to your bath water or simply put a drop on a cotton ball and sniff it.

One interesting herbal compound that has been proved to lower blood pressure is forskolin. This compound is considered a prototype of a new kind of drug to treat low blood pressure, congestive heart failure, blood clotting and asthma and to reduce the pressure in the eye in people with glaucoma. This compound comes from the plant *Coleus forskohli* and was discovered because a closely related coleus is used in the traditional Ayurvedic and Unani healing systems in India. Eventually, this compound will probably be offered both as a drug and as an herbal product.

Rosemary Heart Oil

½ cup olive oil
¼ cup dried rosemary leaves
☙ Pour oil over leaves in a clean jar. Place in a warm location (in the sun or on a radiator, for instance) for 2 days. Strain out the leaves. Use this infusion as a massage oil to rub on the chest.

Low Blood Pressure Tincture

½ teaspoon each tinctures of hawthorn berries and flowers, ginger rhizome, rosemary leaves and Siberian ginseng root
☙ Combine ingredients. Take half a dropperful 2 to 4 times a day.

VARICOSE VEINS AND HEMORRHOIDS

I once thought varicose veins were a problem only for elderly women, until I began discovering road maps on my legs at the tender age of 19. I was in college, spending long hours standing on cement floors in the art room and the library where I worked. Fortunately, I already knew about medicinal herbs and wasted no time in searching for ones that would stop my varicose veins from getting any worse. More than 20 years later, they are smaller than they were in my college days, even though I now spend so many hours sitting at my desk.

Varicose veins and hemorrhoids have a lot in common. They both occur when circulating blood slows down as it fights gravity on its journey back to the heart, and the extra load stretches weak veins. Blood relies on muscles in your legs and pelvis to push it back to the heart, and this is not an easy task if you sit or stand for long periods of time.

If you are overweight, pregnant or constipated, or if you commonly wear skin-tight pants or a girdle, the blood flow through your pelvic area is restricted even more, and varicose veins and hemorrhoids often result. Varicose veins are also quite common during pregnancy; this is not only because a growing fetus pushes on the surrounding veins, but also because rising estrogen levels weaken veins. For the same reason, women generally get varicose veins about four times as often than men. There are also certain enzymes that break down the veins' elasticity. High amounts of these enzymes are found in most people who have varicose veins. Enlarged veins can even indicate liver problems, since surface veins must take on the blood load when the liver becomes congested.

A bad case of varicose veins can cause lots of complications, while the main problems of hemorrhoids are pain and bleeding. Healthy veins produce a substance that breaks down fibrin—the protein that causes blood to clot. Since veins injured by varicosity do not break down as much fibrin, a lot of excess fibrin is deposited around the veins, causing unsightly, hard lumps just under the skin. This creates more problems than just an unpleasant appearance.

Eventually, varicose veins may begin to leak, which can make your skin itch. If enough blood pools in a particular vein, the vein can burst. When this happens, slow-healing ulcers form under the skin. A surgical operation known as sclerotherapy can destroy the offending vein, but other veins must then take on the load, and they too will enlarge.

One of the best ways to stop varicose veins and hemorrhoids from getting any worse is to strengthen your blood vessels and make them less porous. Some of the same herbs used for heart problems, such as hawthorn and ginkgo, can do this. More than 50 studies,

mostly from France and Germany, demonstrate ginkgo's ability to improve blood circulation and reduce the discoloration of varicose veins.

In a study conducted in Italy in 1982, the Indian herb gotu kola improved the structure of varicose veins and increased blood flow through them in 80 percent of the participants who took it for one month. This study also showed that gotu kola strengthens the connective tissue.

Researchers have found that ginkgo and gotu kola are even more effective when used together. Almost everyone who took this combination, many of whom had serious circulation problems in their legs, found that their circulation improved. Some enjoyed their first pain-free walking in months. And in numerous other studies, both ginkgo and gotu kola have been shown to be more effective and better tolerated than tribenoside, the standard drug used for this purpose.

Horse chestnut and butcher's broom—strangely named herbs that are not nearly as well-known in North America as in Europe—can also be used to make veins stronger and less porous. In the seventeenth century, an herbalist wrote that butcher's broom, a Mediterranean shrub, was so named because butchers made brooms from it— the herb's smell kept rodents away. Clinical research conducted in Italy, France and Germany shows that butcher's broom does much more than deter pests—it encourages blood to move up out of the legs, decreases inflammation in the veins and helps to tighten the veins.

Horse chestnut, an ornamental tree that originated in Asia, probably got its name as a corruption of the Welsh *gwres,* meaning "pungent," which was used to differentiate it from the unrelated sweet, edible chestnut. Horse chestnut is one of the few herbs mentioned in this book that needs to be taken with extra care. Small doses (50 milligrams of the plant's active ingredient, aescin) taken two or three times a day are sufficient; very high doses are slightly toxic. European herbalists describe this herb as a "veno-tonic," a tonic that improves the tone of the veins by tightening the elastic fibers in their walls.

Horse chestnut, the enzyme brome-lain from pineapple and gotu kola also stop the enzymes that break down damaged veins. After only 12 days of taking horse chestnut, the level of these enzymes drops by one-quarter. Brome-lain even prevents vein breakage right after surgery, when operations are neces-sary to remove badly varicosed veins. Garlic and pineapple prevent fibrin from forming lumpy deposits around varicose veins.

The compounds known as antho-cyanidins are also beneficial in treating varicose veins—they stop swollen capil-laries from leaking by making them less porous. Several European pharmaceuti-cals sold in France, Germany, Italy and Spain contain anthocyanidins. In Europe these compounds are considered so safe that they are even used during pregnancy. In numerous studies, people with various circulation problems, in-cluding hemorrhoids and varicose veins, who were given anthocyanidins experi-enced dramatic and sometimes total im-

provement in their conditions. In none of the published studies did researchers note side effects.

Similar compounds known as pro-anthocyanidins—currently derived either from grape seeds or from pine nee-dles—support skin and blood vessels in several ways. For one thing, they increase the amounts of intercellular vitamin C and collagen (fibrous protein bundles that form the connective tissue that sup-

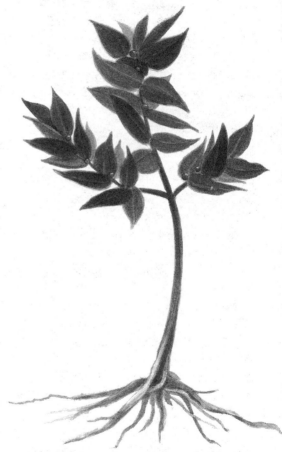

According to legend, butcher's broom was so named because butchers used it to make brooms, primarily because the smell kept rodents away.

ports blood vessels, ligaments and cartilage). Another way to strengthen connective tissue is with the silica-rich herbs horsetail, knotgrass and nettles.

Horse chestnut, butcher's broom, calendula and Saint-John's-wort are used in several European varicose vein ointments and in suppositories for hemorrhoids, to reduce inflammation, pain and broken veins. The witch hazel sold in drugstores and the essential oils of palmarosa, chamomile and cypress have similar properties. If varicose veins break, you can cover them with a cold compress of calendula or Saint-John's-wort with chamomile and carrot seed essential oils. This will decrease the swelling and pain and will deliver healing factors that help repair the veins.

Varicose Vein/Hemorrhoid Tea
¹/₂ ounce each hawthorn berries and flowers, ginkgo leaves and butcher's broom (if available)
Hot water (enough to cover herbs)

Combine herbs. Cover with hot water and steep for 5 minutes. Strain and drink. The same herbs can also be used to make a tincture (they are, in fact, used in several commercial tincture formulas).

Varicose Vein/Hemorrhoid Oil
1 ounce Saint-John's-wort oil
8 drops each essential oils of chamomile, palma rosa and cypress
Combine ingredients. Apply externally.

Varicose Vein/Hemorrhoid Compress
1 cup cold water
1 teaspoon tincture of calendula or Saint-John's-wort
3 drops each essential oils of chamomile and carrot seed
Combine ingredients. Stir a soft cloth in them, wring out and place over itching or broken varicose veins or hemorrhoids as often as practical.

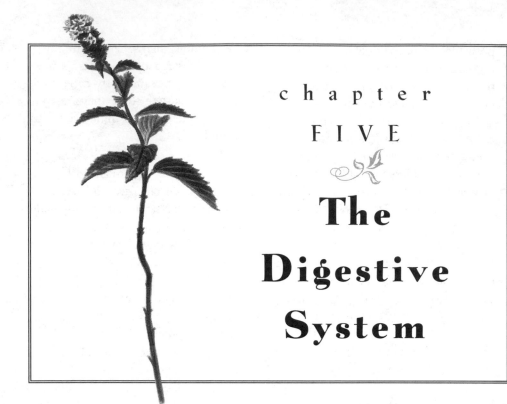

chapter FIVE

The Digestive System

Because of our rich diets and life-styles, most North Americans generally heap liberal amounts of abuse on their digestive systems. Unfortunately, our bodies have ways of exacting revenge. Upset stomach, burping, gas, constipation, diarrhea and other digestive tract disorders are the most commonly voiced physical complaints.

How often have you eaten too much, too little, too quickly, too seldom, too often, while on the move or before bed? Or simply eaten foods that did not agree with you? Even our emotions affect how well we digest food—if you're upset and you eat a big meal, you usually suffer. Stress impairs digestion by restricting the flow of digestive juices and constricting muscles in the digestive tract. Blood also moves away from your digestive tract to feed muscles in case an emergency arises. In addition, most doctors believe that tension contributes to various digestive complaints, including colitis, ulcers and irritable bowel syndrome.

When your digestion is normal, food you eat goes down the esophagus and through a valve into the stomach, where your body starts breaking it down. It then moves into the intestines, which break the food down the rest of the way, extracting the nutrients the food has to offer and sending the waste on to be ejected from the body. Problems can arise at any point in this process. If the stomach is not working properly, for example, you can get peptic ulcers. Irritation of the digestive tract can cause pain and inflammation, and as a result, nutrients sometimes cannot be absorbed.

Bouts of indigestion can ruin not just a meal but your whole day. Herbs can help because they act directly on the digestive system—simply by swallowing an herb, you put it in contact with your entire digestive tract. Be aware, however, that if your digestive problems involve pain or bleeding, you must see a physician to get checked for any serious disorders, such as appendicitis, intestinal blockage or cancer.

APPETITE LOSS

Losing your appetite once in a while is no big deal. A few days of low appetite when you have a flu or fever is not a cause for concern. At such times, it is all right to give yourself a rest from eating so that your body can focus its energies on fighting the illness. And when you feel down emotionally you may not be in the mood to eat much—this is also okay and generally is not something to worry about. But if your appetite loss continues for more than a week or if it happens for no apparent reason, you should make efforts to figure out why you aren't interested in eating. If your problem is due to a simple illness, an herbal appetite stimulant should have your mouth watering and your stomach rumbling in no time at all. But if you lose your appetite as a result of a more serious condition, the underlying problem must be addressed. This will probably require professional help.

Have you ever noticed how the enticing smell of pizza or an herb bread baking in the oven sets your stomach grumbling? The aromas that make foods smell and taste so good also help your digestion even before you take the first bite! The aroma signals the brain, which relays a message to the digestive tract that food is on its way. The digestive tract responds by producing digestive fluids, even though the food hasn't hit your mouth yet. You can stimulate your appetite in a similar fashion, by making an aromatic tea of anise or peppermint.

If a long illness leaves you feeling weak and you are unable to digest solid foods, try making Slippery Elm Gruel (see page 78). This nutritive herbal food will be easily digested by your ailing digestive tract. Slippery elm powder comes from the bark of the slippery elm tree. (Since populations of these trees are dwindling, be sure to insist on slippery elm that has been properly harvested. Careless harvesting results in peeling off so much bark that the tree dies.)

To further spice up your appetite, add a dash of cinnamon. Finally, for people who have been weakened by diarrhea or a debilitating disease, the Chinese suggest astragalus, and Western herbalists use prickly ash to strengthen the digestion tract and improve the appetite.

Appetite Stimulant Tea

1 teaspoon, fresh, grated or dried ginger root

2 cups water

¼ teaspoon each peppermint leaf, anise seed and cinnamon

1 teaspoon honey (optional)

🍃 Simmer ginger in water a few minutes, then remove from heat. Add other ingredients, cover and steep for about 20 minutes, then strain. Drink 1 or 2 cups as needed.

Slippery Elm Gruel
¹/₄ cup slippery elm bark powder
¹/₂ teaspoon powdered cinnamon
2 cups cold water
¹/₂–1 teaspoon honey or maple syrup
    (optional)
🙠 Stir powders into cold water in a
pan and let sit for about 30 minutes.
Slowly heat this mixture for 5 minutes,
gently stirring to prevent clumping. Let
cool, add sweetener if desired and serve
warm or cool.

BOWEL DISEASES

Common bowel diseases, such as ulcerative colitis, Crohn's disease, spastic colon
and irritable bowel syndrome (IBS), are
responsible for nearly half the visits to
digestive tract specialists. The causes of
these diseases are not clear, although
doctors do know that excitement and
stress make them worse.

Regardless of the causes, it is certain
that diet plays a role in bowel disorders.
Surveys show that Crohn's disease is
almost nonexistent in cultures where the
basic diet includes natural, unrefined
grains and plenty of vegetables and
fruits. Surveys also show that the cases
of the disease are rapidly increasing in
technologically advanced countries,
where people tend to eat more refined
sugar, fewer vegetables and less fiber.

Crohn's disease alters your natural
intestinal flora, making it difficult for you
to assimilate important nutrients, particularly protein. The results of a recent
five-year study done in Stockholm
showed that there is an increased risk of
developing Crohn's disease or colitis if
you eat "fast foods" at least twice a week.

Crohn's disease often results in deficiencies in vitamins E and K, copper, niacin
and zinc. And people with bowel problems also tend to be deficient in the important nutrients magnesium, calcium,
vitamin C and folic acid.

Bowel diseases can be both painful
and debilitating. Both colitis and Crohn's
disease produce intestinal spasms,
mucus, and bouts of diarrhea, constipation or both. One difference is that
Crohn's disease tends to cause sharp, intense pain in isolated areas, while colitis
painfully inflames the entire large intestine. And attacks of diarrhea brought on
by IBS are often so unpredictable that
people who have these conditions fear to
stray far from home.

One interesting remedy for various
types of bowel diseases is a grapefruit
seed extract. Although this extract is
generally used to get rid of eczema, researchers testing its effects on skin noticed a curious—but beneficial—side
effect. Grapefruit seed extract not only
cleared up people's skin, it reduced diarrhea, constipation, intestinal gas, bloating and general abdominal discomfort.
The dosages are small, usually only a
couple of drops in a glass of water, so be
sure to follow the instructions on the
package. Grapefruit seed extract is also
available in capsules.

Herbs such as calendula, marshmallow, licorice, Saint-John's-wort, chamomile, peppermint, hops and wild yam
reduce the inflammation that causes the
pain associated with these disorders.
They also relax the nervous constriction
of the digestive muscles and reduce the
general tension that can promote bowel
problems.

It takes only 20 to 40 minutes for a tea or tincture of hops to relax intestinal spasms. In one study on colitis, the pain suffered by almost all the participants disappeared within 15 days of starting a combination of calendula, dandelion, Saint-John's-wort and lemon balm (with fennel seed to relieve gas). Similar remedies that are popular in Europe include salad burnet, agrimony and bilberry. Gamma linoleic acid (GLA), from evening primrose oil, and omega-3, which is found in the herb purslane, also reduce inflammation and pain. The cabbage powder described to treat ulcers also heals the lining of the intestine.

Since psyllium is usually taken as a laxative, you might not think of using it for these various bowel diseases. It has, however, helped many people. In the late 1980s, several studies on psyllium seed were conducted at the department of gastroenterology at Hospital Italiano in Buenos Aires. In one of these studies, people with IBS, diarrhea or painful constipation due to bowel disorders were given psyllium seeds. By the end of the survey, 80 percent of the participants reported a decrease in pain, and all those who had diarrhea or constipation found that the conditions went away.

If you walk into almost any pharmacy in Europe and ask about treatments for chronic bowel problems, the clerk will recommend peppermint essential oil capsules. These specially coated capsules, which are especially effective in treating IBS, do not open until they reach the bowels. In a study conducted in 1984, these capsules were found to cure people suffering from irritable bowel syndrome. Earlier, researchers had re-ported that "peppermint oil in enteric-coated capsules appears to be an effective and safe preparation for symptomatic treatment of irritable bowel syndrome."

Peppermint oil capsules certainly worked for Betty, who suffered bloating and embarrassing episodes of intestinal gas, often accompanied by cramping, as well as bouts of diarrhea that would hit her without warning. Because her bowels were so unpredictable, Betty, a vibrant woman in her seventies, worried about going anywhere, even to visit her doctor. When the loss of her quilter's club meetings, square dancing classes and visits to her grandchildren became too much, she finally made an appointment with her physician. Betty was told she had irritable bowel syndrome and was given a fistful of different prescriptions. She faithfully started taking the pills, but her problem did not improve and she began feeling groggy and out of sorts.

It was only when her daughter examined the fine print on the bottles that Betty realized she was taking some heavy-duty sedatives, which had been prescribed probably because the doctor had blamed her IBS on psychological problems. After visiting various doctors, including several specialists, and spending thousands of dollars on appointments and prescriptions, Betty decided that it was the treatment, not the disease, that was turning her into a nervous wreck. When Betty pointed this out, she was told that, like many of those who have suffered at some time from IBS, she would "just have to learn to live with it."

Then Betty discovered herbs. Her friend Charlotte came to visit from

England and was dismayed to hear Betty's story. While Charlotte had never had IBS herself, two of her close friends and a niece had. Their doctors in England had provided capsules of peppermint essential oil, and they all reported great results. At first, Betty could not find the pills, so she drank plain old peppermint tea. She found it helpful, and when she was able to get the pills, she discovered that they did indeed work wonders—and for a lot less money and with fewer side effects than the drugs.

The inability of researchers to pinpoint the source of many cases of bowel disease has led to a number of theories. One suggests that bowel disease is connected to problems in the immune system and possibly even food allergies. In one study, researchers who looked at a group of people suffering from IBS found that two-thirds of them had food reactions, especially to coffee, alcohol and protein, and that everyone improved when the offending foods were pulled out of their diets.

Some of the best herbs to soothe the bowels, improve immunity and help prevent food allergies at the same time are chamomile, marshmallow and licorice. Chamomile and licorice have even been found to lower the risk of developing colitis. For more information and ways to treat bad reactions to food, see "Food Allergies and Reactions" on page 87.

Some bowel disorders, such as ulcerative colitis, can even result in bleeding, which in turn can cause anemia. Herbalists find that yellow dock helps increase iron levels and also tones the intestinal lining and slows bleeding. For more on anemia, see "Anemia" on page 152.

Bowel Formula

1 teaspoon wild yam root
½ teaspoon yellow dock root
1 quart water
1 teaspoon peppermint leaf
½ teaspoon each marshmallow root, chamomile flower, echinacea root and fennel seed

🍂 Add wild yam and yellow dock to water in a saucepan, bring to a simmer and add other herbs. Steep for about 15 minutes, then strain. Drink at least 2 cups daily. To enhance effectiveness, I like to mix this tea with equal amounts of carrot and celery juice—these vegetables also benefit bowel disorders. This formula can also be made into a tincture by combining the same recommended quantities of tinctures.

CANDIDA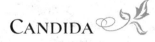

More and more people are tracing various health problems to stubborn, yeast-like fungi called *Candida albicans*. Not a foreign invader at all, Candida occurs naturally in the vagina, on the skin (especially in moist areas such as the armpits) and especially in the digestive tract. Only when it gets out of hand and grows disproportionately in the intestines does candida begin contributing to various health problems, including appetite loss, belching and an overabundance of stomach acid. One of the biggest concerns is graphically termed a "leaky gut." This condition occurs when the intestinal wall becomes too porous, allowing undigested proteins to pass through it into the blood, which increases the risk of developing food allergies.

Candida is usually concentrated in the digestive tract. "Systemic" candidiasis, which occurs when Candida gets into the blood and travels to other parts of the body, is fortunately quite rare—it usually occurs only in people whose immunity is compromised, such as people with AIDS or those undergoing chemotherapy. Unfortunately, many physicians do not see candidiasis as much of a problem until it becomes this serious, and they generally do not diagnose it as such until it becomes systemic. And because Candida has been getting a lot of press in natural health magazines and booklets, many people who are in the habit of diagnosing themselves often think they have Candida simply because they have gas and indigestion, are fatigued or feel fuzzy-headed. So before you jump on the Candida bandwagon, consider that there are many other disorders that produce similar symptoms.

There are a number of herbs that can help control Candida. Studies from Germany, Russia, England and Hungary show that the fungi are inhibited by many plants whose essential oils are potent antifungal agents—cloves, cinnamon, allspice, tea tree, lavender, garlic and chamomile. In one impressive study, the fresh husk of the black walnut was shown to destroy Candida better than a commonly prescribed antifungal drug. Echinacea, valerian and berberine (from goldenseal, barberry or Oregon grape root) have been shown to inhibit Candida in various studies.

My friend David was convinced that Candida had overrun his digestive system. His doctors told him that he did indeed have thrush, an invasion of Candida that was making his mouth sensitive and sore, and they prescribed a common antifungal drug used to treat candidiasis. But David found himself on a healing roller coaster—getting better, then worse, then better and worse again. David decided to concentrate on improving his diet and taking nutritional supplements. But it wasn't until he started taking an herbal tincture similar to the recipe provided below that he saw permanent results. In fact, the herbs worked so well that David decided to enroll in an herbal training program to learn all he could about preventing other health problems.

Candida Tincture
1 ounce tincture of black walnut husk (must be fresh)
½ ounce each tinctures of lavender flowers, valerian root and pau d'arco
Combine ingredients and shake well before using. Take 2 to 3 dropperfuls a day.

You may find similar formulas sold in natural food stores. A tincture is the best way to take black walnut. Tea tree is currently sold only as an essential oil.

CONSTIPATION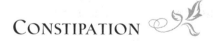

The causes of constipation range from simple—a diet lacking in adequate fiber or water, for instance—to tragic—an intestinal tumor. If you suffer from severe constipation not related to some obvious change in diet, you should see a doctor to make sure that it is not a symptom of a serious health problem. Once your doctor determines that you do not have a serious problem, laxative herbs can rescue you from the occasional bout of constipation. *Warning:* No laxatives, even herbal laxatives, should be used on an ongoing basis. You can become dependent on them.

Laxatives should never be used to compensate for a bad diet. Fiber—indigestible material that the intestines work to push out of the system—is absolutely essential to a healthy digestive system, so make sure you eat lots of it. You can do that by eating lots of fruits, vegetables and whole grains. You should also stay away from pastries and breads made with refined flour, and be sure to drink plenty of water.

Bulk laxatives are the gentlest solution to occasional constipation, especially if you have sensitive or inflamed bowels. Bulk laxatives are often safe to use even when you have intestinal inflammation, hemorrhoids, or colitis or are pregnant or nursing. If you have any of these conditions, ask your doctor if these kinds of laxatives are safe for you to use. Even if you have an iron gut, you should use a bulk laxative as your first choice.

The most popular bulk laxative is psyllium, an herbal remedy that is sold in drugstores. A close relative of the common North American weed plantain, psyllium grows in arid climates and depends upon its seed husks to absorb enough water to sprout. In your intestine, this same action moves everything along like a bulldozer. In a 1987 study, psyllium helped 80 percent of the people whose constipation was due to irritable bowel syndrome. Psyllium products carry warnings about the possibility of developing an allergy to this herb, but

you probably don't have to worry about this if you're planning to use the product at home. The few people who have developed allergies or become sensitive to psyllium were health care workers, such as nurses, who were overexposed to it at work while dispensing it to patients.

Laxative syrups and tablets of the once-popular herbs cascara sagrada and senna are still sold in many U.S. drugstores. Cascara and its European counterpart, buckthorn, are favorites of herbalists and pharmacists alike. After having cascara introduced to them by Native Americans, missionary priests in late nineteenth-century California were so impressed with the herb's action that they christened it *cascara sagrada,* which means "sacred bark" in Spanish. The stronger-acting (but cheaper) senna, a shrub from the Middle East, is the most often purchased laxative herb in North America.

Both of these herbs are considered "irritating" laxatives since they work by aggravating the intestine and causing the body to order an evacuation. They are safe if used in small amounts and for a short period, but remember to go easy with them. Long-term use, especially for more than a week at a time, can make your body forget how to operate on its own and may also encourage hemorrhoids. Nursing mothers should also be careful—these laxatives find their way into breast milk.

Cascara is considered the gentlest of the irritating laxatives since it works primarily through the nervous system and only partly by causing intestinal irritation. Like many herbs, cascara has more than one function—it also helps improve the tone and function of the intestines. Because of this, herbalists suggest it as a tonic to the intestinal tract. In contrast, the irritating laxatives aloe and Turkey rhubarb are much stronger and should be used with care. (Do not confuse the laxative aloe with the healing-enhancing aloe juice. Although these two treatments come from the same plant, the laxative is the yellowish layer right next to the leaf that is removed before making the juice.) And while Grandma may have thought castor oil was a good natural laxative, we now know it should never be used as a laxative because it can produce dehydration and mineral imbalance.

You can take less of any laxative by taking licorice with it. Licorice, which is itself a light laxative, makes the intestine much more responsive to other laxatives. Irritant laxatives should also be combined with an herb to relax the intestines and prevent cramping. Some of the most popular of these are peppermint, ginger and fennel.

If you buy laxative as a syrup or pills, follow the directions on the bottle—the recommended dose is usually a teaspoon of syrup or two capsules. You can also take a tincture. You might even make laxative tea, but it is very bitter.

Be warned that laxatives have a time delay. Irritating laxatives take 6 to 12 hours to work, and bulk laxatives take even longer, 12 to 24 hours. I know of people who took one dose, waited only half an hour for results, then took more and more. Eventually, the laxative did work—and the constipation quickly became diarrhea! I am sure that those people will never make that mistake again.

One way you can make a tasty laxative snack is to soak stewed prunes, figs or dates—all natural laxatives—in licorice tea. This works especially well for children and uncooperative adults who refuse to swallow anything that even vaguely hints of being medicine. Another good laxative technique for the reluctant is a massage oil made with essential oils that are gentle laxatives, such as chamomile, marjoram and peppermint. Use this oil to massage the abdomen for about five minutes. The laxative effect of the massage is not as strong as if you take the herbs internally, but the

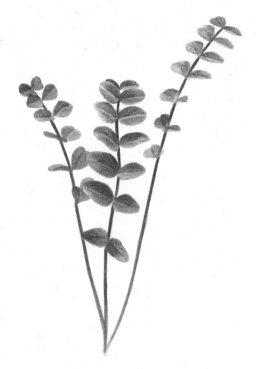

Candy lovers will be surprised to hear that most licorice candy in the United States is not really made from the licorice plant—it's flavored with anise. The real thing actually has a stronger taste than the candy!

massage does help relax intestinal muscles and get them moving.

Another laxative herbal food, which is popular in India, is tamarind pulp. In North America, it is sold in Indian grocery stores and in many natural food stores. This pulp, which comes from the pods of the tamarind tree, is a gentle laxative that improves general sluggishness of the bowels. Take one to two tablespoons of the pulp in the evening, or use it as a flavoring in an Indian dinner.

Licorice-Soaked Prunes

½ teaspoon licorice root
½ cup water
3 stewed prunes, 3 stewed figs or
    2 stewed dates

🌿 Make a tea by simmering the licorice in water for a couple of minutes. Remove from heat and steep for about 15 minutes. Strain and soak fruit in tea for at least a few hours. Eat cold or slightly warmed.

Herbal Laxative Syrup

1 teaspoon honey (or barley syrup or
    some other natural liquid sweetener)
2 teaspoons cascara sagrada bark
    tincture
1 teaspoon licorice root tincture
½ teaspoon tincture of fennel, ginger
    or peppermint

🌿 Warm honey enough to make it liquid. Combine it with remaining ingredients and stir well. Take 1 teaspoon.

Psyllium Seed Bulk Laxative

1 teaspoon psyllium seed husks
1 cup warm water
1 tablespoon lemon juice (optional)
½ teaspoon honey (optional)

🌿 Mix seedhusks in water and stir. Flavor with lemon juice and/or a little honey, if desired. Quickly (before husks thicken) drink 2 teaspoons. Take once a day, preferably in the morning. Drink extra water throughout the day to help the seeds swell.

DIARRHEA

I have found that some of the best diarrhea tonics come from well-known herbs. Although you may not have thought about blackberries, raspberries, blueberries and bilberries as being medicines, the leaves and, to some degree, even the fruit of these berry plants work like magic. Just be sure that the berry remedy you use does not contain seeds, or else it will have the opposite effect and act like a bulk laxative! (Commercial syrups and jellies do not have seeds in them. And if you are making your own, you should use a seed sieve, which is available at any store that specializes in jelly-making equipment.)

Chamomile, fenugreek and meadowsweet also stop light cases of diarrhea. Even more important, they tone the intestine and reduce the pain and inflammation that sometimes accompany diarrhea.

Blackberries are my favorite because they are by far the most potent of these plants. Conveniently, they also grow abundantly around my house. The root bark of the blackberry plant produces the strongest diarrhea remedy I know. You may have trouble, however, finding it in a store, even though it appears on the FDA safety list. This may be because digging up blackberry roots is such hard work! However, if you happen to have blackberries in your yard, as I do, only a few inches of root will give you plenty of medicine! Early American women had an easier solution to stop what they called "the runs"—they served their families blackberry jelly on toast.

In the early twentieth century, North American salesmen carried blackberry wine as they traveled from town to town. In fact, some still do! A few years ago, a man sitting next to me on a plane asked what I did. When I told him I was an herbalist, he opened his briefcase to show me a bottle of blackberry brandy next to the calculator, tape recorder and pens. He said that his father and his grandfather had been salesmen, and of all the tricks they taught him, the secret of blackberry was the best. He added that this trick was why his dad and granddad could pride themselves on never missing an appointment, even when traveling south of the border.

Because your body uses diarrhea to flush out "bad" food and intestinal invaders such as viral or bacterial infections and parasites, so it is not always a good idea to stop it. However, this cleaning attempt is not always successful. In any case, having diarrhea for more than two days can make you weak and cause your body to lose important nutrients. Your best bet is to use herbs not only to stop the diarrhea but also to treat the problem that caused it in the first place.

Fortunately, all the berries already mentioned contain a substance called tannin, which tones and temporarily tightens the intestinal lining. This helps prevent the irritating and

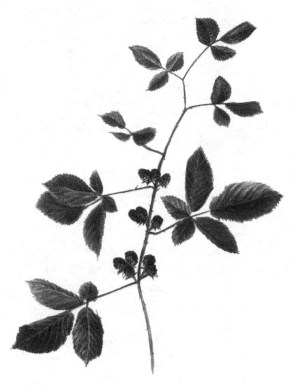

Blackberry, which has a long history as an anti-diarrheal agent, grows wild throughout most of North America.

toxic substances that cause diarrhea from being absorbed back into the bloodstream. Tannins also reduce the bleeding that may result from diarrhea, but if things get that bad, you must see your doctor immediately. You may need to take a dose every half hour or so for a few hours to stop the diarrhea. If the condition persists for more than a few days and the herbs seem to be doing nothing to help resolve it, consult a health care professional.

Do not let diarrhea go unchecked for days, especially in small children. The resulting loss of water and electrolytes can lead to serious dehydration and weakness. If you need to treat your child for diarrhea, you will find more information in "Diarrhea" on page 222. Finally, researchers have found that the herb gentian helps counter the debilitating feeling that sometimes goes along with diarrhea, in part by its action on the digestive tract.

Blackberry Cordial

1 tablespoon chamomile tincture
¼ cup blackberry brandy
3 drops ginger essential oil
2 drops peppermint essential oil
☙ Combine ingredients. Shake well before using. Take 1 teaspoon every 30 minutes.

European Blueberry Remedy

3 heaping tablespoons dried blueberries
1 pint cold water
☙ Put berries in water in a pan and bring to a boil. Let simmer on low heat for about 15 minutes. When the mixture is cool, strain it into a bottle. Take 2 tablespoons every half hour as needed. Stored in the refrigerator, this mixture will keep for a few days.

DIVERTICULITIS

Diverticulitis is a painful condition that occurs when small sacs form in the colon and become inflamed. Although diverticulitis is most common and most serious in the elderly, it can afflict anyone. Susceptibility is greater for people who take prednisone or other drugs with side effects that affect the immune system and increase the chances of developing an infection.

The first indication of diverticulitis is usually pain in the lower left area of the abdomen. You may also develop a fever from the infection, but do not rely on these symptoms to diagnose the condition yourself. You must see a physician to rule out the possibility of several other disorders that have similar symptoms and, if you do have diverticulitis, to judge how serious it is, since bad cases can land you in the hospital.

Doctors believe that the primary cause of diverticulitis is a diet containing little fiber and lots of processed foods. The obvious way to prevent or treat diverticulitis is to improve your diet, although shifting too quickly to a high-roughage menu can irritate your colon even more. Once the problem has cleared up, you must slowly make dietary changes to prevent its return.

If your diverticulitis is not too bad, chances are good that your doctor will send you home to rest and recuperate on a liquid diet and antibiotics to stop the infection. (If you see a holistic or naturopathic doctor, he or she will probably recommend herbal antibiotics.) Once you resume eating semisolid food, usually after a few days, it is likely that even a medical doctor will recommend an herbal treatment—psyllium seed—to keep your bowels loose. See "Constipation" on page 81 for more information on psyllium.

I and other herbalists have found that wild yam can help decrease the pain and inflammation of diverticulitis and promote relaxation in your colon. Chamomile, cramp bark and peppermint are other good additions to your formula. Eating garlic or taking it as pills will directly attack the infection. If you are nervous or stressed, also take herbs that increase relaxation. See "Stress" on page 52 for more tips.

Warning: Do not confuse diverticulitis with appendicitis. An inflamed appendix can produce symptoms that are similar to diverticulitis, with pain in the lower right abdomen instead of the lower left. If you have think you might have appendicitis, you must see a doctor. Once you are on the mend, however, you can follow the same treatments recommended for diverticulitis.

Diverticulitis Tea

2 teaspoons wild yam root
1 teaspoon cramp bark
1 quart water
1 teaspoon each chamomile flower and
    peppermint leaf

Put wild yam and cramp bark in water and bring to a boil. Turn down heat and simmer for about 5 minutes. Turn off heat, add chamomile and peppermint, cover and steep for at least 15 minutes. Strain. Drink 2 or 3 cups a day. You can use the same proportions of these herbs to make a tincture.

FOOD ALLERGIES AND REACTIONS

There is much debate among doctors and researchers about food allergies and reactions. Many define a food allergy strictly as a reaction of the immune system that causes overproduction of histamines with symptoms including hives and difficulty breathing. These allergies can be life-threatening.

Food reactions, however, are much more common but less well-understood and documented. Food reactions create havoc with digestion, causing gas, diarrhea and a long list of seemingly unrelated symptoms not normally associated with allergies, including stomachache. Some physicians totally disregard food reactions, while others claim that they are the cause of up to two-thirds of undiagnosed physical and emotional symptoms. If you have a sensitivity to a particular food, herbs may offer help.

No one knows exactly why some people react poorly to certain foods while others do not. We do know that incidence, or at least reports, of such food reactions has dramatically increased since 1980. Medical experts have theorized that stress, immune system disorders, environmental pollutants, lack of immunity from infant weaning or poor dietary habits might all play a role. Heredity, digestive problems and even emotions may also come into play. If you have impaired digestion, asthma, migraine headaches or an immune disorder, you are more likely to develop bad food reactions than those who don't suffer from these conditions. But it seems that anyone, even healthy individuals, can develop these problems.

According to Joseph E. Pizzorno, N.D., and Michael T. Murray, N.D., authors of *A Textbook of Natural Medicine,* a reference book for naturopaths and even medical doctors who use natural methods in their practice, 60 percent of Americans may react adversely to some food. Many go undiagnosed, however, because few doctors recognize or even think to look for the signs. These include skin rashes, eczema, breathing difficulty, migraine headaches, blurred vision, muscle aches, nervous tension, fatigue, behavior swings, anxiety and even manic depression. Food reactions have been blamed for some cases of paranoia, loss of sight and hearing, hallucinations and catatonic stupors.

Food reactions can be extremely difficult to detect—it can take hours, even days, for symptoms to appear. According to a study conducted in 1973, a delayed reaction is suspected in most such cases. Was the culprit the corn you ate three hours ago or was it that ice cream last night? Could it even be both? Diagnosing food reactions is also tricky for other reasons: It may not be the food itself, but the colorings, additives or artificial sweeteners in the product that cause the problem.

To complicate your detective work even more, the body can respond to food reactions by releasing hormonelike substances that give you a "pick-up." You feel great at first. And when those substances wear off and the unpleasant symptoms kick in, who would think to blame food eaten hours earlier that made you feel so good? In fact, a desire to experience the hormonal uplift can make you unknowingly "addicted" to the very food that is causing your problems. One way to test for problem foods at home is through an elimination diet. Remove one of the suspicious foods from your diet for one week, then start eating it at every meal, for three days if it takes that long, to see if a reaction occurs.

Even after a problematic food has been identified, medical science leaves you with little more than a life of dietary restrictions and a slight hope that the symptoms will someday go away. Herbs combined with temporary diet changes, however, offer something that conventional medicine does not: the possibility of a cure. You could, of course, simply eliminate problem foods from your diet, but remember, the basic concept of holistic healing is to heal the body, not just treat symptoms. It is important that you address the underlying cause as well as the symptoms by improving digestion, liver function and immunity and reducing stress.

One cause of a food reaction is the entrance of poorly digested foods into the bloodstream. When this happens, the foods are treated as invaders and the body reacts negatively. A simple and effective measure is to improve digestion with herbal bitters and natural digestive aids such as papaya, pineapple and ginger. See "Indigestion" on page 91 and chapter 7.

One of the key factors in keeping allergies and reactions in check is maintaining a strong immune system. Allergic symptoms occur when the immune system mistakenly recognizes a food, such as milk or wheat, as foe instead of friend and attacks it. The immune system must be operating at peak efficiency in order to recognize when something is an invader and when it is not. It may seem odd to recommend immunity enhancers when the problem is that the immune system is already overactive, but you must remember that the system works not only to stimulate immune functions but also to keep them in check. Marshmallow, chamomile, licorice and echinacea help the immune system achieve this balance. Since nervousness and stress are known to impair immunity and can make any allergic reaction more severe, you may also want to refer to "Stress" on page 52.

Garlic, onions, licorice and chamomile have all been found to reduce inflammation by decreasing the body's production of histamine, prostaglandins and other inflammatory agents. Chamomile, licorice and marshmallow work not only to stop the inflammation and the allergic reaction, but also to improve digestion and reduce allergic responses in general. Chamomile does this even after the offending food has been eaten. A German study suggests that one way chamomile achieves these results is by stimulating the production of cortisone in the body.

Food Reaction Tincture

*1 teaspoon each tincture of chamomile
    flowers and dandelion root*
*½ teaspoon each gentian rhizome,
    licorice root and marshmallow root*
🍂 Combine ingredients. Take half a dropperful an hour before each meal. You could also use these same proportions to make a tea, although gentian is extremely bitter.

HEARTBURN

Pity the poor heart. It takes the blame for all sorts of upsets. Unrequited love leads to heartbreak. A person who is cruel is said to be heartless. And then there's heartburn, which actually has nothing to do with your heart.

The heat and pain of heartburn occur when your stomach releases acid

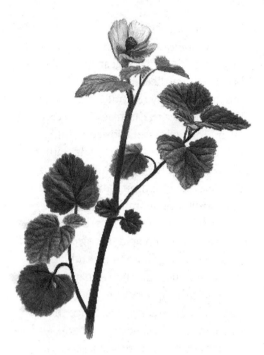

As you might guess from its name, the downy, five-foot marshmallow plant grows in marshes, bogs and damp meadows, and along the banks of streams.

up into your throat—this is called esophageal reflex." The resulting burning sensation and spasm occur next to, but not in, the heart. Heartburn can be caused by several things, but it most commonly happens when there is too much acid in your stomach or you have a hiatus hernia (when your stomach bulges up slightly into the diaphragm, causing belching). Drinking alcohol, smoking cigarettes and eating acidic foods all increase the likelihood of heartburn. However, rather than going through life shunning potlucks and Thai restaurants in fear of what you might accidentally eat, try using herbs to treat this condition.

By the way, if you have not heard already, doctors no longer recommend drinking milk to ease heartburn. This is because it has been discovered that milk only temporarily neutralizes the acidity, then provokes the stomach into secreting even more acid. Antacids containing baking soda are not much help, either. They eventually hinder nutrient absorption, elevate blood pressure and acidity and upset kidney functions.

What does help are herbs that decrease stomach acid: licorice root, meadowsweet, chamomile and lemon. You might also take herbs that absorb excess acid: slippery elm, marshmallow, flax and fenugreek seeds. Since the malic and tartaric acids in carrots and apples also neutralize stomach acid, I like to combine the juices of these vegetables with the herbs to make an extra-tasty tea. Clinical studies have shown that chamomile, marshmallow, licorice, slippery elm, calendula, garlic, wild yam and Saint-John's-wort protect the stomach from its own acid and also reduce inflammation and infection of the lining.

I originally stumbled on a formula for heartburn years ago, quite by accident. When my friends Ed and Carmen had a baby, I sent a basket of herbal baby things, including a tea of chamomile, lemon balm, catnip, fennel and slippery elm to prevent colic. Sometime later, when I spoke to Ed on the phone, he said that he loved the tea and that it relieved his belching from a hiatus hernia that had been plaguing him for years. After some confusion, I realized that the label had fallen off, and he had been drinking the baby's tea!

The most interesting part of this story is that Ed recently asked me if I knew any herbs that were good for treating a hiatus hernia. He said it had not bothered him much for many years and he could not remember why it ever got better. I was not surprised that he forgot, since his "baby" is now 16 years old. I recommended the same tea—and it worked just as well the second time around.

Heartburn Formula

1 teaspoon each chamomile flowers, lemon balm leaves and licorice root
½ teaspoon slippery elm bark
¼ teaspoon each fennel seeds and catnip leaves
1½ cups boiling water
1½ cups carrot or apple juice (optional)
🌿 Combine herbs and pour boiling water over them. Steep for at least 15 minutes, then strain out herbs and add juice. Drink 1 cup after each meal. Stored in the refrigerator, this formula will keep for a few days.

GAS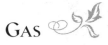

The same spices that improve a poor appetite also relieve intestinal gas. If you suffer from a gas problem, try using coriander, anise, caraway, coriander, fennel and basil when you cook your own meals. Or make yourself a tea of peppermint, thyme, lemon balm or chamomile. Even though many herb books describe all these herbs as digestive "stimulants," researchers have found that most of them actually relax intestinal muscles and relieve cramping. This slowing of the stomach's action gives food more time to be digested, which in turn prevents gas.

Peppermint's versatility has made it the most popular of all these herbs. In 1985 a team of researchers in Germany compared peppermint with drugs that relieved stomach spasms, promoted digestive fluids, killed bacteria and cut down on gas produced in the intestines. In these tests, peppermint proved equally as effective as any of the drugs.

INDIGESTION

Many people assume that their stomach problems are caused by too much acid, as evidenced by the large sales of drug-store antacids. But poor digestion, especially of proteins, can just as easily result from too little stomach acid. Gas and indigestion following a high-protein meal would be an indication of this. Low acidity means that the proteins you eat are not properly broken down. The result is often indigestion and food sensitivities. Tablets of hydrochloric acid are commonly recommended to increase the amount of acid in your stomach, but although these pills provide temporary relief, in the long run they serve only to irritate your stomach even more.

A better treatment for low stomach acid is to take herbal bitters, which encourage your stomach to produce its own acid. The moment these herbs touch your taste buds, a message is sent to your brain, and your digestive fluids, including acids, are activated.

True to their name, these herbs are bitter. But be brave and down your bit-

ters—the health benefits are a sweet payback. One of the best-known bitters is gentian. Appropriately nicknamed "bitter root," this herb remains bitter even at 1 part per 20,000 dilution! When a group of German researchers studied bitters, they found that gentian, combined in a formula with small amounts of cayenne and ginger, cured most cases of general indigestion. You may have already tried gentian without realizing it. It is the main ingredient in the cocktail flavoring Angostura Bitters.

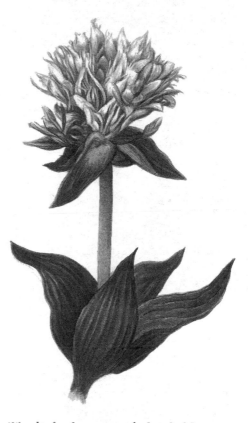

The little-known soft drink Moxie gets its bitter flavor—an acquired taste, no doubt—from gentian, a bitter herb that encourages production of stomach acid.

Campari and vermouth also owe their flavor to herbal bitters.

Bitters enjoy a rather limited popularity in North America, but are quite popular in Europe. Herbal aperitifs, such as the elecampane cordial, are still used to kick off the evening meal in many northern European homes. Greeks dine daily on *horta*, a bitter mix of chicory and dandelion greens sprinkled with olive oil. The French and Italians are certainly no strangers to bitter herbs. Even today, many families enjoy steamed or fried greens such as dandelion every day. The ritual Jewish Passover meal, eaten by Jewish people the world over, includes bitters (in biblical times, these were probably hyssop, wild lettuce, chicory, dandelion and sorrel). In Germany gentian's distant relative, centaury, is used to make a popular bitter drink. And in North America, we drink bitters without even knowing it—the primary ingredient in beer is the digestive bitter known as hops. Other bitters include goldenseal, Oregon grape root and blessed thistle.

The stomach responds to bitters even before they arrive in it. Alerted by the taste receptors, the stomach produces all sorts of digestive juices, which start breaking down fats and proteins in the foods we eat. These juices appear in the intestines within five minutes after a bitter such as gentian is swallowed and remain there for two or three hours. You can forget taking capsules to disguise the bitterness. While it's true that you won't taste the bitterness through a capsule, you also won't get the same results this way. The stomach won't act in the same way as if you took the actual bit-

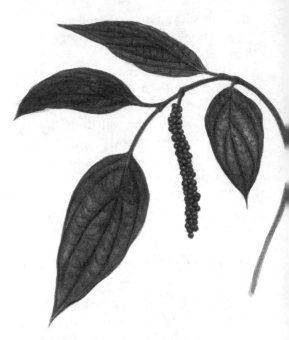

Pepper lovers who suffer from indigestion caused by low levels of stomach acids will be happy to know that black pepper also promotes acid production.

ters because it will be sent a signal that a capsule is on the way, and the digestive requirements are different. What a surprise it must be for the stomach when the capsule opens up and gentian busts out! You can mix bitters with tastier herbs such as orange peel and spices, or even sweeten them. Fortunately, you do not need much of a bitter to enjoy its effects. Just 15 drops of a tincture or a quarter teaspoon of the powdered herb before each meal is enough. You can also take half a teaspoon of Angostura Bitters.

Bitters also encourage the secretion of a digestive hormone called gastrin, which gives hydrochloric acid an extra nudge. If bitters are more than you can handle, try spicing up your meal with a little black pepper or cloves—these will also encourage your stomach to produce acid.

If you often get indigestion after you eat a high-protein meal, this may be because you need more of the enzymes that help your body digest protein. You can find these in papaya peels, pineapples, cucumbers and especially ginger. These digestive enzymes work even when there is not sufficient acid in your stomach. Since they are destroyed by high temperatures, however, you must eat your remedy raw. If fat digestion is your problem, papaya will help your body digest that as well. See chapter 7 for more suggestions on herbs to help you digest fat.

Herbal Bitters

3 teaspoons tincture of gentian rhizome
½ teaspoon tincture of dried orange peel
½ teaspoon tincture of cardamom seeds
Combine ingredients. Drink. You can also purchase bitters at most natural food stores.

NAUSEA AND MOTION SICKNESS

There are plenty of things that can make you feel sick to your stomach, but motion sickness, bad food, the flu, emotional upset and pregnancy are some of the most common causes of nausea. Fear not, however—there are many herbs that can come to your rescue.

Ginger is one of the best natural remedies that I know of, with pepper-

mint and basil close runners-up. Remember, an herbal treatment need not be boring—try some basil in your pasta, soup or salad.

In the 1980s, herbal researcher Daniel Mowrey, Ph.D., came down with a flu and took some ginger capsules. He was surprised how quickly they halted his vomiting and decided to put ginger to the test by giving it to a group of college students and then treating each of them to a dizzying ride in a tilting and rotating chair. Dr. Mowrey's test showed that two 500-milligram ginger capsules are even more effective than Dramamine, the most popular motion-sickness drug.

Since Dr. Mowrey conducted his test, lots of studies have been done on ginger. The results of these studies have often been conflicting, but I will bank on ginger any time. I grew up sailing, and while I have never had much of a problem with seasickness, I have seen plenty of others turn green when they hit the sea. For these people, I always suggest ginger, and so do many of my sailing friends.

David and Barbara first learned of ginger when they were publishing the health magazine *Well-Being*. At the time, they lived on a boat anchored in San Diego and had the opportunity to tell a lot of people about ginger, and also to hear about its results. When they recently took off to sail around the world, you can bet that one of the first things on their list of supplies was ginger to prevent seasickness.

Want to give ginger a try? This tasty herb can be used for any type of motion sickness and lots of other types of nausea as well. In one study, women who were given ginger after they had major surgery experienced much less nausea and vomiting than would normally be expected. If you can, take ginger about 30 minutes before you might experience nausea, then another dose every hour as needed. Unlike most antinausea drugs, ginger will not make you feel sluggish or produce blurred vision and heart palpitations. German researchers think that the difference might be that ginger works via the digestive tract instead of shutting down messages traveling to the brain, which is how many antinausea drugs function. Even the German Federal Health Agency recommends ginger. Delicious ways to use it include baking it into cookies or eating the candied ginger sold in the Chinese section of the grocery store.

I have seen all these herbs in action. Several years ago, when I was at a concert, the promoter sought me out and asked if I had anything for nausea—quick. The band was ready to go onstage, but the lead singer was doubled over behind the curtain, vomiting. Fortunately for her and the anxious crowd, I had a vial of peppermint waters with me. This wasn't anything fancy—it was similar to the peppermint flavoring you can buy at grocery stores. The singer took this remedy and in ten minutes, she appeared onstage, all smiles, and went into her first song. When the promoter returned my vial, now empty, he looked a little dazed. He kept repeating, "What is this stuff? You could make a million on it."

I first learned of how basil can help people who are experiencing nausea as a result of chemotherapy in 1983, when I was researching an article for the *American Herb Association Quarterly*. I found out that Richard E. Anderson, M.D., who was in private practice in San Diego, was giving it to his cancer patients. One of these patients, a woman named Rena, described herself as a skeleton as a result of two weeks of continuous vomiting. After trying every antinausea drug she could find, she tried a tea of basil leaves—and her vomiting ended. Since I wrote that article, I have heard of numerous doctors who recommend basil to stop vomiting. Even eating basil pesto works for some people. (For a recipe for this tasty sauce, see page 340.)

If you find yourself frequently becoming nauseated, you should have your physician check into possible causes. If it is part of chronic indigestion, read the suggestions for using bitters in "Indigestion" on page 91. There is some evidence that bitters help people who tend to get sick to their stomachs.

Natural Ginger Ale

1 teaspoon fresh ginger rhizome, thinly sliced (or ½ teaspoon powdered ginger)
1 teaspoon red raspberry leaves
3 cups water
1 cup carbonated water
1 lemon slice

⚜ Bring the herbs and plain water to a boil, then turn the heat down and simmer for 5 minutes. Remove from heat, and steep an additional 10 minutes. Strain out herbs. Add carbonated water and lemon just before serving. Drink as much as desired.

PARASITES AND OTHER ALIEN INVADERS

Parasites and digestive system infections are common causes of diarrhea and general intestinal upset. The World Health Organization lists 46 infectious agents that lurk in drinking water around the world, but a certain form of the normally friendly bacterium E. coli (called pathogenic) is responsible for at least half of the complaints. In most cases, this particular type of E. coli causes cramps, diarrhea, nausea, fever and vomiting that last no more than a few days. For young children, the elderly, and those weakened by disease, however, pathogenic E. coli infestations can be deadly.

Other unwanted invaders include shigella, salmonella, amoebas and protozoa, including giardia. This last protozoan, which once was a danger primarily for foreign travelers and backpackers, is increasingly becoming a problem even for those who do not stray far from home. Experts estimate that 5 percent of North Americans carry this persistent intestinal parasite. Symptoms of giardia infestation include diarrhea, intestinal cramps, sulfurous belching and sometimes fatigue, decreased appetite, weight loss and difficulty in digesting of fats.

It's up to your stomach acid to kill these invading microbes, so if you have recurring problems, you may have low stomach acid levels. For ways to raise those levels, see "Indigestion" on page 91. There are also herbs that can help get rid of infestations in your digestive tract and herbs to prevent them from establishing residence in the first place. The beauty of these herbs is that, unlike the drugs used to fight intestinal infestations, they interfere very little with your natural intestinal flora. Before you lunge into a self-treatment program, however, it is important to know exactly what you have and how serious it is. Some holistic practitioners blame most digestive complaints on parasites, but I suspect that other problems often cause the symptoms. You should see a doctor to identify the illness and its severity.

Generally speaking, eating garlic and yogurt, and even drinking beer or wine can help ward off invaders—a good thing to remember when you are traveling in foreign countries. Even if your doctor cannot figure out exactly what you have, plenty of studies show that garlic serves as a general cure and overall preventive measure against all sorts of intestinal invaders.

Goldenseal and Oregon grape root fight digestive tract infections, thanks to the berberine they contain. Tablets of pure berberine hydrochloride are sold in Mexico and much of the Orient to destroy parasites. When three Indian pediatricians gave berberine to 40 children infected with giardia, in less than one week about two-thirds of the children showed no traces of the parasite. Other studies from around the world support berberine's ability to fight pathogenic E. coli, shigella and salmonella, as well as several flu viruses, cholera and intestinal parasites such as giardia and other amoebas. South Americans rely heavily on lemon verbena to kill bacterial infections, including pathogenic

E. coli. Hops and nasturtium flowers are also used.

Grapefruit seed extract is also good for fighting the symptoms of various bowel diseases, including constipation, intestinal gas, bloating and abdominal discomfort. In a study conducted in the early 1990s, this same extract was also found extremely useful in treating pathogenic *E. coli,* candida and geotrichum infestations. This remedy is available as a liquid or as capsules; follow the directions on the package.

Traveling almost always increases your chances of infestations and other digestive problems. I've had a few unpleasant experiences traveling in Mexico—I once spent several days in a sagging bed watching a bare lightbulb swing on the ceiling. Montezuma was taking his revenge on my bowels, and the sickness would not end. Once in a while, a matronly woman would peek in, mumbling, *"pobre señorita."*

I have found quassia wood to be one of the best all-around remedies for intestinal infestations. This tree grows in the West Indies and South America, where cups are carved from the wood. I first learned of it when I read how these cups are filled with water and the wood's properties are extracted in a few hours. This drink serves as a remedy for malaria, fever and parasites—these maladies often go hand in hand in the subtropics. Be sure to take it in small amounts, because even a slightly large dose—say, a couple of cups of tea or a couple of dropperfuls of the tinctures—will probably upset your stomach. However, it is so bitter that I have never known anyone to get that much down.

To make quassia more palatable, I borrowed a trick from the Eclectic physicians of the late nineteenth century and added yerba santa, which improved quassia's taste and action. This herb grows wild in the Sierra Nevada foothills where I live, and I pick it every summer. Yerba santa got its name, which means "saintly herb" in Spanish, because it traditionally has been used to treat a number of different disorders. I also add peppermint to this quassia mixture. While neither yerba santa nor peppermint alone is used to treat parasites, both improve general digestion. The mixture I've suggested below still tastes unpleasant, so I suggest you take it as a tincture.

Traveler's Companion
1 ounce each tinctures of quassia bark and goldenseal (or Oregon grape) root
½ ounce each tinctures of yerba santa leaves and peppermint leaves
🐾 Combine tinctures. Even with yerba santa and peppermint, this tincture is rather bitter, so you will have to drink it quickly. Take ½ dropperful about 20 minutes before each meal. If you get sick anyway, double the dose and take 3 times a day.

ULCERS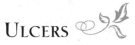

Ulcers are painful sores that occur in the stomach or, more often, in the upper part of the small intestine, which is called the duodenum. As much as 10 percent of North Americans, and four times more men than women, have intestinal ulcers.

There are two types of ulcers: gastric (or peptic) and duodenal. It is very difficult to determine the location of an ulcer by symptoms alone, but almost all ulcers follow a pattern: Pain occurs as acid burns the open sore; food brings temporary relief by neutralizing the acid; pain returns after food is digested.

Ulcers have been thought to be caused by too much stomach acid; more recent research shows that they may be caused by a bacterium called *Heliobacter pylorii*. Overuse of NSAIDS (nonsteroid anti-inflammation drugs)—aspirin, ibuprofen, and the like—also causes ulcers. And stress makes them worse. Nature intended for the intestine to quickly neutralize the acid that is dumped into it from the stomach, but this neutralization does not always happen. Pain from ulcers flares up in response to food entering the system, which causes stomach acid to kick into gear. To know for sure whether you have an ulcer, you need to be tested by a doctor.

Licorice, chamomile, cinnamon, marshmallow, slippery elm, calendula and agrimony are a few of the herbs that herbalists use to lower stomach acid levels. Studies conducted in Germany show that chamomile, licorice and cinnamon decrease the chances of an ulcer getting worse or of your getting another one once the first has healed.

If stress is a problem for you, try taking chamomile, wild yam, Saint-John's-wort and even basil to relax your muscles and nerves, and licorice and marshmallow to stimulate your immune system. In a study conducted in Russia in 1993, a group of alcoholics who had stomach ulcers and chronic inflammation of the digestive tract were treated with a combination of psychotherapy and four to five cups of Saint-John's-wort tea a day. After a couple of months, they had improved and the treatment was pronounced effective.

In the late 1980s, Narendra Singh, M.D., of King George Medical College in India found that a daily tea made of 10 to 20 Indian basil leaves was useful in preventing stress-related disorders such as stomach ulcers and colitis. It is likely that the closely related kitchen spice basil would work equally well and that using it as a spice would be effective.

No matter what your ulcer remedy, there's nothing to stop another ulcer from taking its place unless you make some diet and lifestyle changes. You should also be kind to your ulcer by avoiding irritants such as NSAIDS, alcohol and cigarettes.

Ginger can also be helpful when it comes to ulcers. Japanese researchers who conducted several studies on this spice found that it contains at least six anti-ulcer compounds.

The history of licorice as an ulcer cure is particularly interesting. The ancient Greek physician Dioscorides was using licorice to treat ulcers back in the first century A.D., but over time doctors abandoned the herb. Then, during World War II, the Dutch physician F. E. Revers, M.D., saw a small-town pharmacist prepare a licorice paste for townspeople suffering from stomach ulcers. Dr. Revers could not help trying licorice with a few of his own patients, and he found that it worked just fine. In at least half the patients he tested this paste on, the ulcers were nearly gone within a month. The only real problem that he encountered was that some of his patients developed water retention. In the meantime, doctors have also found that licorice sometimes increases high blood pressure. Researchers have figured out how to remove the compounds that caused these problems, and special licorice preparations that do not have these side effects are available for people with ulcers.

Bruce, a man in his late sixties who has the vibrant energy of a man 30 years younger and an active lifestyle to go along with it, has found licorice to be effective in treating ulcers. After experiencing recurring stomach pain and internal bleeding, he went to the doctor and was tested for stomach cancer. It turned out, however, that the pain and bleeding were due to a severe stomach ulcer, not cancer. Soon after, he started taking herbs.

Months later, I saw Bruce at the movies and waved. He practically skipped up the aisle to where I was sitting and gave me a big bear hug. "They're gone!" he exclaimed. "Who's gone?" I asked. "The ulcers!" After finding out that he did not have cancer, Bruce started an herbal regimen. He took two capsules of licorice three times a day. With a little experimentation, he found that waking up at 4:00 A.M. to take a dose eliminated the early morning feeling in his stomach that, as Bruce said, "can really bite you." When he went back to the doctor after several months, he was given a clean bill of health. As the lights dimmed in the theater, I asked Bruce if I could include his story in this book. Heading back to his seat, he called over his shoulder, "Yes, yes, you should tell the whole world!"

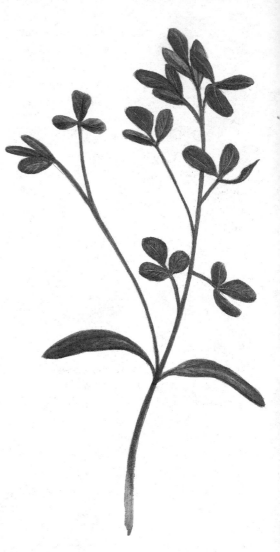

Has the fast pace of today's modern world given you tummy troubles? You'll be happy to know that fenugreek soothes inflamed stomach tissue.

Meadowsweet, aloe vera, mullein and fenugreek all soothe inflamed and bleeding ulcers. Meadowsweet is a known pain reliever and is good for treating ulcer pain. In a study conducted in Russia, compounds in aloe vera juice healed every participant's ulcers so completely that the researchers responsible for the study compared aloe vera favorably to cimetidine, one of the most popular anti-ulcer drugs. In Bulgaria, doctors successfully treat intestinal ulcers with a pharmaceutical preparation called Verbascan, which is made from mullein.

Classic European remedies whose effectiveness has been verified by medical research include raw cabbage and potato and celery juices. Drinking a cup of cabbage juice four times a day can heal stomach ulcers in only ten days. If juicing cabbage does not fit into your busy schedule, you can purchase dehydrated, raw cabbage powder at natural food stores.

The magic ingredient in cabbage is sometimes called the anti-ulcer U factor. Its technical name is glutamine, and this compound is also available in capsules. Glutamine has proved to be a better ulcer cure than antacids. In one study, the ulcers of half the participants disappeared in only two weeks, and those of almost all the rest were healed in four weeks.

One herbal combination with a long history of curing ulcers is Robert's Formula. Not much is known about Robert. He was probably a physician, but legend has it that he was a sailor who suffered from severe stomach ulcers. Robert tried various herbs to cure his ulcers. Some had minor effect; others didn't work at all. Every time he visited a new port, he added a new plant to his formula. The final concoction healed his ulcer. There have been some revisions to the formula since Robert's time, but it is basically the same. Some of its main ingredients are marshmallow, slippery elm and dried cabbage powder, with echinacea and baptisia to help enhance immunity and fight infection.

With Robert's Formula in mind, I concocted this tea to combat ulcers. Friends have found it very helpful.

Ulcer Tea

*1 teaspoon each licorice root,
marshmallow root and chamomile
flowers*
*½ teaspoon each Oregon grape root,
hops strobiles, echinacea root and
cinnamon bark*
1 quart water

🍃 Put herbs and water in an uncovered saucepan. Bring to a boil, then turn down heat and simmer for about 15 minutes. Remove from heat and steep for about 10 minutes. Strain herbs and store the tea in the refrigerator. Drink 2 or more cups a day.

If you have ulcers, there are some natural substances that you should avoid: papaya and pineapple. The digestive enzymes made from papaya, which are used in most commercial meat tenderizers, will corrode the areas in the stomach that have been injured by your ulcer. Pineapple can make your ulcer worse in the same way.

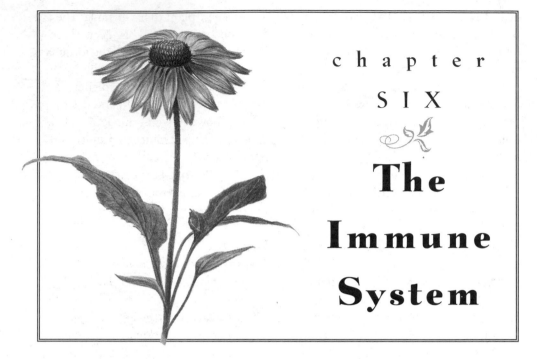

Avoiding viruses, bacteria and the like is nearly impossible in the modern world. Potential infections are everywhere, and new ones spring up all the time, or at least find their way beyond previously insurmountable geographic and biological barriers. You can almost hear some of those exotic viruses singing, "It's a small, small world."

You have probably noticed how often I talk about the importance of building up your immune system. This is because your general health is based on your ability to fend off disease. I'm not just speaking about the common cold, flu viruses and allergies. As our understanding of immunity increases, so does the list of serious immune-related diseases, among them psoriasis,

asthma, multiple sclerosis, cancer, Epstein-Barr virus and chronic fatigue syndrome. Even arteriosclerosis and chronic infections like nephritis and colitis may belong on this list. With some conditions, such as allergies and asthma, the problem is not that your immune system is suppressed, but that it is overactive and responding overaggressively to harmless foreign substances such as pollens or dust.

Several autoimmune disorders actually cause your immune response to work against itself. The immune system is composed of many different parts working together to protect the body. This system has built-in regulators that tell it when to turn on and when to shut down. Autoimmune disorders occur when your immune system falsely identifies normal substances in the body as invaders and attacks them, injuring tissue. Examples of such disorders include lupus, rheumatoid arthritis; pernicious anemia, a severe blood disease; and Addison's disease, which is caused by partial or complete failure of the adrenal glands. According to medical researchers, it is quite possible that some cases of diabetes and infertility, chronic hepatitis, atopic dermatitis (an intensely itchy swelling of the skin caused by an allergic reaction), some cases of asthma and many other inflammatory and several degenerative disorders with no other known causes may also be autoimmune problems.

The term "immune stimulant" was coined by German researchers to describe herbs that help put your immune system in gear. It may seem that immune herbs simply crank up your immune system, but this is not necessarily true. The immune system is complex, and immune herbs can play many different roles. German scientist Hildebert Wagner, Ph.D., who has studied immune herbs extensively, prefers the term "immunoregulator." These herbs not only stimulate an underactive immune system, but also help prevent the immune system from overreacting to invaders or to substances the body falsely identifies as invaders.

Many of the herbs discussed in this chapter increase the production and activity of macrophages—cells that the immune system sends to digest foreign invaders. Some herbs also stimulate the production of defense substances, such as interferon, which protect noninfected cells from viruses. Herbs can also enhance the production and function of T-cells, vital immune cells that kill viruses, fungi and certain bacteria. There is even a special type of T-cell called a natural killer that is in charge of destroying cells already infected with a virus or a cancer.

Your natural immunity is lowered by emotional or physical stress, poor diet, smoking cigarettes and drinking too much alcohol. Of course, laughter and positive imagery can boost your immunity. Be on an immune alert when the chances of getting sick are high—say, when the kids go back to school or when you visit a foreign country. Also look out for a stressful situation on the horizon, such as school exams, a job change, a move or a legal battle. Even "good" stress, like a vacation or getting married, can lower your immune response. Use herbs at these times to bolster your immune system.

BOOSTING IMMUNITY

Herbalists of bygone days may not have understood how the immune system works, but they did know that certain herbs make the body more resistant to disease. If you have a chronic disorder or if it seems that you get sick more often than you should, your immune system probably needs some attention. My suggestion is to use herbs to build up your natural defenses. The beauty of immune system herbs is that they do more than simply hand out temporary instructions for your body to follow—they can actually teach it how to operate better.

ECHINACEA—THE KING OF IMMUNE HERBS

Without a doubt, the most popular immune herb in North America today is echinacea. At last count, more than 300 echinacea products were being sold worldwide. Although this herb is native to North America, most of the research studies have been done in Germany.

Echinacea was introduced to American physicians in 1887, when self-proclaimed doctor H.C.F. Meyer of Nebraska asked Eclectic pharmacist John Uri Lloyd, Ph.D., to endorse his Meyer's Blood Purifier. Meyer told Dr. Lloyd that, just to prove the effectiveness of his Blood Purifier (of which echinacea was the primary ingredient), he would have a rattlesnake bite him in Dr. Lloyd's office, then take the remedy. Dr. Lloyd was unimpressed with Meyer's extravagant claims and declined the demonstration. His opinions changed, however, when he himself began studying echinacea, which quickly became one of the Eclectics' favorite remedies for fighting all sorts of disorders.

In the 1950s, the German pharmaceutical company Madaus began studying echinacea. Since then, nearly 400 studies have shown that echinacea can be used to improve the immune system in numerous ways. These include increasing activity of three of the immune system's workhorses—T-cells, interferon and natural killer cells. Echinacea also destroys many types of viruses and bacteria. Echinacea even makes cells stronger and more resistant to invasion. That's a pretty impressive list of abilities for one herb, and those are only the highlights.

Echinacea is not only versatile; it's extremely safe. And it's especially effective for children. One story demonstrating echinacea's power for kids is that of a young boy named Jason, who was born with such low immunity that he practically lived in a bubble. His dishes, clothes and chair were kept separate from those used by the rest of his family, so that germs wouldn't be transmitted from his folks to him. He had to be home-schooled, and he even had his own bathroom. His doctors had suggested that it might be best for everyone if he lived in a special, sterile home for children like him, but his parents, Mary and Jack, simply could not bear to send him away. Instead, they lived in constant fear of his encountering a bacteria or a virus. In fact, a packed suitcase was always waiting by the door—if he so much as sneezed or coughed, they would rush him to the hospital without a moment's hesitation. Unfortunately, they lived in the country, and the nearest hospital was an hour away. By the time they arrived there, he often had already developed pneumonia and had to be hospitalized.

When I first heard about Jason's problem, I had my doubts about whether herbs would actually help the little guy, but I agreed that they were certainly worth a try. Mary started by giving him a tincture of echinacea. A few weeks later, Jason started coughing. "So much for echinacea," she thought, as she flew out the door with Jason and his suitcase. A couple of hours later, she was in the hospital staring at her son. He had a runny nose and a sniffle that the doctor had diagnosed as a cold. Mary called me, sobbing, "He has a cold, a cold!"

At first, I could not figure out who it was. I thought this mom sounded much too hysterical over a simple cold. Then it dawned on me. It was Jason's mother and she was excited, not worried—this was the first cold that her son had had that had not progressed into pneumonia. The echinacea had worked. And it continues to work to this day. Now a teenager, Jason attends public school and, although he must still be careful when it comes to germs, he lives a nearly normal life.

In my herb classes, I am asked lots of questions about how echinacea works and how to use it. Research from Germany shows that it probably works best as a preventive if you do not use it continuously. For example, you might take it for two weeks, then not take it for a week. It also seems to be best in small doses (up to a dropperful of tincture, or two pills) taken several times a day rather then all at once. Echinacea is not toxic, however, and there is nothing wrong with taking it continuously if you are fighting an active infection.

There is a good deal of confusion about the several varieties of echinacea. Although the different kinds do not all have the same chemistry, they all work. The real concern is that the rarer ones are being overharvested. See chapter 15 for more on this topic. The roots and seeds of this herb have the strongest immune properties, but the leaves are also fairly potent, so some companies use the entire plant.

In a study conducted in China in 1990, even people who were perfectly healthy found that echinacea temporarily increased their immune response, even raising their levels of interferon. Echinacea is often used in China with the herb ligustrum in an immune restorative therapy called *fuzhung*. This treatment, which has been found to increase the manufacture of immune cells in the bone marrow, is sometimes referred to as a deep immunity reaction because it creates more disease-fighting cells, rather than simply stimulating existing ones.

OTHER IMPORTANT HERBS FOR IMMUNITY

Echinacea may be the best-known immunity-enhancing herb, but it is not the only one. In China, astragalus is traditionally used to promote vitality and healing.

Licorice is another great immunity enhancer. This herb is right out there on the front lines, strengthening the very first defense put up by an immune system under siege. A tincture of licorice root is effective against candida and several types of bacteria, including the notorious staph infection. According to laboratory studies done in the 1970s and 1980s, a compound in licorice increases interferon production. Another compound impairs the ability of viruses—including herpes—to survive.

Another important Chinese immune herb is bupleurum. It is a main ingredient in a popular combination called *shosaikoto*, which Chinese researchers believe improves immune system activity. The other ingredients in the formula are licorice, Chinese skullcap and ginseng. Studies conducted in China have shown that Chinese skullcap stops the development of certain viruses and makes uninfected cells more resistant to invasion.

The results of several studies show that when healthy adults are given either capsules of ginseng or a tincture of Siberian ginseng for a few weeks, a whole range of positive changes occurs—in one case, the researchers even referred to them as "drastic" changes. Even greater improvement was seen in volunteers who took a ginseng extract daily for eight weeks in a 1990 study.

Siberian ginseng was not widely used in Russia until the 1960s, when Professor Itskovity Brekhman began studying it. This herb proved to be amazingly versatile, and soon after Brekhman's studies, Siberian ginseng was taken into space with cosmonauts and to the Olympic games with athletes. In time, its use spread to the general population of the Soviet Union. Brekhman dubbed ginseng and Siberian ginseng "adaptogens" since they help the body adapt in so many ways. Most important, they improve immunity and counter the effects of stress, which are commonly implicated in the immune system's becoming deficient.

Preliminary results of studies conducted by Dr. Wagner and his colleagues in Germany show that the Ayurvedic herb ashwaganda from India may also be an adaptogen. Called Indian ginseng, this herb is another known immunity enhancer.

Another possible adaptogen is the immune herb Chinese shizandra. This herb is very important in China, where it appears in many different types of formulas.

According to Dr. Wagner, in German-speaking countries several medicinal herbs are used to enhance

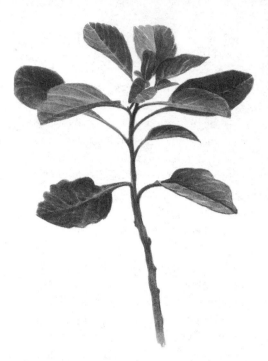

If you get sick often, you may want to check out the Ayurvedic herb ashwaganda, or Indian ginseng, which enhances the immune system.

the immune system or bring it back up to normal levels folllowing an illness. To return the body to health naturally, the Germans use a treatment called *Reizkörpertherapie*. Preliminary scientific evidence shows that some of the herbs in this remedy, including calendula, chamomile, burdock, baptisia, red clover and marshmallow, have immune-enhancing properties similar to those of echinacea. Yellow dock and yucca have similar properties.

All of these herbs increase immune system responses and decrease the number of cancerous cells, at least in the laboratory. They also have a long history of use in treatments for immune-related problems. Burdock, for example, has been used around the world to inhibit and slow the growth of cancerous tumors. It also contains a compound shown to inhibit tumor growth. Other herbs or herbal compounds that have pronounced effects on the immune system include garlic, shiitake mushrooms and gamma linoleic acid (GLA), which is found in evening primrose oil.

In 1960, American herb researcher Kenneth Cochran, Ph.D., of the University of Michigan, launched studies on the properties of shiitake mushrooms. He discovered that shiitake has a strong antiviral compound called lentinan that stimulates the immune system. In follow-up research conducted in Japan, shiitake proved more effective than the powerful prescription drug amantadine hydrochloride in fighting viruses. It was also effective against many types of viral infections. Researchers found that one reason for this is that lentinan apparently increases interferon activity.

Italian researchers have found that thyme, lavender, bergamot and lemon stimulate immunity. After conducting numerous studies, researchers have added eucalyptus, tea tree, rosemary, black pepper, cardamom and ginger to this list. Other herbs historically used to inhibit tumor cells in the laboratory are gotu kola, kelp and dandelion. Depending on the herb, the active ingredient may be the essential oil or some other compound.

The more we learn about the immune system and about herbs, the more immunity enhancers we recognize. Consider the Peruvian rainforest herb uña de gato, or cat's claw, which got its name because of its clawlike

stems. Although this herb did not gain wide acceptance in the United States until 1994, Peruvian Indians have been using the root bark for centuries. Like most immune herbs, cat's claw can be used to treat a wide array of disorders related to the immune system, including rheumatoid arthritis, gastric ulcers, colitis, Crohn's disease, inflammation, allergies, herpes, candida, the leaky bowel syndrome associated with many food allergies, cancer and AIDS. Today, cat's claw is sold in pharmacies throughout Peru.

In one study, cat's claw improved immunity in people with cancer by increasing the amount of disease-fighting immune cells in their blood. In 1989, a U.S. patent was issued to Klaus Keplinger, M.D., of the Immodel laboratory in Austria, for a cat's claw–based product to help the immune system. The report that explains how the product works states that compounds in the bark are "suitable for the unspecified stimulation of the immunologic system."

Cat's claw, which is available mostly in tincture and pill formulas that also include other herbs, seems to be especially useful for treating urinary tract problems associated with poor immunity. This may be due to its ability to reduce spasms in the bladder, as reported in a 1979 study.

This use of cat's claw is demonstrated by the story of Phillip. While gathering information for an article on cat's claw that I was running in my herbal newsletter, I found one person who had had great success using cat's claw by itself. Phillip said that he had been plagued by a chronic urinary tract problem for about 20 years. This problem involved an unspecified inflammation that was probably related to his enlarged prostate gland. Over the years, Phillip had visited a number of different doctors, both holistic and conventional, and had tried numerous nutritional and herbal combinations with minimal results.

Finally, an herbal importer suggested that he try taking cat's claw. After only three days of drinking three cups of cat's claw tea a day, Phillip noticed that his symptoms were starting to diminish. And by the second week, they were gone. Enthused about the herb, he continued to take it and noticed that his resistance to colds, flus and other types of infections also seemed much better.

My friends Sylvia and Dale have had lots of success with immune herbs. Their story is a tale I hear over and over again from many people. Sylvia and Dale sell hand-made items at craft fairs throughout the West. When I first met them, they told me that the extensive amount of traveling they did was not so bad, but getting sick was. All the late nights at motels and stressful days working fairs were not helping their immune systems at all. They seemed to pick up a cold or flu everywhere they went.

Then they started taking an immune tincture similar to the one below. At first, they noticed only a little difference, but later they both realized that they had not been sick for months. This was a definite first for them. As time went on, they got fewer and fewer colds and flus. Dale even said that he felt he had more energy. By now, they have been taking immunity-enhancing herbs

for several years and do not use them on a regular basis—they don't have to. But they do make sure to stock up before a trip.

Immune Tincture

½ teaspoon each tinctures of echinacea root, pau d'arco bark, Siberian ginseng root, licorice root, astragalus root and bupleurum root

Combine ingredients. Take 1 dropperful of formula twice a day for a few weeks at a time to build up your immune system, or 4 to 6 times a day during an active infection or other immune-related problem.

SWOLLEN LYMPH GLANDS

One important part of the immune system is the lymph. This clear liquid flows through the body through its own extensive system of porous channels, passing into the blood vessels and surrounding cells. It empties into strategically placed lymph glands, which filter out foreign materials, particularly bacteria. The tonsils, which are located in the throat, are the best known of these glands.

The extra workload these glands have during an infection can make them swell. That is why swollen lymph glands anywhere in your body indicate that there is probably a nearby infection. Also lymph glands work to stop cancer cells from spreading, but when they do, they become vulnerable to cancer themselves.

Unlike the blood, lymph does not have the luxury of having a heart to pump it around the body. Since lymph relies on the body's movements to get around the body, regular exercise is important. When you are bedridden and unable to exercise, periodically elevating the legs and arms will help. So will alternating hot and cold treatments using a sponge bath or compresses.

One of the many jobs performed by most immunity-enhancing herbs is to assist the lymph system in collecting toxins in the body. Herbs that have traditionally been used to encourage lymph flow and to reduce swollen glands include red root, red clover, cleavers, mullein, prickly ash, lemon peel, baptisia and echinacea. With the exception of mullein and echinacea, these herbs have not been well-studied, but herbalists have been using them to help drain infections for hundreds of years.

Herbalists consider baptisia, also called wild indigo, one of the first options in treating swollen lymph conditions such as tonsillitis and laryngitis. They have found that this herb enhances immune cell destruction of viruses and bacteria, stimulates production of lymph cells, and then gives them a kick in the pants to get them going.

Baptisia is often used for sinus infections. Unlike most herbs mentioned in this book, baptisia must be used with some care. Regular doses of half a dropperful or a tablet or two a day for a week are fine for an adult, but larger doses should be avoided. Baptisia is commonly used in Sweden, but it is classified as a drug there.

Use the lymph-draining herbs when you have a severe or chronic infection or whenever your lymph glands become swollen—when you have tonsillitis; mumps, which swells glands on the sides of the neck; or Epstein-Barr virus, which includes infectious mononucleosis. The lymph herbs are also safe to give

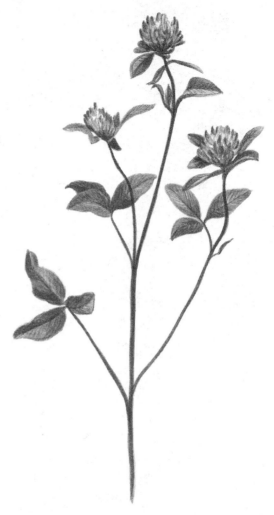

Some poker trivia: Red clover was the model for the clubs suit in every deck of cards.

to children who are plagued by constant ear infections.

The spleen is the largest lymphatic tissue in the body. This organ produces lymph and small immunity-enhancing compounds called peptides. It also helps destroy bacteria and cellular debris such as worn-out blood cells. According to studies done in India, the compound

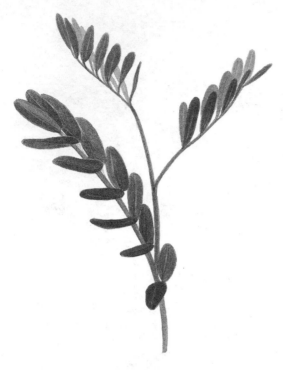

In China, astragalus is used to promote vitality and healing.

berberine, which is found in goldenseal, Oregon grape root and barberry, enhances blood flow through the spleen and thus is thought to improve spleen function. Berberine also increases the activity of certain immune cells. There is also some evidence that astragalus and ligustrum improve spleen activity.

During an infection, a lymphatic massage that uses deep strokes up the arms and legs helps with drainage. Aromatherapy oils, particularly a lemon massage oil, make a lymphatic massage even more effective. The essential oil of bay is another good one, but it is difficult to find. Most of the bay sold in North America is actually pimiento bay, which is related to allspice and is used to make bay rum cologne.

Lymph Drainer

½ teaspoon each tinctures of mullein leaves, echinacea root, prickly ash bark, red clover flowers and cleavers leaves

Combine ingredients. Take half a dropperful 4 to 8 times daily during an active infection. This formula can be taken along with the Immune Tincture on page 106.

CANCER

Although there is still no cure for cancer—pharmaceutical or herbal—medical researchers are busy searching the plant world for an answer to this plague. Medical science already uses compounds derived from the Pacific yew tree to treat ovarian cancer and from mayapple for certain lung and testicular cancers. While these toxic herbs are not suitable for home remedies, there are many herbs that can help you ward off cancer in the first place.

Researchers at the National Cancer Institute's Designer Foods program are currently investigating cancer-fighting compounds in foods and herbs. Researchers there and elsewhere are coming up with some interesting findings. Research conducted at the University of Illinois in Chicago, for example, has shown that thyme contains 40 cancer-preventing substances and sweet basil has more than 30. And this research is not limited to the United States.

In a study conducted at the National Institute of Nutrition in Hyderabad, India, chronic smokers took turmeric daily for a month. Their bodies converted and eliminated three to eight times more carcinogens than smokers who did not eat this spice. Because of this study, researchers are encouraging Indians—whether they smoke or not—to increase their consumption of turmeric. In New Jersey, researchers at Rutgers University speculate that regular use of even small amounts of culinary herbs like thyme, basil and turmeric can reduce your risk of cancer.

Garlic may also protect against some forms of cancer. A survey of 4,000 Italians and Chinese was reported at the First World Congress on the Health Significance of Garlic in Washington, D.C., in 1990. The results of this survey led researchers to conclude that people who eat lots of garlic and its relatives, including onions, leeks, chives and scallions—at least 25 to 50 pounds a year over 20 years—have fewer cases of stomach cancer.

Other studies lend support to the healing powers of garlic. Mei Xing, M.D., of Shandong Medical College, for example, found that the residents of two towns in China had similar lifestyles and diets with one exception—the inhabitants of Gangshan ate about six cloves of raw garlic daily while their neighbors in Qixia ate none. The residents of Gangshan also reported ten times fewer cases of stomach cancer than those who live in Qixia. In the laboratory, both raw and dried garlic have been shown to destroy tumor cells. It takes about three hours for garlic compounds to enter the cell, but once in place they get to work almost immediately.

HERBS FOR TREATING CANCER

If you do get cancer, there are some herbs that can be used to reduce the effects of chemotherapy and radiation. Keith Block, M.D., medical director of the Cancer Care Program at Edgewater Medical Center in Chicago, is researching how herbs can be used in conjunction with standard cancer treatments. He has found that cancer patients undergoing standard treatment have fewer side effects, such as hair loss and nausea, when they take herbs that benefit the immune system (see "Boosting Immunity" on page 101).

So far, Siberian ginseng has not been proven to have any direct effect on

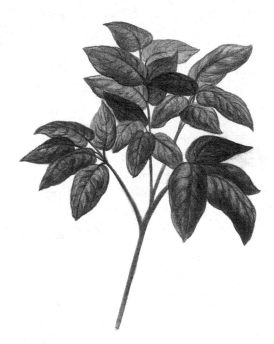

Siberian ginseng is not true ginseng, but it does contain similar active compounds and so is lumped together with Korean and American ginseng.

cancer cells, but it can increase general resistance and improve side effects resulting from chemotherapy and radiation. In Russia in 1964, a tincture of Siberian ginseng was given to 38 people with similar types of cancer of the mouth an hour before they went through 14 days of radiation therapy. They experienced numerous benefits, including better sleep, an improved appetite and even a renewed interest in life, as well as normalization of blood pressure, pulse and breathing rates. Also, the wounds that resulted from the cancer healed approximately one month before those of the people in a similar group not taking the herbs. The researchers concluded that Siberian ginseng can counter the harmful effects of radiation treatment and increase the rate of healing. Two years later, another Russian experiment showed that Siberian ginseng decreased the toxic effects of chemotherapy used to treat breast cancer.

Laboratory studies in China and thousands of years of experience have paved the way for various herbs to be used in combination with Western drug treatments in Chinese hospitals. The herbs given to people with cancer include astragalus, ligustrum and Siberian ginseng.

In numerous studies on astragulus and ligustrum, these two herbs improved the immune response in most of the people with cancer who took one or the other or both. Researchers even concluded that astragulus contains "one or more extremely potent naturally occurring immune stimulants." At the M.D. Anderson Cancer Center in Houston, researchers have found that immune cells taken from people with AIDS and cancer became more active in the test tube and that these people felt physically and emotionally strengthened after being treated with astragalus.

Medical doctors in Japan are also more open to using herbs than are their counterparts in North America. After the National Cancer Research Center in Tokyo discovered in the 1980s that shiitake mushrooms could be used to shrink cancerous tumors, Japanese hospitals began giving their patients a shiitake concentrate to increase their immune response. Japanese doctors also used an extract of a mushroom called polporus to improve the expected cancer survival rate by a few years.

One herb that has had a lively history is pau d'arco. This medicinal plant has been used since the time of the Incas and the Aztecs to treat various immune-related problems, including poisonous snakebites. In the 1960s, the Brazilian press published reports that included hundreds of testimonials that declared pau d'arco a cancer cure, and people were soon ripping the bark off trees throughout the country, even climbing into the Botanical Gardens in Campinas to do so. These people were spurred on by the miraculous story of a young girl in Rio de Janeiro who was cured of cancer after an angel visited her and told her about the bark. A newspaper account also told of University of São Paulo botanist Valter Accorsi, Ph.D., who daily dispensed the bark for free to crowds that sometimes numbered 2,000 people! Unfortunately, the sensational stories made most scientists cringe, and the little research that was done at places like the São Paulo Hospital of Clinics was short-lived.

A colleague of Dr. Accorsi, however, was also reporting success using pau d'arco. The award-winning botanist Teodoro Meyer, Ph.D., had been a professor at the Miguel Lillo Institute and Herbarium in San Miguel de Tucumán, Argentina, where he had supplied herbs for study by pharmaceutical companies in the United States. He developed an alcohol-free elixir that he distributed as a treatment for immune-related disorders, including cancer. He observed the effects of this elixir on the people he gave it to, and reported an improvement in their "general state and their spirits." Dr. Meyer died in 1972 after years of frustrated attempts to convince the world of pau d'arco's healing abilities. One of the few clinical studies on pau d'arco, done in 1980 in South America, showed that this herb reduced most of the symptoms, especially the pain, in people who had various types of cancer. The only reported side effect was a few cases of nausea.

When researchers at the National Cancer Institute studied pau d'arco for use as a cancer treatment, they found that it contained only moderate tumor-inhibiting abilities, but did produce a definite immune response. Other research has shown that the herb is sometimes effective in fighting cancer, malaria, viruses and bacterial infections. Herbalists use it to treat such immune-related disorders as asthma, rheumatism, eczema, psoriasis, shingles and yeast infections. Some success has also been reported with diabetes. For more on the history and science of pau d'arco, see Kenneth Jones's book *Pau d'Arco*.

For suggestions on dealing with side effects you might experience while undergoing chemotherapy or radiation, such as digestion problems, nausea and headaches, see pages 76, 93 and 34, respectively.

CHRONIC FATIGUE, MULTIPLE SCLEROSIS AND OTHER SERIOUS DISEASES

There are some serious immune disorders, such as chronic fatigue syndrome (more accurately known as chronic fatigue and immune disfunction syndrome, or CFIDS), multiple sclerosis (MS) and lupus, that are not well-understood. One thing we can assume about these disorders is that they are also related to problems of the nervous system. These serious illnesses require professional diagnosis, but as far as treatment goes, often all you can do is treat the symptoms. Partial relief can be provided through herbal treatments and other therapies such as diet improvements, acupuncture, stress reduction and nutritional supplements such as pantothenic acid, vitamins C and B_6 and magnesium.

In 1987, a study was done on a group of individuals who had been experiencing uncomfortable fatigue and sporadic fevers for at least six months. Blood tests showed that these people had especially low levels of the important T-cells known as natural killers, a condition that occurs with chronic fatigue syndrome. Antibiotics and conventional fever drugs had no effect. It was not until these people took lentinan, a compound found in shiitake mush-rooms, that their energy levels rose and their fevers subsided.

GLA has also been found to alleviate symptoms in many people who have chronic fatigue and also those who suffer from MS or lupus. If you suffer from any one of these disorders, you might also consider trying a variety of immune and nervous system herbs, including wild oats, skullcap and especially Saint-John's-wort—try adding ½ ounce tinc-ture of each of these to the Immune Tincture (see page 106). An herbal for-mula will not cure the disease, but it can certainly improve your quality of life. I know several people with these disorders who have used this tincture and have told me that they are happy to have found something that makes their lives a bit better.

Warning: If you have lupus, avoid alfalfa, even the sprouts. Herbal researchers believe that this herb can encourage relapses of the disease after remission.

If you are HIV-positive, some immune herbs are not appropriate. It has been observed that stimulating T-cells sometimes only encourages this terrible virus. Since several herbs used to improve immunity stimulate T-cell activity, there is a possibility that herbal treatments would hinder more than help. If you are HIV-positive or have AIDS and wish to treat yourself herbally, it is important that you work with a professional health care practitioner who is knowledgeable about their effects, especially when combined with the vari-ous drug treatments available for these conditions.

There are several herbal compounds currently being studied that do show anti-HIV activity in the laboratory. These include high amounts of concentrated compounds from Saint-John's-wort, licorice, astragalus and the Chinese gourd *Trichosanthin kirilowii.* In studies organized by the University of Califor-nia, San Francisco, Medical School and the Hagiwara Institute of Health in Japan, the shiitake compound lentinan has been shown to inhibit HIV by stop-ping its reproduction and by keeping the T-cells from fusing.

A paper presented at the 1988 Pro-ceeding of the National Academy of Sci-ences showed that compounds from Saint-John's-wort appear to disrupt the virus. And GLA was approved for AIDS trials in 1995. Infected cells are not capa-ble of producing their own GLA, but when they are bombarded with it, they break up and die without harming the normal cells.

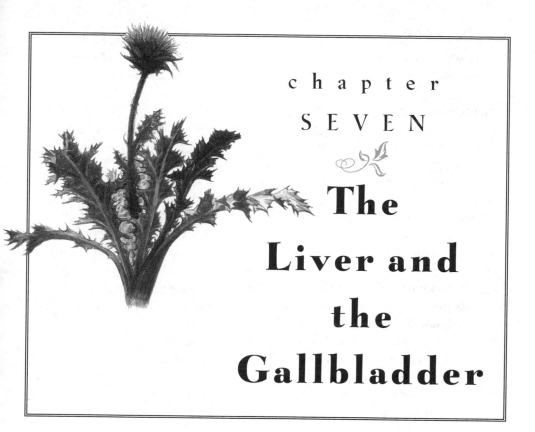

The Liver and the Gallbladder

Have you ever wondered just what functions your liver and gallbladder perform? The liver and the gallbladder serve as a team, working to eliminate toxins and other potentially harmful agents that are taken into the body. It is the liver, however, that does most of the work; the gallbladder is primarily a backup organ—it stores the bile that the liver produces and empties that bile into the small intestine where, with additional enzymes from the pancreas, food is further broken down for absorption. The liver is also responsible for metabolizing various foods and producing certain substances needed by the body.

LIVER DISEASES

Unless you have had a liver problem, chances are that you barely give the organ much thought. A liver is easy to ignore. It never grumbles, thumps, burps or makes itself obvious like other organs. However polite it may be, do not underestimate your liver's importance. This organ performs an amazing assortment of tasks as your body's manufacturing plant.

Through eating, breathing and even absorption through the skin, we all take in quite a smorgasbord of substances, ranging from life-sustaining foods to toxic chemicals. The liver's role is to break down and neutralize a wide array of potentially toxic chemicals, including such things as food additives, environmental pollutants, petroleum, paint and solvents. Even many natural substances, such as hormones, need to be broken down. Toxic levels of the hormones estrogen and testosterone circulate through the blood and increase the risk of hormonally related cancers if they are not transformed by the liver. The liver also converts protein into usable amino acids. Nutrients such as fats, carbohydrates and vitamins A, D, E, K and B_{12} are metabolized by your liver. Several vitamins are stored in your liver. And as if your liver is not busy enough, it also manufactures antibodies for the immune system, produces agents that allow blood to clot when you get cut, and even helps control blood sugar levels.

Liver problems are easy to shrug off at first because the typical symptoms tend to be the last things you would think of being related to your liver. Headaches, irritability, fatigue, aches and pains, indigestion, bloating, constipation, hormonal imbalances, PMS and menstrual irregularities are just a few examples. However, if you ask an herbalist for advice on how to clear up chronic skin problems, including rashes, boils, eczema and psoriasis, she will probably give you a list of herbs for the liver.

Hepatitis and cirrhosis are two diseases that can badly damage your liver. Hepatitis is an inflammation of the liver brought on by certain viruses or by overexposure to a toxic substance. This disease commonly causes a fever that is often accompanied by vomiting. About 20 percent of alcoholics can count on developing hepatitis after five to ten years of too much alcohol, but the disease can also result from poor nutrition, a viral or bacterial infection or toxic poisons.

Cirrhosis is a serious disease that changes the structure of the liver so that it cannot function properly. One of the biggest problems with cirrhosis is that less blood flows through the liver, and the toxins that are normally eliminated can now poison the body. About 20 percent of heavy drinkers eventually develop cirrhosis, and alcoholic hepatitis is often a precursor of cirrhosis. This condition can also be caused by poor nutrition (especially too little protein), poisonous substances, or a previous viral or bacterial infection that inflamed and weakened the liver.

The good news is that even a damaged liver retains an incredible ability to regenerate itself. The even better news is that herbs can help. Thanks to many scientific studies, mostly from Germany and the United States, we know that dandelion, burdock, chamomile, licorice and especially milk thistle can heal a damaged liver and protect it from further destruction. Clinical studies show that with these herbs, symptoms from liver damage, especially digestive problems, begin to improve in only two weeks. And as added benefits, people in the studies reported increased feelings of well-being and improved appetites.

Milk thistle most impressed the medical world when G. Vogel, M.D., used it to save lives in the 1970s. A leading milk thistle researcher, Dr. Vogel

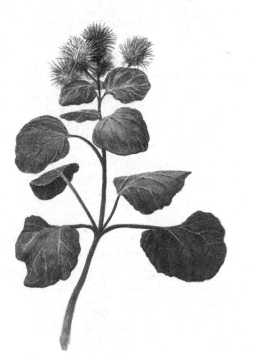

Liver-healing burdock is a really "sticky" plant. Even if you just brush past it, you leave with several of its small flowers attached to your clothing or hair.

brought to his clinic 60 people suffering from severe mushroom poisoning. He gave them a compound called silymarin that was extracted from milk thistle and found that "results ranged from amazing to spectacular," even though most of the people were not treated until a full day after eating the bad mushrooms.

Dr. Vogel and other well-known plant researchers, including Hildebert Wagner, Ph.D., have found that the antioxidants in milk thistle called flavonoids are some of the most potent liver-protecting substances known. (Antioxidants prevent cell destruction and damage caused by the harmful compounds known as free radicals.) Studies

conducted by these experts show that flavonoids work even better than the well-known antioxidant vitamin E. So do ginger and garlic, according to the results of numerous studies conducted all over the world. Similar flavonoids that improve liver function are also found in rosemary and grape leaves, which are used in Greek cooking. All of these herbs protect the liver from damage and increase the production of beneficial liver enzymes so that the liver can do its job better.

One important function of antioxidants is to protect the liver against damage from heavy metals and other toxic substances in the air and the food we eat. In case you think that heavy metal exposure is nothing to worry about, consider that more than 600,000 tons of lead are put into the atmosphere every year in the United States alone. Heavy metals are all around us—lead solder in tin cans, lead and cadmium in cigarette smoke, mercury in dental fillings and some cosmetics, and aluminum in antacids. Research conducted in Germany has shown that milk thistle helps protect the liver from drug and heavy metal poisoning. As a result, milk thistle is the basis for a number of German drugs used to treat liver problems.

Milk thistle is available in a number of preparations, but you can also sprinkle it onto your cereal or soup or incorporate it into other meals. To make milk thistle powder, buy whole seeds and grind them in a coffee grinder. Keep the powder on the table in a spice shaker.

Milk thistle is not the only member of the thistle family to come to the aid of the liver. If you like artichokes, you are in luck. While few American doctors consider artichoke a medical herb, European doctors regularly prescribe artichoke extracts to patients with liver problems. In fact, they have been using artichoke to treat jaundice and other liver complaints since as far back as the eighteenth century. Artichokes protect the liver from damage and help it regenerate—and yes, eating them for dinner counts. However, before you make up your shopping list, be aware that most commercial artichokes are highly sprayed, and if you are trying to heal your liver, pesticides are among the last things you want to eat.

It was not until the 1930s that German and French researchers began to study artichokes in their laboratories. Later, Italian researchers joined them to produce a substantial amount of research. In one study, dozens of Polish workers who were exposed to the toxic chemical fumes of carbon disulfide were given an artichoke extract for two years. The results of this study were presented in 1960 at the Symposium on Drugs Affecting Lipid Metabolism in Milan, Italy. Because of the artichoke, the workers did not experience the changes in their blood that would normally occur from inhaling this pollutant. The researchers found that artichoke is also useful in treating hepatitis because it helps reduce bile levels in the liver, thus decreasing congestion in the liver and the consequent risk of damage.

Licorice has been found to neutralize liver toxins. The Chinese may have been the first to use licorice to treat the liver. In modern times, licorice has been studied by the Research Group of Liver

Disease at the Shanxi Medical College in China. Since the 1950s, medical doctors in both the East and the West have used a compound derived from licorice to treat chronic hepatitis. In Japan, glycyrrhizin, a compound extracted from licorice, was found to be so successful in treating hepatitis that it was written up in at least three scientific journals. One of these reported that licorice increased the production of interferon, which is commonly used to treat hepatitis B.

The Chinese herbs astragalus, shizandra and bupleurum also neutralize liver toxins. Studies conducted in China show that all these herbs work in several ways, including serving as antioxidants, to protect your liver and keep it healthy and strong. In one clinical study with shizandra, a tincture was given to a group of people with chronic hepatitis. Another group received vitamin E and a liver extract. After six months, almost 75 percent of those who were taking shizandra had normal blood tests, indicating that their problems were over. Those taking the vitamin E and liver extract improved only half as quickly and not as much. Of the more than 100 people who took shizandra, only 4 reported side effects: mild headaches and nausea. Shizandra was recently developed into a new drug by the Pharmaceutical Research Institute of the Chinese Academy of Medical Sciences. This herb has been proven to diminish hepatitis B in less than a month.

Bupleurum has also been the subject of some study. The organizers of one study described a compound found in this herb as remarkable in its ability to stop liver damage. Because of these findings, Japanese physicians who use modern Western medical methods have recently taken a hint from Japan's herbal doctors—they are now turning to traditional formulas that contain bupleurum. Their renewed interest in this herb has sparked several studies, which have shown that bupleurum can even help people who have had hepatitis for several years.

A whole list of herbs used in the Orient—ginger, turmeric, cardamom, ginseng (especially red ginseng), the Japanese plant ukon, reishi mushroom and psyllium seed—have been shown to reduce liver damage. In one Chinese study, about 75 percent of a group of people with chronic hepatitis were successfully treated with reishi mushroom, shizandra and *Astragulus baicalensis*. Their liver swelling went down, and their appetites improved.

Ginger actually gives other herbs a boost by improving the body's ability to assimilate them. Since the liver is responsible for breaking down substances in the blood, it eventually deactivates medicinal compounds in herbs. Ginger actually protects herbal compounds from being destroyed, making it possible for them to pass through the liver unchanged and thus continue circulating in the blood for a longer time. According to a 1981 study on the bioavailability of herbs, this is probably why ginger is found in so many traditional Ayurvedic and Chinese formulas. Research has shown that ginger, along with black pepper and the closely related long pepper, also improve the intestines' absorption of other herbs. These three herbs are the ingredients of the popular Ayurvedic formula called *trikatu*.

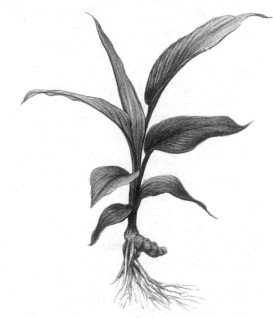

During the nineteenth century, turmeric was used in place of litmus paper—turmeric paper was used to test the pH of various liquids.

Turmeric is what gives the Eastern spice known as curry (which is actually a mixture of several different ground herbs) its yellow color. You get a healthy medicinal dose of this herb every time you eat foods seasoned with curry powder. Because the compounds found in turmeric are not water soluble, this herb is best taken as a pill or, even better, as a tincture.

Tamalaki, another herb from India, has been used by practitioners of Ayurvedic medicine for more than 2,000 years to treat liver disfunction. Recently, it has come to be used to treat hepatitis B. One study showed that even those who still had the virus had less chance of developing liver cancer if they continued to take tamalaki.

Of course, one of the best things you can do for your liver—and your general health—is to go easy on alcohol consumption. If you do overindulge, however, there are herbs that seem to help the liver. For example, ginseng can lower the alcohol level in your blood in 40 minutes, according to research on alcohol-lowering enzymes done by the Korean Ginseng and Tobacco Research Institute. Gamma linoleic acid (GLA) from evening primrose, borage and black currant seeds may prevent hangovers and poisoning and depression from alcohol, and may ease alcohol withdrawal. According to Brian Leonard, Ph.D., a researcher at the University College in Galway, Ireland, GLA also encourages regeneration of alcohol-damaged liver cells. Also, many herbalists have found that fennel seeds help reduce alcohol's effects.

Liver Tea

1 teaspoon each dandelion root, milk thistle seeds and roasted chicory root
½ teaspoon each sarsaparilla root, licorice root and ginger rhizome
1 quart water

❧ Combine ingredients in a saucepan and simmer for a couple of minutes. Turn down heat and let steep for about 15 minutes. Strain and drink at least a cup a day.

GALLBLADDER PROBLEMS

Think of the gallbladder as the liver's sidekick. In comparison to the much larger liver (under which it appears to nestle for protection), the gallbladder has comparatively little to do. Primarily, it stores bile manufactured by the liver. When you eat a fatty meal, the gallbladder contracts and releases bile into the first section of the small intestine, which is called the duodenum. In fact, two signals of gallbladder problems include stomach pains and a bloated feeling after eating high-fat foods. Bitter herbs like gentian are the best way to stimulate bile-production and improve fat digestion.

Most North American physicians are not very concerned about bile defi-

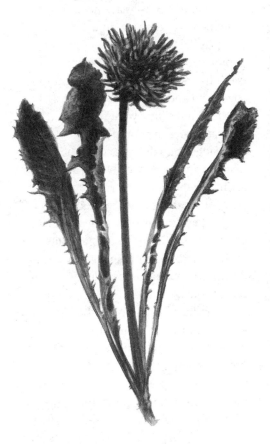

European herbalists use the juice of the dandelion root to treat diabetes and liver diseases.

ciency, but European doctors do worry about this problem. If a patient of a European doctor is diagnosed as being bile deficient, chances are, the physician will prescribe an herbal formula to correct the problem. Several European drugs contain one of the most potent bile stimulants in the plant world—dandelion. When the German over-the-counter drug Hepatichol—which is made mostly from dandelion—along with nettle and a few other herbs, was tested, the results were impressive. A study conducted in Germany in 1952 showed that all the people with gallbladder problems who took Hepatichol improved within only a few days.

Several compounds in turmeric increase bile and also help other bile stimulants do a better job. In the early 1970s, German researchers found that when turmeric was taken with milk thistle and celandine, it increased bile flow about six times more than when the herbs were used without it.

One of the most common—and most unpleasant—gallbladder problems is gallstones. These little "stones" are usually formed from concentrated bile and cholesterol combined with minerals and pigments. Gallstones do not create much trouble until they journey out of the gallbladder through the narrow duct that leads into the small intestine. If the stones are large, this can be very painful. Even worse, if the stones get lodged in the duct, they can block the flow of bile, upset the digestion of fats and cause inflammation, infection and even jaundice.

Because of these serious consequences, any gallstone treatment should be conducted only under the expert care of a health care professional. Any herbs that increase the production and flow of bile will encourage gallstones to move along. However, if the stones are moved out into the duct or are already blocking it, you could make things worse instead of better by taking herbs. This is particularly true of "the liver flush"—a popular home treatment for gallstones. If someone recommends drinking this unappetizing combination of olive oil and lemon juice, be wary. I have heard many people describe the

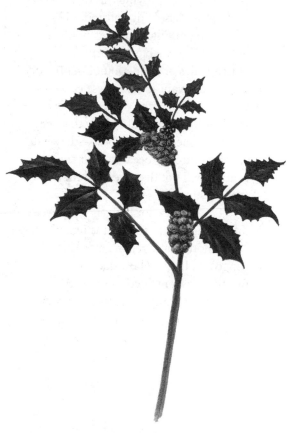

The flower of the Oregon grape, also known as mountain grape and holly-leaved barberry, is the state flower of Oregon.

impressively large "gallstones" that they magically passed with no pain. According to Michael Murray, N.D., and Joseph Pizzorno, N.D., the authors of *The Encyclopedia of Natural Medicine,* these are not gallstones at all, but rather balls formed when a chemical reaction causes oil and lemon to combine with minerals in the intestine.

British physicians suggest the over-the-counter drug Rowachol, which contains a mixture of compounds from numerous herbs, including peppermint. Several studies proving this drug's effectiveness in dissolving gallstones have been done in England. This product is not readily available in North America, but capsules of peppermint essential oil are. If you want to take these capsules, you should take one or two with each meal. Also, you should know that the enteric-coated ones are best—they will act most directly because their special coating will not dissolve until they reach the intestines.

The best use for herbs is for preventing gallbladder attacks in the first place. Dandelion root, Oregon grape root, fringe tree bark, yellow dock, wahoo and radish root were once considered so effective in treating stones that they were listed in the U.S. Dispensatory, a common doctor's prescription guide. Milk thistle, artichoke and turmeric all help prevent gallstones by making bile less saturated. Whatever route you choose to treat your stones, you can reduce the inflammation with marshmallow, chamomile and an old Russian folk remedy, nettle. And you can use cramp bark to help prevent painful spasms.

A diet that contains too much refined food and too little fiber may be at least partially responsible for gallstones. With such a diet, the gallbladder secretes less acid into the bile fluid. The body needs this acid to dissolve cholesterol. Without sufficient acid, cholesterol builds up into stones. One reason that vegetarians hardly ever get gallstones may be that they eat so much fiber.

Gallbladder Formula

1 teaspoon each dandelion root, Oregon grape root and marshmallow root
1 quart water
½ teaspoon each chamomile flowers and nettle leaves

❧ Combine roots and water and simmer for about 5 minutes. Turn off heat, add remaining herbs and steep for about 20 minutes. Strain herbs. Drink at least 1 cup daily. This formula can also be used to make a tincture or pills.

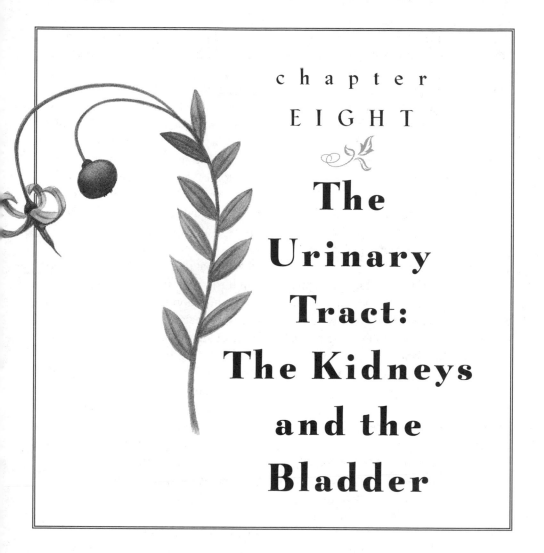

The Urinary Tract: The Kidneys and the Bladder

In Chinese medicine, the kidneys are the seat of longevity and health. This is not surprising, considering the kidneys' responsibility. The urinary tract is an elaborate filtration system—the kidneys alone contain about a million tiny filters that remove waste products from the blood. When your kidneys are working well, this refuse is diluted in a watery bath to make it less toxic to the body, then sent to the bladder, which serves as a holding tank, keeping this waste until the body discards it as urine.

Filtering wastes from the body is an essential job, but your kidneys perform an amazing assortment of other tasks as well. For example, they recycle important nutrients like glucose and amino acids out of the urine and back into the blood. They also control your blood pressure and the balance of electrolytes—important minerals such as potassium and sodium—in your body. Your kidneys are also responsible for telling the body when more red blood cells need to be produced.

Because the kidneys have so many jobs to do, many seemingly unrelated disorders and symptoms can be traced back to these organs. These include water retention, poor circulation, anemia, electrolyte imbalance and high blood pressure. Even a puffy face, dark circles under the eyes, a pale complexion, dizziness or tension can indicate kidney problems.

What causes your kidney problems in the first place? The urinary tract is the unfortunate victim of modern civilization—while the liver pulls toxins out of the blood, the kidneys eliminate toxins through the bladder. So the kidneys are responsible for eliminating the toxins we inhale and ingest. Solvents, gasoline, paint, synthetic fragrances and colors, preservatives and even the nitrogen waste that results from a high-protein diet put stress on the kidneys. In addition, infections anywhere in your body—even tooth decay—contribute to kidney problems. If diagnosing urinary tract problems sounds confusing, that's because it is—and it is a job best left to your doctor.

If you want to introduce herbs alongside a conventional remedy for kidney problems, you should seek the advice of someone knowledgeable about the relationship between herbs and your particular condition before embarking on an herbal program. If, however, you are already on the road to recovery after a bout with kidney stones or a kidney infection and you want to strengthen your kidneys, or if you have a simple bladder infection, there are herbal remedies that you can turn to without professional guidance. In fact, if urinary infections are a recurring theme in your life, do not wait until the next infection to start a maintenance program.

Herbs that serve as general urinary tract tonics for long-range health include rose hips, fennel, dandelion, marshmallow, oat straw and nettles. These herbs rarely conflict with other kidney treatments, but you should take into consideration that they are all diuretics—they will flush water from your body.

In addition to taking beneficial herbs, to maintain the best kidney health I suggest that you eat a high-fiber, low-fat diet based on unprocessed foods. I also recommend avoiding coffee, black tea and alcohol, especially if you have had urinary tract problems in the past. These substances are all strong kidney and bladder irritants. If incontinence and frequent urination are a problem for you, see "Bedwetting" on page 214.

General Urinary Tonic

½ teaspoon each dandelion root, oat straw, nettle leaves and rose hips
¼ teaspoon each fennel seeds and marshmallow root
1 quart water

🍂 Put herbs in water and bring to a simmer. Turn off heat and steep for about 30 minutes. Strain, then store in the refrigerator. Drink 1 or 2 cups daily, as desired. These herbs can also be taken as a tincture or pills, but a tea is the preferred way to take this tonic because water helps flush the urinary tract.

BLADDER INFECTIONS

The urinary tract is supposed to be a one-way system, but sometimes traffic goes in through the out door—the bladder serves as a gateway for bacteria to enter the body, and urinary tract infections are the result. Because the path from bladder to exit is shorter in women than in men (since the penis is part of the urinary tract), women are 20 times more likely to contract urinary tract infections. One out of five North American women can expect to have at least one urinary tract infection in her lifetime. The notoriously long lines in women's restrooms are also frequently blamed; all that delay distorts and weakens the bladder and invites infection. Tight pants, synthetic underwear, vaginal powders and deodorants and even deodorant soaps can be irritating and can encourage infection.

Two early signs of bladder infection are cloudy urine and a burning sensation when you urinate. You may also experience pain or a sense of heaviness in the bladder, especially when it is full or has just been emptied. As the infection progresses, false alarms from irritated nerves can send you running to the bathroom unnecessarily. If the symptoms of your bladder infection grow to include a dull ache in the lower back and a fever, consult a doctor immediately—these symptoms are warning signs that the infection has spread to the kidneys, and kidney infections are very serious problems.

Several years ago, I was at a New Year's dinner party and got to talking with a man named John. I'm not sure how we got on the subject of bladder infections, but I think it started with the cranberries we were eating. I listened with interest to John's bladder infection odyssey. It began in California as he embarked on a long drive to Canada. It was obvious from his story that the trip would have been much less eventful had it not been for a persistent bladder infection that got worse the farther north he drove. He met people he never would have met and had adventures that never would have occurred without the infection, in part because he had to make so many "pit stops." In time, the situation became rather dire, but by that time he

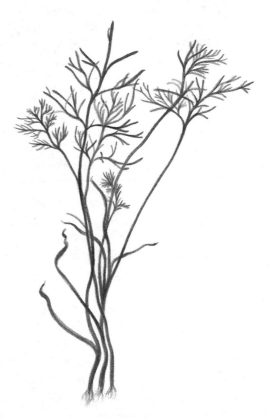

In medieval England, the seeds of the fennel plant were believed to be an appetite suppressant.

was working in the wilderness in Canada's remote Northwest Territory.

Far from any doctors, he suffered with his problem for a few months. When he returned to California, his doctor immediately put him on a high dose of the antibiotic tetracycline. Thinking the problem would finally be resolved, John returned to his job in Canada. Unfortunately, the drug did little to help the infection, though it did permanently stain his teeth (an unfortunate side effect that sometimes occurs with this antibiotic). During his next trip back to California, John received a prescription for a second, stronger round of antibiotics, also with no results.

By this time, poor John was ready to put himself in the hospital because he could barely urinate, was suffering tremendously and feared he was becoming impotent. He was saved when someone told him about cranberry juice (and pumpkin seed oil for his reproductive system). To his complete amazement, the juice began to improve his infection in only a couple of days. Not knowing I was an herbalist, he turned to me after finishing his tale and said that I probably found that hard to believe. I smiled and said, "Not at all." Actually, I had heard dozens of similar stories.

An increasingly common source of bladder infection is chlamydia, a sexually transmitted disease (see "Vaginal Infections" on page 181). The culprit behind most bladder infections, however, is E. coli, a bacteria normally found in the bowels that all too easily finds its way into the bladder.

One way to discourage bladder infection is to keep your urine too acidic

for bacteria like E. coli to survive. Cranberry juice is famous for this, and it is so well accepted that your physician may already be prescribing this folk remedy. You can also acidify your urine the Japanese way, by eating umaboshi plums. In Japan, one or two plums are added to a pot of rice or some other dish. For convenience, there is also an umaboshi plum concentrate sold in natural food stores.

Recently, researchers working at the Weizmann Institute of Science and Tel Aviv University in Israel discovered that cranberries and blueberries do even more than simply increase urine's acidity. They also contain compounds that keep bacteria from attaching to the bladder's wall and so prevent infections from

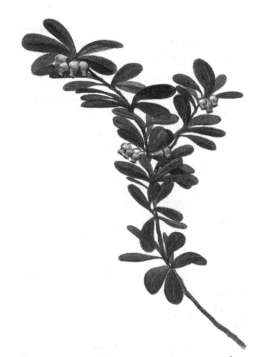

Bears are said to enjoy the taste of uva ursi's berries, but humans find the bright red fruit quite bland.

taking hold. The recommended dose is three to six ounces a day of cranberry juice or 1½ ounces of the berries. Since commercial cranberry juice is laden with sugar, it is best to make your own remedy from raw berries or to buy unsweetened cranberry concentrate or capsules of dried cranberry, both of which are sold in natural food stores. If you have ever tasted raw cranberries, you already know that they are much too tart to eat raw, but they can be cooked into a tasty medicine—see the recipe on page 345. Unlike cranberries, blueberries can be eaten raw.

I have seen the herb uva ursi work on bladder infections that even cranberry could not defeat. This groundcover from the southwestern United States contains a powerful antiseptic that is activated when it reaches the urinary tract. Once there, it kills bacteria, removes infectious material, reduces inflammation and probably even strengthens the urinary tract lining. Interestingly enough, medical researchers have found that this herb works best in the alkaline environment produced by bacteria. Uva ursi enjoyed official recognition in the prescription guide known as the U.S. Pharmacopoeia as late as 1950, when it was replaced with sulfa drugs (antibiotics). In Germany, this herb is still used by doctors to treat urinary tract infection and inflammation. On the advice of herbalist and author Michael Moore, I use manzanita, a close relative of uva ursi, since it grows abundantly where I live in the northern California mountains.

For all its good, uva ursi can slightly irritate the kidneys and upset your stomach if used for more than a week or so. However, this should give you plenty of time to knock out even the most stubborn bladder infection. One way to mellow out uva ursi's harshness is by adding marshmallow to your formula. Marshmallow soothes the urinary tract and also fights urinary tract infection in a way similar to uva ursi, although it is not quite as powerful. Your best bet is to take these herbs as indicated below, then, when the symptoms have subsided, switch to cranberry, blueberry or umaboshi. You can also use a massage oil on the bladder area that contains an antiseptic essential oil such as tea tree, for extra soothing.

Other urinary tract infection fighters that you can put on your dinner plate include garlic, nasturtium and rose hips (which is high in the infection-fighting vitamin C). And next time you dine out, you should think twice before leaving your parsley garnish on your plate. One of the compounds found in parsley seeds is a basic ingredient in pharmaceutical drugs used to treat urinary infections. Since parsley seeds can be toxic in large amounts, however, you should stick to using the leaves and the root. One food that contains plenty of both parsley and garlic is the Middle Eastern salad known as tabbouleh. You can purchase this salad already prepared at many delis or you can make your own.

Several herbs reduce the inflammation and pain that often accompany a bladder infection. Marshmallow, cramp bark and especially goldenrod are good choices. Another herb that can be used to soothe irritation is purslane. Although you may not find purslane in stores, you may find this "weed" growing in your garden. This sprawling succulent is so healthful, in fact, that some vegetable gardeners have taken to planting it in their gardens. To use it, simply chop it up and add it to salads and vegetable dishes.

If you suffer from urinary tract spasms and constriction, both of which make it difficult to urinate, try taking meadowsweet, fennel seed and

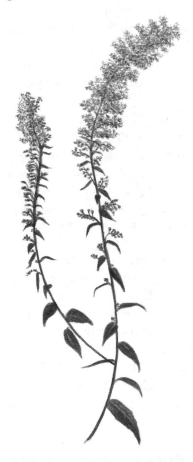

In British folklore, goldenrod is both a healing herb and a sign of wealth— this plant was said to point the way toward hidden gold and hidden springs.

hydrangea. European herbalists suggest drinking a "tea" of lemon and barley water as a soothing diuretic. You can make barley water by cooking barley with a whole chopped lemon, then straining and drinking the water. Or you can get the same health benefits by dining on barley soup (see page 335). For other recipes to allow you to eat your way to good bladder health— tabbouleh and dishes that include parsley, nasturtium flowers and garlic— see chapter 18.

Urinary Infection Tea

1 teaspoon uva ursi
½ teaspoon each corn silk, cramp bark,
  marshmallow root and rose hips
1 quart water

🌿 Simmer herbs in water for a couple of minutes, then steep them for 20 minutes. Strain herbs. Drink 2 to 4 cups daily. To make sure the infection is gone, continue taking the herbs for 2 days after the symptoms disappear.

Urinary Massage Oil

⅛ teaspoon tea tree essential oil
4 ounces vegetable oil

🌿 Combine ingredients and it's ready! Rub directly over the bladder twice a day to relieve the pain resulting from urinary tract infection.

KIDNEY STONES

About the best that can be said of kidney stones is that once you go through the experience, you may find yourself willing to go out of your way to make sure they do not come back again. For most people I know who have had kidney stones, one bout was enough to persuade them to start drinking herbal teas and to make some radical changes in their diets.

Unfortunately, about half the people who get kidney stones will suffer them again, along with the symptoms of sudden, sharp waves of pain, nausea and profuse sweating that accompany this problem. Severe cases are also accompanied by bleeding and, if there is an infection, even fever. As with any kidney condition, you must see your physician to determine the exact cause of your symptoms and the severity of the condition.

Kidney stones are mineral deposits made up of calcium, uric acid or the amino acid cysteine. There are numerous theories as to how these "stones" form, but no one knows for sure how it happens. Medical experts agree, however, that diet is certainly a factor. For instance, kidney stones develop in vegetarians and other people who eat plenty of fresh vegetables only about half as often as in those whose diet does not include these important foods. Obesity and repeated kidney infections are also risk factors. Even after an infection has passed, a small amount of debris remains in the kidneys—medical researchers suspect that the stones form around this debris. You are also at greater risk of developing this problem if there is a history of kidney stones in your family.

In some herb books, it is said that lemon juice reduces the size of kidney stones, but most herbal remedies, including those based on lemon juice and hydrangea, do not actually dissolve

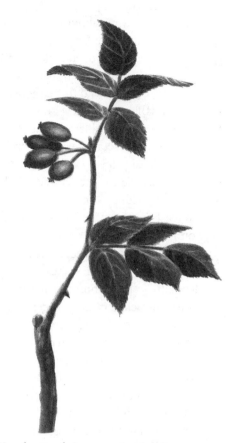

The fruit of the rose bush, the rose hip, is a great source of vitamin C—it has more of this vitamin, ounce for ounce, than an orange.

stones. Instead, they help eliminate the stones and reduce or relieve the pain that occurs as they are eliminated. The larger the stone, the more uncomfortable this can be. Herbs that reduce infection, pain and spasms are cramp bark, goldenrod and joe-pye weed, aptly nicknamed "gravel root" for its ability to get rid of stones.

Goldenrod has received official recognition in Germany for its effectiveness in getting rid of kidney stones.

Several species of the plant are used for this purpose throughout Europe, although it is not as popular in North America. This is too bad, considering that goldenrod is an excellent urinary tract herb that grows wild throughout much of North America. Several scientific studies support goldenrod's action.

Agrimony, horsetail, yarrow, shepherd's purse, Saint-John's-wort and nettles can also be used to reduce bleeding caused by kidney stones.

At least 75 percent of kidney stones are composed of calcium combined with phosphate or oxalic acid. Medical experts believe that these stones result from an accumulation of unused calcium, and lack of exercise is generally thought to be a factor. A study conducted in 1973 showed that cranberries help prevent stones in some people by reducing the excessive amounts of calcium commonly found in the urinary tract. There is some scientific evidence that this may also be true of rose hips, which have traditionally been used to ease various urinary tract infections. Since the calcium-phosphate stones are most common in alkaline urine, cranberries and other herbs that acidify urine also help prevent stones.

Levels of the enzyme urease, which contributes to kidney stones, are increased by bacteria and the alkaline urine they produce. Studies on rosemary conducted in Paraguay, where this herb is an important folk medicine, showed that it almost completely inhibits urease.

If you are prone to kidney stones, play it safe and avoid such foods as rhubarb, spinach, beet greens, sorrel, green tea and chocolate. All of these are rich in oxalic acid. If you do eat these foods, try not to eat foods high in calcium at the same time—this means that spinach and cheese soufflé or chocolate milk are especially problematic.

Uric acid stones are found in urine that is too acidic. If you get this type of stone, eat cherries, strawberries, apple juice, asparagus and nettles to make your urine more alkaline. Also consider changing your diet. One thing that can cause overly acidic urine is an overabun-

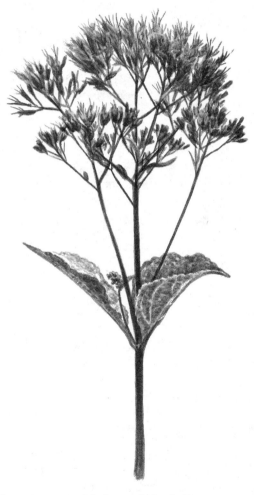

Joe-pye weed helps rid the kidneys of excess uric acid.

dance of protein. The herbs meadow-sweet, sarsaparilla, joe-pye weed and plantain (which is widely used by the Chinese to treat kidney problems) help rid the kidneys of excess uric acid. This use for meadowsweet was acknowledged in a French medical journal in 1942.

Kidney Stone Tea

2 teaspoons hydrangea root
1 teaspoon wild yam root
1 teaspoon cramp bark
1½ quarts water
1 teaspoon joe-pye weed
½ teaspoon each corn silk, plantain leaf
*   and yarrow leaf*

Add hydrangea, wild yam and cramp bark to water in a saucepan. Bring to a boil, then turn down heat and simmer for 15 minutes. Remove from heat, add other herbs, cover pan and steep for at least 20 minutes. Strain and keep refrigerated. Drink 3 to 4 cups daily. If bleeding occurs, add 30 drops shepherd's purse tincture to each cup of tea.

A tea is especially appropriate when treating a kidney infection because you should already be drinking plenty of water to keep kidneys flushed and help prevent the stones from forming. For convenience, you can also take this formula as a tincture; take 2 to 3 dropperfuls a day.

WATER RETENTION

Water retention may sound like a simple enough problem to remedy—just take a diuretic to eliminate the excess water. But water retention can be a symptom of a serious heart or kidney problem. And leaky capillary walls, malnutrition, bacterial toxins and hormone changes such as PMS can also be the cause of this problem. If your body is retaining water, be sure to see a doctor and find out exactly what is causing this problem before trying to treat it.

If a simple diuretic will solve your problem, dandelion and corn silk are two of the best choices—these are some of the safest diuretics ever to grow in the wild. And they also counter some of the negative effects of commercial diuretics. Most pharmaceutical diuretics pull potassium out of the body, creating a harmful imbalance that requires you to take potassium supplements. But dandelion and corn silk contain high amounts of potassium and even help the body retain this important mineral. Studies have shown that dandelion is as effective as the often-prescribed diuretic drug Frusemide. If you want to collect your own dandelion leaves and roots and corn silk, go right ahead. Just make sure they have not been sprayed with pesticides!

Diuretic Tea

1 quart boiling water
2 teaspoons dandelion root
½ teaspoon each nettle leaf, oat straw,
*   fennel seed and corn silk*

Pour boiling water over herbs, then steep in a covered container for 20 minutes. Strain herbs. Drink 1 or 2 cups as needed.

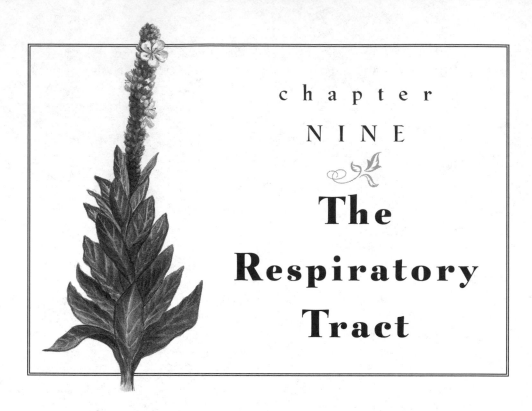

The Respiratory Tract

Sore throats, lung problems and sinus discomfort are as common as the air we breathe. That's because the air contains pollutants, allergens, bacteria and viruses that can easily invade the lungs. Your respiratory tract's main line of defense consists of delicate nasal hairs and a protective mucous lining. But because the warm, moist environment in your lungs and sinuses is such a wonderful place for microbes to grow, your defenses sometimes are not enough.

If it seems that nature gave the respiratory tract a bum deal, consider the herbs it has also provided as treatment. Respiratory problems such as a chest cold, laryngitis or hay fever usually respond quickly to herbal medicine. Just remember that any breathing problem is serious enough to warrant a visit to a health care professional.

The health of your lungs depends on how you breathe. Only about one-fifth of inhaled air is oxygen. Remember to take deep, slow breaths that fill your lungs and to relax while you do so. Also, try to reduce stress whenever you can—stress weakens the immune system, thereby opening you to infection.

COLDS AND FLU

If you don't have personal experience with cold and flu symptoms, you must be from another planet. First comes the tired feeling, followed soon after by crankiness, runny nose, sore throat, cough and head and body aches. Fever and nausea often join in.

A word to the wise—spending a day or two in bed nursing a cold or flu is a necessity, not a luxury. Getting over a cold or flu is a full-time job in itself. Most of the healing of the virus-damaged cells occurs between midnight and early morning. It is also a good idea to eat lightly, since a semi-fast enhances immune activity.

Your cold symptoms are a sign that your immune system is hard at work throwing off an infection. That's why you should try not to suppress certain symptoms. When you have a fever, for example, you should think twice before trying to lower it, even with herbs. Fevers are one of your body's natural defenses.

Heat deactivates viruses even better than antibodies. In fact, scientists at Johns Hopkins University found that symptoms cleared up a couple of days sooner in cold sufferers who did nothing at all than in those who took aspirin. Even worse, while aspirin and acetaminophen work well to relieve pain, they can impair the immune system, putting people who are already in poor health at risk for more serious sinus infections, sometimes even pneumonia. And conventional cold medicines such as antihistamines are not much better. In fact, these remedies have little to offer the bleary-eyed cold or flu sufferer other than suppressing their symptoms and prolonging the misery.

So if you have a cold or flu, try using herbs. While your symptoms may not disappear overnight, chances are you will get well sooner, and probably more completely. Since pharmaceutical drugs are not very effective against viruses, medical researchers are investigating medicinal plants as alternatives. In time, compounds from these herbs will probably be synthesized by pharmaceutical companies, the resulting formulas will be classified as prescription drugs, and consumers will have to pay a fortune to take advantage of them.

But why wait? And why pay through the nose? If you can go direct to the source for less money, why not do so?

In one study, medical researchers looked at more than 50 medicinal herbs. Once the results were in, the strongest flu fighters were found to be eucalyptus, sage and licorice. Lavender, tea tree, rose geranium, bergamot, lemon balm and hyssop also scored high in numerous studies testing their ability to inhibit the most common types of flu. As it turned out, these were also effective against cold viruses.

You can even eat your way to good health. Popular kitchen spices that are also cold and flu fighters include cinnamon, black pepper, lemon, thyme, marjoram, rosemary, basil, garlic and peppermint. These natural antibiotics can also be taken directly into infected lungs and sinuses by inhaling an herbal steam made using their essential oils. An easy way to do this is to add the essential oils to a commercial humidifier (first make sure that your unit can handle the oils—if it can't, it will say so in the manual).

If you do not own a humidifier, you can create a steam by simmering a few drops of essential oil in a pan of water. Of course, when you are away from home, it is usually inconvenient to steam. So if you are traveling, you should carry with you a nasal inhaler containing essential oils. You can buy these inhalers at most natural food stores or you can make your own—see the Homemade Nasal Inhaler recipe on page 142.

Essential Oil Steam
3 cups water
¼ teaspoon eucalyptus or peppermint essential oil

◈ Bring water to a simmer and turn off heat. Add essential oil. Set pot where you can sit down next to it. Place your face over the pot and drape a towel over the back of your head to form a mini-sauna. Breath in the steam, coming out for fresh air as needed. Do at least 3 rounds a few times a day. If you can't find the pure essential oil, fresh or dried herbs can be used instead.

If you tend to get flus or colds often, Siberian ginseng, echinacea, shizandra and astragalus are some of the immune herbs that will help you build up a natural resistance (see "Boosting Immunity" on page 101 for more helpful herbs). These herbs seem to have a special ability to help the lungs.

When researchers who wanted to confirm the usefulness of Siberian ginseng, they surveyed residents of the cold regions of northeastern China. They found that those who took this herb regularly got far fewer colds and reported fewer cases of bronchitis. In a Russian study, children in the town of Chirchik who were given shizandra were more resistant to a serious flu epidemic that swept through their town. Astragalus increases the body's production of inter-

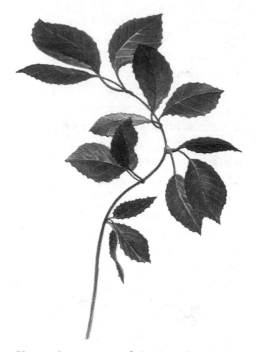

Shizandra is one of the best herbs nature offers for building up your immunity.

feron, which protects cells from invasions of viruses. It has been used to prevent both viral and bacterial lung infections. In a huge study conducted in China in 1981, when more than 1,000 people were given a combination of interferon and astragalus, they came down with far fewer colds than with interferon alone.

Echinacea, that wonderful immunity enhancer, also stops cold and flu viruses from reproducing once they have gained access to a cell. Licorice works in much the same way. Most of the investigation into the workings of echinacea as a powerful immune-system enhancer is being done in Germany. This research has shown that echinacea stimulates cells in the immune system called macrophages. These cells, whose name means "big eaters," quickly go to the site of infection to literally gobble up the microbes causing the problem.

Three studies conducted in Germany in 1992 emphasize echinacea's power. When an echinacea root tincture was given to people who were coming down with a flu, all of their symptoms— weakness, chills, sweating, sore throat, muscle pain, joint aches and headaches—decreased. Those taking echinacea also got fewer colds, and when they did get sick, their symptoms were less severe. This herb especially helped anyone who had a tendency to get more than their share of colds.

Herbalists use mostly the roots of echinacea, but even the tops of the plant are potent. One German company even sells the juice from the fresh flowers and leaves. In one study, as little as one-half teaspoon of this juice daily reduced risk of catching the common cold.

Madeleine Mumcuoglu, Ph.D., began studying elder berries after her mentor Jean Lindenman, Ph.D. (who discovered the immune-system enhancer interferon), mentioned that elder berries had long been used as a folk remedy for flu. Sure enough, subsequent research at the Hebrew University Hadassah Medical Centre in Jerusalem found that more than one compound in the berries prevent the flu virus from invading healthy cells in the laboratory.

To prove that this worked in the natural world, the researchers gave an elderberry syrup to some of the local kibbutz members during a flu epidemic. Those who took the syrup got better much sooner than those who opted for more standard treatments. Continuing

research leads scientists to conclude that elderberries may even inhibit more serious viruses such as herpes and Epstein-Barr.

Elderberries can easily be made into a tea, but you are more likely to find them sold as a tincture, as a syrup or in pill form. If you are interested in making elderberry syrup, see chapter 18. The flowers of the elder plant are also beneficial—they not only lower a fever, but also ease symptoms such as sinus congestion, sore throat and headaches. They also improve circulation and act as a diuretic, so herbalists use them to help flush toxins produced by cold and flu viruses out of the body.

Cold and Flu Tea
½ teaspoon each echinacea root, peppermint leaves, hyssop leaves, yarrow leaves, elder flowers and shizandra berries
1 quart boiling water
Combine herbs and pour boiling water over them. Steep for at least 20 minutes. Strain and drink frequently throughout the day. I prefer teas for treating colds and flus since it is important to drink lots of fluids to thin congestion and flush out toxins. If you can't find the herbs, you can make instant tea with tinctures (use the same proportions as above) or buy a commercial tea with similar ingredients. A hot tea is the most effective way to take these herbs, but you may find tinctures or pills more convenient (take them with hot water or tea). If you're using a tincture, just add half a dropperful to half a cup of water, juice or tea. And don't forget to drink plenty of water as well.

Still feeling lousy after taking these herbs? You can ease uncomfortable symptoms such as muscle aches with a natural aspirin—tea or pills of willow bark. Osha, a southwestern herb that I grew particularly aware of when I lived in New Mexico, eases the pain and discomfort of lungs that are sore as a result of coughing or congestion. It also relieves the indigestion that often accompanies colds and flus.

It is a well-known medical fact that antibiotics do not kill viruses, only bacteria. But doctors still prescribe them for colds and flu in case a bacterial infection gains access to your already weakened system. I think that antibiotic drugs are overused. And I'm not alone in this; many laypersons and even some doctors will agree. For information on natural herbal antibiotics, see the suggestions in Coughs, Sore Throats and Laryngitis.

COUGHS, SORE THROATS AND LARYNGITIS

I often speak in public—about herbs, of course—and have had quite a few untimely sore throats myself. Fortunately, a demonstration on treating laryngitis fits in the middle of most of my lectures. I generally start by whipping out a vial of lavender essential oil, putting two drops into a pan of steaming water and inhaling its vapors. The students think I've taken the treatment for their benefit, but sometimes the therapy is all that allows me to complete the lecture.

A cough, sore throat or laryngitis— which simply indicates that your sore throat involves your vocal cords—are really more symptoms than actual illnesses. They can be caused by anything from an infection or simple irritation in the throat to a tumor, so do not assume that a sore throat or cough is a minor problem. Most likely, they are the result of a cold or flu virus or a bacterial infection like strep throat, which is caused by the bacterium Streptococcus. If you have strep throat—to find out, go see your doctor—you should probably treat it with antibiotics to prevent the onset of rheumatic fever.

If you are coughing because you have a relatively minor cold or an irritation that would normally send you running to the drugstore for over-the-counter medication, you can easily switch to an herbal alternative. Even the more serious viral laryngitis is medically considered "self-limiting"—that is, it will eventually go away on its own without any kind of treatment.

Coughing can actually be beneficial—it's the body's way of clearing the airways so that you can breathe better. After a while, though, it irritates your throat. Coating your throat by sucking on a cough drop or drinking syrup reduces the irritation that makes you cough and also diminishes the pain. Sucking on a cough drop will also stop the natural reflex to cough. It does this by stimulating the flow of saliva so that you swallow more often and simply do not need to cough as often. All of these methods bring herbs into direct contact with your throat and coat and soothe it better than a tea or tincture.

Anise, eucalyptus, fennel, peppermint and thyme are some of the favorite herbs used in cough medications. They make a syrup or cough drop very tasty, but their real purpose is to stop your coughing. It is probable that one way these herbs work is by shutting down the brain's coughing center.

Other coughing and wheezing preventives that soothe the throat include marshmallow, licorice and slippery elm. Marshmallow was suggested as a cough remedy back in the fourth century B.C. by the Greek physician Theophrastus, and licorice has been a cough syrup favorite for a long time. Native Americans have long used the bark of the slippery elm tree to stop coughs. This practice worked so well that it was eventually adopted by white settlers. Native peoples of the Northeast made a tea of slippery elm, created a slippery elm gargle using a thick decoction of the plant, and even chewed on small pieces of the bark when they had sore throats.

Plantain, another good cold remedy, is quite popular in Germany, China, India and Russia. Research conducted in those countries has shown that this herb stops coughing, wheezing and chest pain, even from bronchitis. Another herb that helps relieve wheezing and chest pains is osha.

And how about getting rid of the source of all the coughing and soreness? Many of the same essential oils used to knock out a cold or flu—eucalyptus, lavender, cinnamon, black pepper, lemon, thyme, marjoram, rosemary, basil and peppermint—also inhibit infections caused by Staphylococcus and "strep."

Numerous scientific studies support herbalists' claim that garlic is a "natural antibiotic." Researchers have found it to

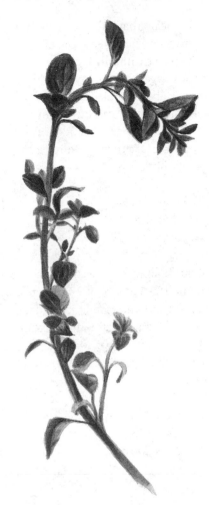

The ancient Greeks coated their hair and eyebrows with a pomade made of marjoram.

be particularly good for fighting strep infections. Still more antibiotic action is found in the compound berberine, which comes from goldenseal, barberry and Oregon grape root. Researchers have done studies verifying berberine's specific ability to counter strep.

My favorite laryngitis remedy is the Essential Oil Steam on page 132. Both lavender and eucalyptus work so well with the steam that I always need to re-mind myself to not overdo the talking until my voice can fully recover. For centuries, sage, hyssop, thyme and marjoram have been gargled to relieve laryngitis and tonsillitis, and European singers still follow a tradition of preserving their voices with marjoram tea sweetened with honey.

Sage Gargle
1 cup boiling water
2 teaspoons sage leaves
Salt
❧ Pour boiling water over sage leaves, cover and steep for about 20 minutes. Strain and add salt. Gargle as needed. Stored in the refrigerator, this mixture will keep for a few days. Marjoram, thyme or hyssop can be used instead of sage.

Honey Cough Syrup
1 tablespoon each licorice root,
*   marshmallow root and plantain leaf*
1 teaspoon thyme leaf
1 pint water
4 tablespoons honey
4 ounces glycerin
⅛ teaspoon anise essential oil (optional)
❧ Prepare a triple-strength tea by simmering the herbs in water for 10 minutes, then steeping for 20 minutes. Strain the tea, then stir in honey and glycerin while the tea is still warm. Finally, add essential oil, if you're using it. Take 1 tablespoon at a time. (This recipe is suitable for children, but not for infants, who should not have honey.) Stored in a cool place, this syrup will keep for 2 weeks. Stored in the refrigerator, it will keep for several months.

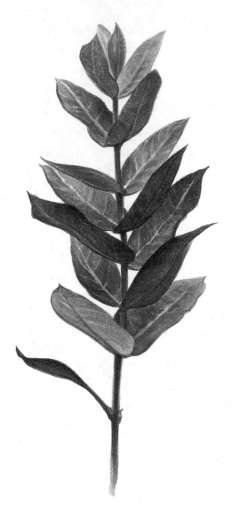

Most everyone knows that eucalyptus leaves are a favorite snack of koala bears, but did you know that eucalyptus oil is a powerful antiseptic and astringent?

Laryngitis is not usually a cause for alarm, but there are times when you really have to talk—like that crucial business presentation or to say your wedding vows. A couple of years ago, I attended my friend Tim's wedding. While I was happily chatting with the other guests, I was surprised to see Tim run up to me looking like anything but a happy groom. "What's wrong?" I whispered. "Please," begged Tim, "Do you have your first-aid kit?" I dashed out to my car as quickly as possible. Upon returning, I was directed to Heather, a pale, distraught bride who pointed to her throat. I quickly got the message and sent the bridal attendants into action finding a pan, water and towels to protect her dress. I managed to locate a quiet place for Heather to sit down, and I set a steaming pot of lavender in front of her. The ceremony started a little late, but no one seemed to mind. I have to admit that it was the only wedding I have attended where the entire assembly broke out in a light applause after the bride proclaimed "I do."

HAY FEVER

Ah, the glory of spring—warm weather, singing birds and fragrant flowers; not to mention, sneezing, runny nose, watery eyes, and depleted energy. If this sounds familiar, you probably have allergies. Hay fever got its name because so many people are allergic to pollen from hay and grass, but many types of pollens, as well as dust, animal dander and other airborne irritants can cause an allergic reaction, or allergy attack. Unfortunately, the more exposure you receive to the offending substance, called an allergen, the worse your allergy can become. And short of moving to the Arctic or wearing a filter mask, escape is impossible.

You can, however, use herbs to relieve lung and sinus congestion and to build up your immune system. Allergic reactions such as hay fever occur when your immune system mistakes an innocent substance like pollen for a threat and attacks it. When an attack occurs, several substances, including histamines, are released; these substances produce inflammation and make your sinuses run and your eyes tear.

Many people throughout the world have allergies, and I am one of them. I used to sneeze constantly as I worked in my herb garden, and I ended up giving my springtime garden tours with red, tearing eyes. Once, while trying to take a publicity photo in the garden, I could not stop sneezing long enough to smile. Looking around, I realized that most of the medicine I needed was within picking distance, and I immediately went to work harvesting it.

My hay fever did not disappear overnight, but every year it became a little less severe. I always suspected that I beat my allergies in large part because I started taking herbs, along with supplements of pantothenic acid (one of the B-complex vitamins), long before hay fever season hit. My suspicions were confirmed when I moved to a lower elevation and was caught off guard by an early spring, accompanied of course by hay fever. The herbs that I took began helping immediately, but it was a week before I completely stopped sneezing.

For my anti-allergy program, I turned to natural antihistamines such as chamomile, peppermint, ginger, anise and feverfew. Since sniffing essential oils sometimes makes people with hay fever sneeze even more, I concentrated on teas, tinctures and pills. I also used herbs that relieve congestion and stop sneezing, such as elder flowers and yarrow, which are described in "Sinus Congestion" on page 141. Echinacea and chamomile decreased the congestion and slowed the allergic reactions.

Occasionally, I hear warnings about using chamomile to treat hay fever because it is in the same family as ragweed, which is notorious for causing hay fever. This huge family actually includes echinacea, daisies, feverfew and hundreds of other flowers grown in flower and herb gardens. Personally, I have seen chamomile do much more good than harm in treating hay fever for dozens of people, but you may want to take care.

Another hot tip for treating hay fever is using onions, garlic and hot peppers to inhibit the inflammation that often comes with allergic attacks. Capsaicin, the compound that gives cayenne and other peppers their distinctive "hot" flavor, desensitizes the respiratory system to irritants. You can also try stinging nettles. In a 1990 study, tablets of freeze-dried nettles successfully reduced hay fever symptoms. Of course, using nettles to treat hay fever is nothing new. These spring greens were once a popular "old country pot herb"—an herb that was thrown into pots of soups or stews. Stinging nettles taste something like spinach. And don't worry about those stingers on the nettle's leaf—they dissolve when the plant is cooked.

So far, I have only discussed getting rid of your symptoms. Of course you want to feel better, but it is equally important to fix the imbalance that is causing your hay fever in the first place. Although you certainly need to enhance your immune system as a start, hay fever may involve seemingly unrelated organs such as your liver. Stress can also be a big factor. Stress can worsen hay fever and most other allergies. Likewise, the allergy itself causes a lot of physical and often emotional stress, which can affect your adrenal glands.

There are three Chinese herbs that you can use to improve an immune system hampered by hay fever. Siberian ginseng is a good choice as an immune herb because it also clears bronchial passages, reduces inflammation and counters fatigue. Although many people erroneously consider don quai only a woman's herb, Chinese herbalists have long used this herb to treat allergies, especially those related to the lungs. While it is generally used to treat certain women's conditions, research shows that this multipurpose herb also reduces the number of antibodies manufactured by your immune system. Fewer antibodies mean less reaction to allergic substances like pollen. Chinese skullcap is another excellent choice to treat hay fever because it cuts down on the swelling and puffiness caused by allergies. As an added plus, both don quai and Chinese skullcap also improve liver functions. If you cannot find these herbs sold individually, they are available in pills and as part of Chinese remedies.

I find that a combination of herbs with vitamins is usually in order. This combination produces faster results than just using the herbs by themselves. Rose hips, which are high in vitamin C and will thus help detoxify irritating allergens, and pantothenic acid (100 to 200 milligrams daily) will help support your adrenal glands. You might also try taking herbs for the immune system and for the liver, nervous system and sinus congestion. For example, since hay fever and sinus congestion go hand in hand, I have added both elder and peppermint to the following formula.

Hay Fever Preventive

½ teaspoon each tinctures of Siberian ginseng root, nettle leaves, elder flowers, peppermint leaves and Chinese skullcap leaves (if available)
❧ Combine ingredients. Take half a dropperful at least 5 times daily. It is best to start when you experience the earliest signs of hay fever season approaching. Because of the frequency with which you need to take this formula, most people find that a tincture is most convenient, but you can also use these herbs to make a tea.

LUNG CONGESTION

Lots of things can cause lung congestion, but the big three are asthma, pneumonia and bronchitis. These three disorders produce similar symptoms—congestion, wheezing and difficulty in breathing— but their origins are different. Asthma is an allergic reaction, pneumonia is a bacterial or viral infection, and bronchitis is usually an infection in your bronchi— tubes in your lungs that can become swollen and clogged. These lung conditions are often serious, and you should seek professional help before starting an herbal program.

Lung irritants such as dust, smoke, fumes and airborne allergens can aggravate any of these lung problems. So can breathing cold air. A common cold can lead to bronchitis or pneumonia, especially if your lungs are already below par or are often congested.

When you are congested, it's a good idea to go easy on strenuous exercise, which demands more air intake than your restricted lungs may be able to handle. If you have chronic lung congestion, there are probably underlying problems that need to be addressed. Use immune herbs such as shizandra and Siberian ginseng to build up your resistance to infection and allergies. For more information on asthma, see chapter 13.

Herbs graphically called expectorants loosen congestion and help clear your lungs so you can breathe better. The most popular herbal expectorants— mullein, thyme, horehound and elecampane—are found in most herbal lung formulas, and for good reason. These expectorants also enhance the immune system. In Europe, even physicians recommend these herbs for treatment of bronchitis and other lung conditions. Their historical use has been supported by the results of numerous scientific studies. They are best combined with soothing herbs that relieve inflammation, such as marshmallow and licorice.

Used for centuries in Germany, mullein is officially regarded there as an effective treatment for bronchial spasms and bronchitis. In addition to its other attributes, mullein reduces the swollen glands that may accompany bronchitis.

Horehound was originally sold as cough drops, so you may already be

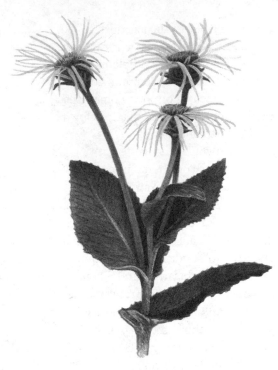

The flowers of elecampane, one of nature's best "lung herbs," look very much like daisies.

familiar with it. That is how I was introduced to it as a child. I was dismayed to discover how bitter it is, and was sure the name was short for "horrible." (It actually is derived from *hoar*, Old English for "white," because of its downy-white leaves.) While the Food and Drug Administration (FDA), the federal agency that oversees the sale of drugs in the United States, decided in 1989 that there was not enough evidence to enable horehound to be classified as medicine, the German equivalent of the FDA holds it in more esteem. They recently approved horehound for bronchial congestion. In fact, horehound and derivatives from it are used in hundreds of bronchial medications throughout the world. There is

evidence that part of the way it works is by influencing the areas in the brain that control respiration. A slightly less bitter alternative to horehound is hyssop, which is very similar in chemical makeup and use—they actually share the same major compound.

You may have never heard of elecampane, but until about 1920 the root was a common flavoring in English sugar cakes and was itself sold as a candied treat. People with asthma would chew a piece every morning and evening. And people passing by a polluted waterway would chew a piece of the root to keep their lungs from becoming irritated or infected.

If you want to take any of these bitter herbs in sweet form, take a teaspoon of the powdered herb and mix it into one or two teaspoons of honey. Take a quarter teaspoon a couple of times a day. You might want to forgo the sweetener and just tough it out. Since the action of these herbs is helped along by a chain reaction that starts with their bitter taste, they are best used as a tea or as a tincture added to water.

Other lung decongestants that counter infection are the same herbs suggested for clogged sinuses: eucalyptus, peppermint and thyme. To reduce congestion, essential oils of these herbs can be used in a steam or made into a vapor balm to rub on the chest. The balm increases circulation and warmth in the chest—both of these are important factors in fighting infection. We are also sure to hear more in the future about traditional antihistamines and bronchiodilators (herbs that open up the breathing passages, called bronchi) from around the world, such as khella from Egypt, which was a model for the asthma drug disodium chromoglycate.

If you like Mexican, Chinese and Thai food, you are in luck. Spicy-hot herbs make it easier to breathe by watering down lung secretions. Cultures that habitually eat hot spices, such as Mexican and Szechwan and Hunan Chinese, have less chronic lung diseases than the British, whose diet is more bland. Even eating foods spiced with cayenne, horseradish, garlic, black pepper, mustard or ginger will do the trick. Researchers at the University of California at Los Angeles suggest eating enough cayenne or ginger "to cause tingling of the nose and sneezing." And they actually recommend gargling with these herbs if your stomach is too sensitive for spicy foods!

One old-fashioned remedy to take seriously is onions. These vegetables are as potent a cure as they are smelly. Make them into a homemade, inexpensive cough syrup or chop them into a poultice to lay on your chest.

Lung Tincture

2 teaspoons tincture of mullein leaf
1 teaspoon each tinctures of chamomile
*   flowers and elecampane root*
½ teaspoon each tinctures of thyme
*   leaves and Oregon grape root*
*   (or barberry or goldenseal)*
❧ Combine ingredients. Take ½ dropperful (using a 1-ounce dropper) or ¼ teaspoon added to ½ to 1 cup of water or juice 3 to 5 times a day. You can use these herbs in the same proportions to make a tea (though I don't suggest it, because they're quite bitter). Or you can take them as pills.

Vapor Rub

¼ teaspoon eucalyptus essential oil
⅛ teaspoon each peppermint and thyme
*   essential oils*
¼ cup olive oil
❧ Combine ingredients in a glass bottle. Shake well to mix oils evenly. Gently massage into chest and throat.

Cayenne Gargle

⅛ teaspoon cayenne powder
¼ cup warm water
❧ Stir cayenne into water and gargle.

Onion Syrup

1 onion
2 cups water
3 tablespoons honey
❧ Gently simmer onion in water for about 20 minutes, then blend it with the water. Mix in honey. Take a tablespoon at a time, as warm as possible.

Onion Poultice

1 chopped onion
1 cup water
Cloth
❧ Lightly cook onion in water, enough to soften. Mash or blend and apply to the chest while still warm. Cover with a soft cloth.

SINUS CONGESTION

Sinus congestion can stem from many different problems, but viral or bacterial infection, allergy and irritation from airborne substances are the most common causes. Don't worry if your nose is constantly stuffy or running, however. There is hope. Some of the best herbal treatments for chronic sinus problems are yarrow, elder flowers and peppermint. Yarrow and elder flowers reduce inflamed sinuses and, along with peppermint, help drain them.

For quick relief, thin out congestion with eucalyptus, peppermint and bergamot. These essential oils can be combined with steam to help you breathe easier. If steaming with herbs is not practical, then carry an herbal nasal inhaler. These are available in natural food and drugstores, or you can make your own.

Homemade Nasal Inhaler

1/4 teaspoon coarse salt
5 drops eucalyptus essential oil

Place the salt in a small vial (glass is best) with a tight lid and add oil. The salt will absorb the oil and provide a convenient way to carry the oil without danger of spilling it. Open the vial and inhale deeply, as needed. This same technique can be used with any essential oil.

Though it is not nearly as appealing, another thing you can do when you do not have time to steam is to sniff a small pinch of powdered barberry or Oregon grape root up your nose. You might also try herbal antihistamines, such as peppermint, ginger, anise and chamomile, and hot spices like cayenne pepper. These will help clear a stuffy nose as well as congested lungs.

Mark is a good example of someone who has greatly benefited from using herbs for his sinus condition. When I first met him, he described how the wastepaper basket next to his desk at work filled up a couple of times a day with tissues as he constantly blew his nose. His co-workers began giving him all sorts of advice. But it was not as if Mark's doctors had not already investigated every possibility they could think of. The best they could finally offer was a powerful antihistamine for constant use.

At that point, Mark figured nature probably knew best and it certainly would not hurt to try some herbs. For convenience, he settled on a tincture that he could carry to work and to the gym, as well as on weekend jaunts. Along with lung herbs, it included some of the herbs well-suited for the immune system, such as echinacea, Siberian ginseng and shizandra. It did not take long for Mark, as well as everyone around him, to notice a difference. The waste basket contained less and less tissue.

Mark is still trying to get to the source of the problem, but meanwhile the herbs are relieving his symptoms and making life much easier. I suspect that some insult to his immune system, such as undiscovered allergies or simply stress, is at play here.

Sinus Congestion Tea

1 teaspoon each yarrow flowers, elder flowers, peppermint leaves and elecampane root
1 quart boiling water

Pour boiling water over herbs and steep for at least 20 minutes in a covered container. Strain out the herbs. Drink the tea a few times a day, or every half hour when severely congested. This same formula can be taken in tincture or pill form.

chapter

TEN

The

Skin

Your skin is your body's most visible tissue, which means that when you have a skin problem, it's generally impossible to ignore. Skin tissue is not endangered only by cuts, scrapes, bruises and other wounds—it can also be subject to various diseases. In chapter 17, I discuss herbal cosmetics, treatments designed to help improve the way your skin looks. Here's a look at skin problems that can become serious health matters.

PSORIASIS, ECZEMA AND OTHER SKIN DISEASES

One hot summer day at my herb shop, a woman named Laura arrived looking for a skin salve. The temperature was well up into the nineties, yet she was wearing a long-sleeved turtleneck shirt. I politely said nothing about her attire, for I suspected she was covering up a skin problem. It turned out I was right, and Laura was more than anxious to roll up her sleeve. When she did, I saw a terrible case of eczema and asked if she had seen a dermatologist. She nodded, but then explained that except for keeping her on cortisone, her doctors were ready to give up. In spite of this poor prognosis, she hoped that a skin salve might help. She chose one that contained comfrey and calendula.

A month passed and I forgot about Laura, until I received an order for more salve and some traditional herbs used as a tea for the liver, such as burdock, yellow dock, sarsaparilla and dandelion. Then, one day in the fall, I was at a laundromat sorting clothes when a slender woman wearing a spaghetti-strap blouse practically jumped over my laundry cart, spilling my clothes in the process. She gave me a huge bear hug. As she stepped back, wearing a huge smile, I saw that it was Laura, thanking me for helping her. Actually, I had done nothing, but I was certainly impressed with what the herbs had done for her. Her skin was smooth and clear—I could see why she had chosen the blouse she was wearing. Equally impressive was her slender figure—in addition to clearing up her scaly, oozing skin, she had lost a great deal of weight. She said that she felt so much better about herself that she no longer binged on food.

If you're confused about the difference between psoriasis, eczema and dermatitis, I'm not surprised. Even dermatologists sometimes have trouble identifying these skin problems. Actually, both eczema and psoriasis are types of dermatitis, which simply means "inflammation of the skin." Eczema is considered more of a symptom than an actual disease, and is best treated by dealing with the underlying cause. Psoriasis can be controlled by prescription drugs, but these are hard on the liver and therefore must be carefully administered, especially considering that impaired liver function is thought to contribute to psoriasis.

Most types of dermatitis result in inflamed, red skin that is often itchy and may develop into lesions. Eczema can include crusty sores, scabs, thickened skin, pimplelike eruptions and sometimes even lesions. The skin can be either oozing or crusty and easily becomes infected. Psoriasis produces reddish lesions with a characteristic silvery scaling that flakes off, causing the skin underneath to bleed. These scales are actually excess skin generated when certain substances in the body that are responsible for directing skin cell growth go out of control and make the cells grow too quickly—sometimes 1,000 times faster than the normal rate of growth.

The exact cause of these skin conditions is often difficult to determine. We do know that you are more prone to get them if you have thin, dry skin. According to researchers, dermatitis is often caused by allergies and sensitivities to particular foods. Eliminating the foods most likely to cause allergies often decreases eczema.

Most people with eczema test positive to some type of allergy, have elevated levels of antibodies in their blood (a sign of an allergic reaction) and often do not have enough stomach acid, a common cause of food sensitivities. People with psoriasis usually have high levels of polyamine, an undesirable, toxic type of amino acid that is formed during poor protein digestion, another cause of food sensitivities.

To combat psoriasis and eczema, first try the Cleanser for Dry Complexion (see page 310). Do not use soap, because it can irritate your skin. Another natural way to treat psoriasis is by exposure to direct sunlight and heat. Secondary skin infections, which often occur with eczema, need to be treated with antiseptic herbs such as those suggested for acne on page 179. To make a salve for eczema or psoriasis, you can start with a standard salve and add a few essential oils.

Dermatitis Skin Salve

½ teaspoon each tinctures of pau d'arco bark and goldenseal root (or barberry bark)

8 drops each tea tree and chamomile essential oils

2 ounces skin salve (buy a comfrey salve from a store, or use the Herbal Healing Salve on page 257)

Using a toothpick, stir the tinctures and essential oils into the salve. This will make the salve semi-liquid. Apply throughout the day.

HERBS FOR HEALING THE SKIN

Many internal remedies for dermatitis start with the herb sarsaparilla. Michael Murray, N.D., and Joseph Pizzorno, N.D., authors of A Textbook of Natural Medicine, believe that this herb aids people with psoriasis by binding toxins in the intestine and stopping the production of polyamines. For centuries, sarsaparilla was regarded as an important "blood purifier." Doctors and herbalists used it to treat all sorts of serious skin problems. Doctors were still using it in the 1940s when an article in the New England Journal of Medicine described it as "dramatically" successful in helping cure psoriasis. Little research has been done since, but herbalists continue to use this herb for psoriasis and eczema.

Psyllium and berberine, a compound found in barberry and goldenseal, can also halt production of polyamines. Bitter melon, a Chinese plant that is a relative of cucumber, also interferes with the production of this chemical.

Psoriasis and eczema often respond to herbs used to enhance the immune system's function and to herbs that help the liver do its work. Indeed, researchers have found that outbreaks of eczema lower immunity, making people who have this skin condition more likely to get viral diseases like herpes and warts. Burdock root and the Chinese herb bupleurum have long been recommended to treat dermatitis, especially eczema.

Studies have shown that the popular liver herb milk thistle also helps combat psoriasis. Another herb that is potent against both liver and skin problems is the Indian plant gotu kola. According to French studies, compounds in gotu kola, which has long been used to treat leprosy, rapidly heal broken skin. The Rudolf Stiftung Hospital in Vienna uses a salve and also an injection of these compounds to help wounds heal faster.

An immunity-enhancing herb with a particularly good track record for improving dermatitis is pau d'arco, the bark of a South American tree. For other ways to improve immunity, see "Boosting Immunity" on page 101, and for other herbs to help improve liver functioning, see chapter 7.

Licorice root may seem a surprising choice for helping the skin, but researchers find that it combats many types of dermatitis, improves liver health, reduces skin inflammation and is useful in treating symptoms of stress and allergies.

Numerous studies show that gamma linoleic acid (GLA), which is found in evening primrose oil, and compounds in licorice and chamomile can reduce skin inflammation even better than cortisone. In one study of almost 100 adults and children with eczema, evening primrose oil significantly reduced the itching, redness and severity of the problem within three months. Other studies show that GLA also helps in treating impetigo, a crusty outbreak of pustules that usually occurs around the mouth and nose and is caused by a bacterial infection. I have also heard reports that GLA helps fight ichthyosis, a condition that makes the skin dry and scaly, resembling that of a fish.

Stress seems to play a big role in many skin disorders. Over one-third of the people who have psoriasis say that their initial outbreak happened within a month of a very stressful event. In Laura's case, she realized which stresses in her life—exams at school, a visit from her in-laws and pressure at work—set off her skin condition, and that those stresses needed to be controlled. For herbs to combat stress, see "Stress" on page 52.

Dermatitis Tea

½ teaspoon each sarsaparilla root, licorice root, burdock root, pau d'arco bark and bupleurum root (if available)
3 cups water

Gently simmer herbs in water for 10 minutes. Turn off heat and let steep for another 10 minutes. Strain. Drink a cup of tea 3 or 4 times a day. This combination of herbs can also be taken as a tincture, using the same proportions as the tea. Or you can purchase a similar tincture formula at a natural food store. Take half a dropperful 3 or 4 times each day.

Sending Parasites Scurrying

So you think you're feeling lousy today? The next time you use this expression, think twice. It is derived from "louse," the singular of lice. Originally, a person who felt lousy had, you guessed it, lice.

The expression may be an old one, but parasitic infections are more common today than ever. They began increasing in the 1970s—incidence of head lice in North America doubled during a two-year span. There are many myths surrounding head, body and pubic lice. The truth is that they are not caused by a lack of hygiene and they have no respect for social class—everyone is at risk. Lice are most frequently transmitted by hairbrushes, hats and bedding. The tiny eggs of these parasites have an uncanny resemblance to dandruff, except that they cling tightly to hair. Because of this, they often go unnoticed until the lice themselves start your scalp itching.

The U.S. Center for Disease Control in Atlanta does not label lice a health hazard. Although lice have at various times carried such serious infections as typhus and trench fever, currently they transmit no diseases in North America. Even so, people find these parasites unnerving. Lice may not be considered a serious health problem, but getting rid of them can be more than irritating—it takes something mighty powerful to do away with the little buggers.

The poison of choice for more than 30 years has been lindane, a cousin of the infamous and now banned pesticide DDT. Lindane, available only by prescription, is toxic to people as well as lice because it is readily absorbed by the skin and can cause nervous system problems, even convulsions. This chemical is not exactly what you want to put on your preschooler's head when he or she comes home from school infested with lice. To make matters worse, strains of lice are becoming resistant to lindane, so there is a chance that it may not even work.

A better choice is an insecticide made from pyrethrins, a compound most commonly found in chrysanthemums. While this more natural option is no gentle substance either, it is much safer, and it is not readily absorbed through the skin like lindane.

Another way to fight lice is with a homemade remedy made up of a strong concentration of essential oils. This formula will have to be very potent, so use it carefully. Do a skin test first. Apply a drop of the oil to the inside of the elbow and leave it alone for several hours. If there is no sign of irritation, go ahead and use it. Keep the treatment away from the eyes and shampoo it off at the first sign of irritation, especially with children.

The oils will usually do the trick, but the eggs are more resistant than the lice themselves and you may need to repeat treatment after a week to eliminate newly hatched lice. Whatever method you choose to treat lice, be sure to wash clothes, bed linens and anything else that comes in contact with the person's head—and don't forget to vacuum the backs of chairs and couches.

Lice Treatment
2 ounces vegetable oil
20 drops tea tree essential oil
10 drops each essential oils of rosemary, lavender and lemon

Combine ingredients. Apply to dry hair and cover with a plastic bag or shower cap. Wrap the head in a towel. Leave on for 1 hour. Then put shampoo on dry hair to help cut the oil. Work the shampoo into hair, rinse, shampoo again and rinse.

Part III

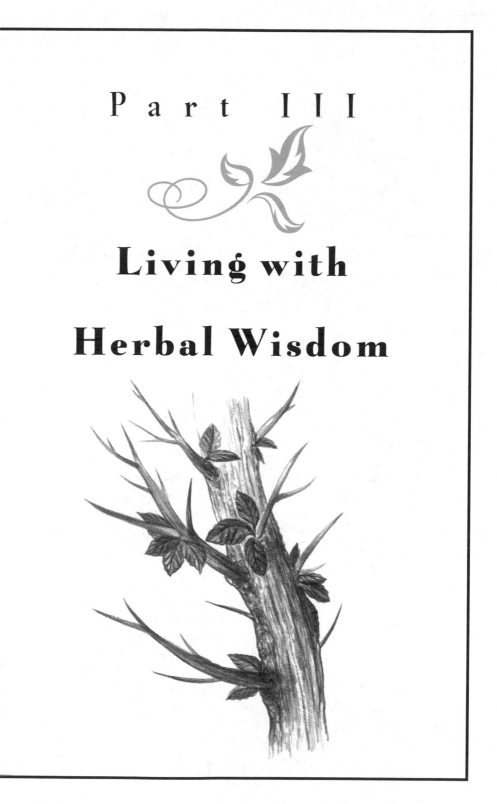

Living with

Herbal Wisdom

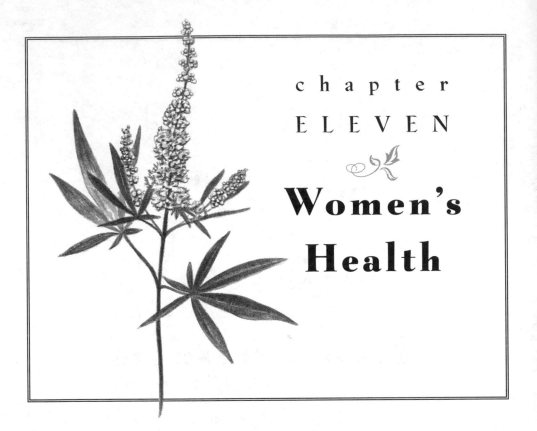

chapter

E L E V E N

Women's Health

Most of the health problems that are specific to women can be traced to our endless cycle of hormones. Some of us ride natural hormonal changes like crests of a wave, while others feel more as though they are being pulled into the undertow! If you fall into the later group, keep in mind that you have plenty of company. In fact, estrogen, the name for the primary female hormone, comes from the Latin word *oestrus,* which means "frenzy" in English.

For those of you whose hormonal cycles drive you into a frenzy, I have good news: Almost every woman I know who has tried herbs and supportive nutrition gets some relief. And though natural remedies may involve some trial and error to discover which herbal formula works best for you, finding the right combination will help you move gracefully through most health problems specific to women, from monthly cycles to menopause. You must be patient, though—it may take a while before you begin to see real improvement.

Before plunging into an herbal healing program, you need to determine what is wrong. Your gynecologist or a health care clinic can help you do this. You may even have a local clinic that specializes in female problems. If you discover that yours is a serious disorder, be sure to work on the treatment with a professional health care practitioner.

Female hormones are indispensable—they help maintain physical and emotional well-being, as well as physical endurance and sex drive. If you alter their delicate balance, your body will let you know in a variety of ways. At times, hormonal problems can seem very complicated, since an increase in production of one hormone can lead to a decrease in others. This can place you on a hormonal seesaw! To make it even more puzzling, your hormone levels fluctuate throughout the month and even throughout the day.

Fortunately, herbs can help still the seesaw. While herbs do not contain the hormones found in our bodies, some of them do contain substances that influence our hormonal activity. How they do this is not completely understood—in fact, there is much that medical science still has to learn about hormones—but we do know that herbs sometimes mimic, activate or block natural hormonal activity. And some herbs make your body more or less sensitive to its own hormones.

THE ESTROGEN STORY

Estrogen is the most well-known female hormone. It helps improve your complexion, makes your hair silky and your skin soft, and discourages wrinkles. It even helps keep you feeling spunky and energetic. But when estrogen levels soar too high, nervous jitters, insomnia, memory impairment and overly sensitive or tingly skin can result. Stress, cortisone and some antidepressant drugs increase estrogen levels. So do fatty or fried foods, sugar and alcohol.

An overabundance of estrogen also leads to other problems. It can slow the body's ability to break down fat, cause water retention, throw off blood sugar levels and even reduce the amount of oxygen the lungs and cells take in. In the 1980s and 1990s, medical researchers discovered that excessive estrogen can cause even more far-reaching complications—endometriosis, uterine fibroids, uterine cancer, cervical dysplasia, breast cysts and many breast cancers are all thought to have some connection to high estrogen levels. To further complicate matters, there is more than one kind of estrogen in the body, and not all types are carcinogenic (cancer-causing). A specific problem may not be related to all types of estrogen, but specifically to one troublesome kind that tends to be more carcinogenic than the others.

THE PROGESTERONE STORY

Progesterone is an equally important female hormone. It helps you feel content and emotionally balanced in a number of ways. It reduces stress, uterine spasms, water retention and muscle weakness and helps the body to handle alcohol, sugar and food cravings. As with estrogen, high progesterone levels also pose problems—they can lead to sluggishness, tiredness, muscle aches, low blood sugar, increased appetite and weight gain.

It is a medical fact that progesterone and estrogen keep each other in balance. In fact, premenstrual syndrome (PMS), irregular menstruation, menstrual cramps and a tendency toward miscarriage may be at least partially caused by an imbalance of these two hormones—too much estrogen and too little progesterone. For this reason, women with PMS or uterine fibroids are sometimes given progesterone to adjust this imbalance. In a study conducted at the Johns Hopkins University, in which a group of women were given 800 International Units of vitamin E for ten weeks, results showed that vitamin E corrects the progesterone-estrogen ratio, increases a woman's libido and normalizes her menstrual cycle.

While we are on the topic of hormonal balance, let's not overlook the liver. Ask any herbalist: Liver herbs such as burdock and dandelion often help women with hard-to-treat health problems. This is because the liver deactivates estrogen, especially the carcinogenic form, which tends to settle in breast and uterine tissue. For more information on herbs to help maintain the health of your liver, see chapter 7.

Anemia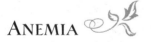

Anemia is not really a disease, but a symptom of an underlying problem. It is most common in women—because of blood loss due to menstruation. About 10 percent of North American women are iron-deficient during their childbearing years. The typical woman with anemia is pale and often finds herself weak or dizzy and falling asleep easily. She usually describes herself as feeling tired most of the time. She may be prone to

headaches and digestive disturbances and may also experience heart palpitations. If this sounds like you, you should ask your doctor to check your iron level. This involves a simple blood test that takes only a few minutes.

If your doctor determines that you are low in iron, it will not take long to correct the problem. But the most obvious choice for treatment—iron supplements—are never my first recommendation. These supplements do not help all the women who take them. Even when they do help, they often cause constipation and stomach distress, as well as rob your body of vitamin E. The fear of anemia leads most doctors to prescribe iron supplements to pregnant women. However, according to the U.S. Preventive Services Task Force (a nongovernment panel sponsored by the U.S. Public Health Service, a federal agency), "There is currently little evidence to suggest that routine iron supplementation during pregnancy is beneficial."

Instead you might want to try yellow dock root, a more easily assimilated source of iron. Yellow dock contains only a small amount of this important mineral, yet herbalists consider it one of the most effective herbs for raising your iron level. Although the way that this herb increases iron remains a mystery, the proof is in the results. I cannot count how many women with anemia have told me how amazed their doctors were when yellow dock brought their iron count up to normal in only a few weeks. Many physicians are not aware that an herb can be so effective, especially a humble weed that grows throughout most of the United States.

Sara, who is fifteen years old, is a perfect example of how effective this herb can be. A classic case of anemia, Sara felt worn out and listless and never seemed to have enough energy. But after taking a tincture of yellow dock every day for a month, she found herself feeling energetic enough to try out for the high school track team.

Karen is another example. At one point, when Karen was six months pregnant, her iron count was so low that her doctor was threatening drastic measures, starting with hospitalization. Iron supplements weren't helping much, so she turned to yellow dock. Within two weeks, her iron count had returned to normal.

In my years of working with herbs, I have met literally dozens of other women who felt so run-down and sluggish that they described themselves as having only "half a life." All of them started taking yellow dock and received such a boost that they are now living very full lives. For some of these women, yellow dock brought up their iron levels permanently and they were able to discontinue using the herb. Others found that they needed to continue taking it to maintain their iron count at a healthy level.

Even if your anemia is so stubborn that it does not respond to yellow dock, a few additional herbs will usually do the trick. Studies conducted around the world have shown that the roots of burdock, sarsaparilla, dandelion, cooked Chinese rehmannia and Chinese wild yam increase the assimilation of iron, as do carrots and most green vegetables. (Although Chinese herbs like rehmannia and wild yam were once restricted to the realm of Chinese medicine, they are now available in most natural food stores.) German researchers were so impressed with how anise, caraway, cumin, mint and linden flowers improved iron absorption that they suggested that anyone with an iron deficiency drink tea made with at least one of these herbs. Iron-rich herbs include parsley, watercress and the seaweed dulse.

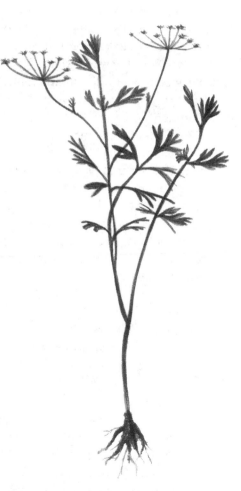

Caraway seeds were so revered by sixth-century Persians that citizens used them to pay taxes.

If these herbs seem like the ingredients for the start of a delicious soup or stew base, you're right! Throw in a few beet roots to add even more iron, and dine on this soup at least twice a week. The Chinese traditionally prescribe soups made from healing herbs like rehmannia, wild yam and burdock. When you wish to incorporate medicinal herb roots into your meals, all you need to do is finely chop or grate them, then treat them like carrots. Caraway and cumin can also be used to spice up beans and vegetables. For recipes, see chapter 18. By the way, if you suffer from anemia, you will want to avoid black tea, which slows down iron absorption.

Women who experience heavy menstruation frequently have a low iron count. If this is true for you, you should not only follow the above suggestions, but also see "Heavy Periods" on page 162. Anemia can also signal several other problems, such as a blood disorder, so consult a physician before treating with herbs.

Iron Tea

2 teaspoons yellow dock root
½ teaspoon each nettle leaves, dandelion root, beet root, licorice and cooked rehmannia root (if available)
3 cups water

🌿 Bring herbs and water to a boil, then turn down heat and simmer for 5 minutes. Turn off heat and let steep for 20 minutes. Strain out herbs. Drink 2 cups a day. This formula can also be taken as a tincture or in pill form. To take yellow dock by itself, you will want to use a tincture since the taste is so bitter.

CERVICAL DYSPLASIA

Cervical dysplasia occurs when cells form irregularly on a woman's cervix, which is located at the mouth of the uterus. Since this unusual growth is considered a precondition to cancer, physicians generally suggest burning, freezing or cutting off the problem cells. However, the condition progresses so slowly that your doctor will probably wait a month or two, then retest you. Take advantage of this time to try an herbal remedy.

My neighbor Nancy had cervical dysplasia more than once. When her doctor first noticed irregularities on her cervix, he conducted a series of laboratory tests that led him to conclude that her dysplasia was at "stage three"—not a good sign, considering that stage four is cancer. The treatment he used was to freeze the problem cells. Three years later, Nancy was again diagnosed as having cervical dysplasia. This time, she chose a particularly vigorous herbal therapy, as her doctor now said that the most effective treatment would be surgery.

With only one month to turn around her dysplasia, Nancy was committed to healing herself. She placed castor oil packs over her abdomen, sat in sitz baths filled with a strong tea of sage, eucalyptus and comfrey leaf tea and used a tampon soaked in a strong solution of calendula tea. She faithfully did each of these treatments at least once a day, more often when she could manage it (and got lots of reading done at the same time!).

When Nancy told me the results of her next test, I was as impressed as she was with the herbs. The baffled doctor found far fewer signs of dysplasia and, although he was apprehensive about discussing herbs, sent her home to "continue doing whatever you are doing." The next three times she was tested, she came up completely clean; so she stopped taking the herbs. That was years ago, and following her doctor's advice, she continues to get tested regularly—at least twice a year. She also follows her herbalist's advice to keep estrogen down to normal levels and her immunity up. She does not expect the dysplasia to return, but if it ever does, she knows what she will do.

Cervical dysplasia can be caused, or at least promoted, by the same virus responsible for genital warts (human papillomavirus) and possibly by those viruses that cause herpes (herpes simplex types 1 and 2), although not all women with warts or herpes necessarily develop dysplasia. Another contributing factor is excessive amounts of the more carcinogenic form of estrogen that is manufactured by the body. In addition, women whose mothers took a synthetic estrogen called diethylstilbestrol (DES) in the 1940s and 1950s to prevent miscarriage were overexposed to estrogen and often develop dysplasia. (Unfortunately, until 1979, much of the meat sold in the United States also contained small amounts of DES.) The American Cancer Society also lists estrogen-based birth control pills, multiple sexual partners and smoking as risk factors for dysplasia. Researchers have reported that smoking even two or three cigarettes a day seems to concentrate carcinogens in the cervix.

You can treat the problem cells and at the same time stimulate your immune system with a tea or tincture of echinacea, calendula and false indigo, an immune system herb with properties similar to echinacea. While most people may not think of calendula (which is known to gardeners as pot marigold) as more than a pretty garden flower, it is a potent immunity builder that seems to have a special affinity for healing the cervix.

Among the most important herbs for treating gynecological problems are the berries from vitex, an attractive tree from the Mediterranean. Vitex is one of the few herbs known to balance a woman's hormones, and so has become invaluable for many different formulas. To help keep excessive estrogen in line, you should also take herbs that are good for the liver, such as burdock.

You can also put herbs directly on your cervix—as Nancy did—by using vaginal suppositories or a tampon soak of goldenseal, calendula and tea tree. Tea tree suppositories are also available in natural food stores.

I know quite a few women who have conquered cervical dysplasia using herbal teas, tinctures and suppositories alone, but you can speed along the process by also taking herbal sitz baths and applying castor oil packs. These techniques are explained in "Endometriosis" on page 156. These treatments require a little extra time, but the end results are worth it.

Folic acid, which is not an herb per se but is found in green, leafy vegetables, can also play a role in treating cervical dysplasia. Many women with cervical dysplasia have a folic acid deficiency, especially if they take birth control pills. According to one study of women on the Pill, three weeks of folic acid supplements reversed the risk of cervical cancer for a significant number of women. Joseph E. Pizzorno, N.D., and Michael T. Murray, N.D., authors of *A Textbook of Natural Medicine,* a natural healing reference commonly used by naturopathic doctors and medical doctors who use natural methods, suggest that women who have cervical dysplasia take 2 milligrams of folic acid a day for three months, then reduce the dose to 0.5 milligram a day. Along with your herbal therapy, vitamins A, C and the B-complex can be extremely helpful.

While Nancy's story attests to the power of herbs, do not get discouraged if you try them and you do not experience Nancy's success. Herbs sometimes work quickly, sometimes not. Another friend of mine, Dora, was given three weeks to self-treat cervical dysplasia that had nearly reached stage four. She was diligent about taking sitz baths and applying castor oil packs and taking an herbal tincture similar to the tea recipe given below. She even made her own herbal suppositories. Three weeks later, Dora's test results did not look any better, and her doctor advised removing the cells right away.

At least Dora knew that she had done what she could in that short amount of time. She also felt that the herbs prepared her body better for the doctor's procedure. (She also decided to quit smoking.) Even if you decide on medical treatments, you can do as Dora did and take these herbs once a day for one week every month to prevent the dysplasia from returning.

Cervical Dysplasia Tea

2 teaspoons vitex berries
1 teaspoon each burdock root and false indigo root
½ teaspoon each calendula flowers and echinacea root
5 cups water

Bring herbs and water to a boil in an uncovered pot, then simmer gently for 5 minutes. Remove from heat, cover pot and let steep for 20 minutes. Strain out herbs. This can also be taken as a tincture or in pill form.

Tampon Soak

1 heaping teaspoon dried calendula flowers
½ teaspoon goldenseal rhizome powder
1 cup water
5 drops tea tree essential oil

Put herbs and water in a pot, place on stove and bring to a boil. Turn off heat and let steep for about 30 minutes. Strain and add essential oil. Soak tampon in mixture, stirring well to distribute the oil. (Be sure to use a tampon that comes enclosed in a cylinder inserter or the soaking will expand it too much.)

ENDOMETRIOSIS

Endometriosis occurs when tissue from the lining of the uterus—the endometrium—attaches itself elsewhere in the abdomen. This creates havoc throughout the pelvic area, especially just before menstruation, when the misplaced lining expands along with the normal uterine lining.

Endometriosis, which is well known to almost 10 percent of U.S. women, can be quite painful. Its symptoms include severe cramping, excessive menstrual bleeding, and intestinal gas, sometimes accompanied by depression and insomnia. The scarring that results from the misplaced tissue can lead to infertility and bowel inflammation.

The causes of endometriosis remain a mystery. Curiously, European women rarely get it. We do know that one of the risk factors is an abundance of estrogen. That is why endometriosis occurs mostly in women between the ages of 25 and 40, when estrogen accumulates at its highest levels. Endometriosis is exacerbated by anything that irritates the uterus, such as a pelvic infection, constipation, uterine fibroids or cancer, or the presence of an IUD or a tampon. Even ingesting caffeine, alcohol or fried foods increases the problem.

Medical science offers us many theories about the cause, but no cure for this poorly understood disorder. Often, the recommended treatment for endometriosis is quite drastic—either a hysterectomy or hormone therapy with a drug such as danazol, which suppresses estrogen and initiates a false menopause—complete with hot flashes, vaginal dryness and a decreased sexual drive. Understandably, many women are reluctant to take this drug.

Thankfully, many cases of endometriosis can be treated with herbs, but you must be patient—most of the women I know who chose to treat this disorder

herbally found that successful treatment took many months. For best results, work with a natural health care professional who has experience with this disorder and can help you develop a complete healing campaign that includes dietary changes, massage and possibly acupuncture.

Since an overabundance of estrogen is one contributing factor of endometriosis, vitex berries, which balance a woman's hormones, are a valuable herb in any endometriosis formula. When I discuss the treatment of this disorder with other herbalists, they always say that vitex is the most important herb in their formulas.

And since hormones are a major factor in the development of this disorder, it is generally a good idea to also treat your liver with herbs, particularly burdock. Remember, the liver helps clear estrogen from the body. For more information on herbs to help the liver do its job, see chapter 7.

If you suffer from endometriosis, it is also important for you to reduce the bleeding, inflammation, muscle cramps and pain that generally accompany this disorder. The first herbs that I turn to for easing these symptoms are cramp bark and wild yam. For herbs to stop cramping and other menstrual pain—evening primrose oil and ginger, for instance—see "Menstrual Cramps" on page 171. Red raspberry reduces bleeding and is thought to strengthen the uterus—herbalists and midwives have been using it for these purposes for at least a thousand years.

Horsetail also reduces excessive bleeding, especially menstrual bleeding.

And it may do more than that for women with endometriosis—herbalists believe that it keeps scar tissue flexible, thus preventing further scarring. During the tuberculosis outbreaks of the early twentieth century, horsetail was used to reduce the amount of scarring on people's lungs. Pills containing horsetail are commonly sold to strengthen nails and hair, and may also strengthen connective ligaments such as those that hold the uterus in place.

Medical science is now realizing that endometriosis is a signal that you need to build up your immune system. Taking echinacea is a good way to do this because this herb not only improves immunity, but also helps repair connective tissues and fibers.

Castor oil packs are also very helpful in treating endometriosis. No one can explain exactly how they work, but experience has shown me time and again that they often make the difference between the success of a natural treatment and its failure. A recent study from Washington University in Washington, D.C., showed that castor oil packs can improve the function of the immune system in the pelvic area. For directions on how to do a castor oil pack, see page 159.

Any woman with endometriosis can tell you that the disorder can make life very difficult, but I felt particularly sorry for my friend Cathy. She performs and teaches Middle Eastern dance—probably one of the hardest things in the world to do when suffering from endometriosis. In the middle of one performance, the pain became so bad that she barely finished the show. She made an appointment to see her gynecologist the next day.

The minute her doctor suggested that she take hormonal drugs, she hesitated. Nevertheless, she figured that taking them would be better than having a hysterectomy. Cathy is also a registered nurse, and one of her jobs when she worked in a gynecology clinic was to check in patients who were to undergo hysterectomies. She learned that almost every woman she admitted was there because of painful menstruation, often from endometriosis.

Cathy started having problems with her medication from day one—she was suffering every side effect in the book—and her gynecologist kept switching her from one drug to another. Finally, Cathy became fed up with the drugs and started reading up on herbal alternatives. She had been studying herbs for years, but to her dismay had discovered very little information about endometriosis. Piecing together what she did find, she made a customized formula. The primary herbs she chose were echinacea, vitex, wild yam, red raspberry, motherwort and nettles, with burdock and milk thistle added for her liver. All the while, she kept searching for more information.

Figuring that it was going to take a lot to solve her problem, she tried castor oil packs and hot and cold sitz baths with a few drops of lavender or chamomile essential oil (in the hot bath only) to increase circulation in the pelvic area. Since her apartment did not have a bathtub, she used two large plastic tubs that she had bought at a hardware store. She really had me laughing as she described the looks that came across the faces of the other customers as they watched her sit in the tubs to find the right size.

She also noticed that stress and anything that lowered her immunity, such as not getting enough sleep or not eating well, made it much worse. Just one cup of coffee started the cramping again. It took lots of discipline, but Cathy managed to change her habits and improve her endometriosis dramatically. Now she is dancing again, with only a little twinge of pain when she eats or sleeps poorly or feels stressed.

Cathy describes her recovery using herbal treatments as "amazing." You can imagine her reaction when she heard her friend Judy complaining that endometriosis was preventing her from getting pregnant. Judy had been following her gynecologist's advice to a T for more than two years, but her condition was no better, possibly even a little worse. Cathy designed for Judy a formula that was similar to the one she herself had used, and gave Judy a list of lifestyle things to watch out for. Because Judy lives in another town, the two did not see each other for more than a year, but when they did, Judy gave her benefactor a huge hug—as best she could considering she was seven months pregnant!

Endometriosis Tea
1 teaspoon each vitex berries, echinacea root, wild yam rhizome and cramp bark
½ teaspoon each horsetail stalks, red raspberry and motherwort
1 quart water

Combine herbs and water in an uncovered pot and bring to a boil. Turn down the heat and let simmer gently for about 5 minutes. Remove from heat, cover and steep for 15 minutes. Strain out herbs. Drink at least 2 cups daily. This formula can also be taken as a tincture or in capsules.

Castor Oil Pack
¼ cup castor oil
8 drops lavender essential oil
Soft cloth

Combine castor oil and lavender essential oil. Soak cloth in this mixture, then fold it and place it in a baking dish in a 350°F oven for about 20 minutes— it should be quite warm, but not uncomfortably so. Place the folded cloth directly over the afflicted area and cover it with a towel to keep it warm. (A hot water bottle on top of this also works well.) Use the pack once a day for 30 to 60 minutes. Rinse off the oil after each application.

Sitz Bath
10 drops rosemary essential oil

Add essential oil to a bathtub and stir well to distribute. Sit in tub with hot water up to your waist for 5 to 10 minutes (this is a good time to read a book). Then sit in a tub of cold water, also up to your waist, for at least 1 minute. (The large plastic tubs sold at hardware stores work fine.) Continue for 2 to 5 rounds. Perform this treatment every day, if possible. Lavender or chamomile essential oils could be used in place of rosemary. If you want, you can make a strong tea of these herbs and use that instead of the essential oils.

FIBROCYSTIC BREASTS

Fibrocystic breasts plague about one-third of U.S. women in their childbearing years. Women with this condition have breasts that usually swell and become painful just before menstruation. In some cases, women become so uncomfortable that they find they can sleep only on their backs, must forgo aerobics classes and cannot even hug their kids! Nonetheless, if you have lumpy breasts, do not despair. For one thing, most specialists agree that this condition does not lead to breast cancer. However, since any breast lump can be worrisome, have your gynecologist or a health clinic check any new lump just to be safe. (If you do have breast cancer, you can use the herbal treatments for fibrocystic breasts as part of more comprehensive therapy.)

Too much estrogen is the most common cause of breast cysts, but it is not the only one. One of the functions of estrogen is to control another hormone called prolactin, whose job is to prepare a woman's body, specifically her breasts, for possible pregnancy. When prolactin levels rise too high, problems occur: breast tenderness and cysts, as well as water retention. Prolactin is also stimulated by stress, lots of fat or protein in the diet, alcohol, marijuana and prolonged pain.

Doctors can surgically remove breast cysts or shrink them with a drug that blocks prolactin, but I am sure that you will be relieved to know that herbs offer a much less drastic approach. From reading reports on numerous studies,

and from my own observations, I know that evening primrose oil (sold in capsules at natural food stores) almost always reduces breast cysts within three months, often sooner.

If you are one of the few women whose breast lumps don't disappear that easily, try taking 400 International Units of vitamin E along with the evening primrose. We do not know exactly why combining vitamin E with herbs is so effective, but it probably has to do with this vitamin's ability to detoxify and to

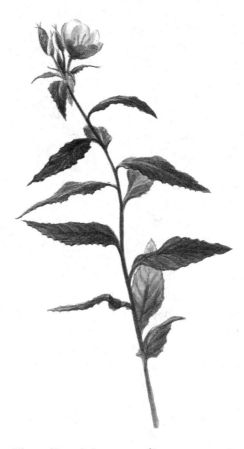

The tall and dramatic flowering stalk of evening primrose makes this herb one of nature's most easily identified medicinal plants.

increase circulation. Vitamin E encourages the cysts to drain and helps the blood and lymph systems to carry excess fluids away from the cysts. Its use to eliminate breast cysts is backed up by numerous clinical studies from Mount Sinai Hospital in New York, the Boston School of Medicine and various other medical institutes.

For the most stubborn cases of fibrocystic breasts, try using treatments of prickly ash bark, which also increases blood circulation, and burdock, calendula, cleavers, mullein and dandelion, which improve lymph drainage. Each of these herbs can be taken as a tea, as a tincture or in pill form. For more information about these multipurpose herbs, see chapter 4 and chapter 6. Meanwhile, to ease the inflammation and pain, alternate warm and cold compresses over the area. The warm compress should be made using calendula, chamomile, ginger and lavender; the cold compress should be plain (just water).

Many women have found herbs to be helpful in treating this condition. Sue, for example, complained that her breasts would swell so much each month that she needed a bra that was a whole size larger. She had heard that drinking coffee could be the source of the problem, but even after she swore off caffeine, the swelling did not completely subside. Evening primrose oil helped, but she had to take almost double the recommended dose of six pills a day, so she started looking for a less expensive alternative.

Sue found that taking 800 International Units of vitamin E daily allowed her to drop down to two capsules of evening primrose oil. In addition, she started drinking the herb tea described on page 162. Two years later, Sue no longer drinks her tea, but she still takes one capsule of evening primrose oil and 400 International Units of vitamin E daily. She seldom slacks off her routine because if she does, a slight swelling returns, along with persistent pain.

Medical experts believe that it's important to avoid caffeine and related substances called methylxanthines because they apparently confuse chemical messengers in the body. According to John P. Minton, Ph.D., of Ohio State University, these messengers responsible for making protein, fluid or fiber in the breast do not get shut off. They tell breast cells to keep producing more cells and to retain fluid long after they should have stopped. The result can be fibrous cysts. Methylxanthines are found in coffee, colas, tea, chocolate and the herbs maté and guarana. Also check with your doctor to see if they might also be lurking in any pharmaceutical drugs you take.

No one knows why one woman who drinks coffee develops cysts and another doesn't, but the results of several studies show that almost 75 percent of the women with fibrocystic breasts who eliminate caffeine from their diets are spared biopsies and breast surgery. In one study, Dr. Minton gave a choice to 47 women with fibrocystic breasts who had imbibed the equivalent of four cups of coffee a day for several years: have a biopsy or go off methylxanthines and see what happens. Twenty of the women accepted the challenge by cutting out coffee, and in two to six months, the cysts of two-thirds of them completely disappeared. Of the 27 other women in the study who continued to drink coffee, only one had her cyst recede and the rest had to have surgery.

So if you suffer from breast cysts, try to muster up all the willpower you can to eliminate these substances from your diet, at least for a few months. Dr. Minton has found that the older a woman is, the longer it takes for cysts to recede. Some women in their fifties wait a year after they stop drinking coffee before their cysts completely disappear.

Breast Cyst Tea

1 teaspoon each burdock root, mullein leaves and dandelion root
½ teaspoon each prickly ash bark and cleavers leaves
1 quart water

🍃Combine ingredients. As soon as your breasts begin to feel uncomfortable, try to drink at least 2 cups daily. This formula can also be taken as a tincture or in pill form.

Breast Compress

½ teaspoon tincture of calendula flower
10 drops lavender essential oil
3 drops each ginger and chamomile essential oils
1 cup warm water
2 cloths

🍃 Combine ingredients in a shallow bowl. Swish a small, soft cloth in the solution. Wring cloth out over the bowl and fold it into several layers. Place over swollen breast while the cloth is still warm and leave it on for 5 to 10 min-

utes. Run another cloth under cold water and wring it out. Exchange the warm compress for the cold one, and leave on about 2 minutes. If you have the time, alternate the cloths a few times.

HEAVY PERIODS

Heavy menstrual periods (or menorrhagia, as doctors call this condition) are blamed on a long list of imbalances, including too much of the hormones estrogen and prolactin, as well as an excess of a hormonelike substance called prostaglandin 2. A sluggish thyroid also increases menstruation. So can endometriosis, uterine fibroids, the presence of an IUD, and drugs that inhibit blood coagulation. Some medical re-searchers believe that an iron deficiency stimulates bleeding, which in turn leads to an even greater deficiency of iron.

Weakness and a great deal of inconvenience often accompany heavy menstruation. Menstruation normally causes a decrease in physical energy, and if you bleed heavily you may find that respiration is impaired and blood pressure lowered—some women become light-headed and exhausted. Since excessive bleeding can indicate several serious problems, be sure to have a physician investigate the cause before embarking on self-treatment.

Of course, "heavy bleeding" is a relative term. Watch for changes in your own cycle. One survey from Scandinavia found that almost 50 percent of the women with what doctors consider heavy flow considered their flow moderate, while more than 10 percent of those with a light flow judged their periods to be heavy.

Yarrow, nettles and especially shepherd's purse lessen menstrual bleeding by directing blood away from the pelvis. Although mainstream medical science never adopted the use of shepherd's purse, scientists learned in the late 1930s that this herb effectively decreases heavy periods. Where I live, all three of these herbs grow wild. In my garden, I also grow other herbs to slow menstrual bleeding—agrimony, used by the Chinese for this purpose, lady's mantle, vervain and red raspberry, which is thought to strengthen the uterus. Another herbal treatment is to rub on the lower belly a massage oil containing sage essential oil.

These herbs are good for a quick fix while you are bleeding heavily, but for long-term results treat the source of the problem by adjusting out-of-balance hormones with vitex. In the late 1950s, researchers began investigating how this herb helps women who have menstrual disorders. They used a product called Agnolyt—a tincture of dried vitex berries—which had been developed and patented in the 1930s by a German doctor, Gerhard Madaus, M.D. When women who had short but very heavy periods took Agnolyt, almost half of them started having completely normal menstrual cycles, and even more of them found that their periods were much more regular. Dr. Madaus wrote a manual on the use of vitex in which he described numerous studies that have been conducted on this herb. In the late 1980s, this book and accounts of other

German studies were translated by herbal researcher and licensed acupuncturist Christopher Hobbs, who has also written a booklet about this herb called *Vitex: The Woman's Herb*.

When heavy bleeding leaves you feeling weak, see your doctor to make sure that it is not making you anemic. If you are suffering from anemia, see "Anemia" on page 152. If you experience cramping along with heavy bleeding, use the same herbs suggested for alleviating menstrual cramps—wild yam root, false unicorn root, cramp bark and American spikenard—to reduce the severity of both of the problems.

Menstrual Bleeding Tincture

1 teaspoon each tinctures of shepherd's
*   purse leaf and yarrow flower*
½ teaspoon each tinctures of red
*   raspberry leaf and vitex berry*
Combine ingredients. Take half a dropperful every 15 to 30 minutes. This formula is most effective when made with fresh shepherd's purse. When dried, shepherd's purse loses some of its strength.

Sage Massage Oil

2 ounces vegetable oil
12 drops sage essential oil
Combine ingredients. Massage into lower belly a few times a day.

INFERTILITY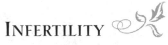

Infertility is a heartbreaking situation for many women. Many leap too soon to the conclusion that they may be infertile. But you shouldn't even begin to consider that you might be infertile until you have tried to get pregnant for at least one year. Even then, do not despair—it sometimes takes even longer to conceive.

Herbs are most successful in treating a woman's infertility when the problem is the result of a hormonal imbalance. An imbalance can occur for a number of reasons, including the menstrual cycle being disrupted by birth control pills. Herbs also help the estimated one-twelfth of women in the United States who are infertile due to uterine fibroids or pelvic inflammatory disease, as long as there is no scarring or other structural damage. Structural problems, such as a blocked fallopian tube, are difficult to treat with herbs—they usually require surgery.

Before you can treat infertility, you must first determine the root of the problem. To start, rule out the most obvious possibilities, along with some not-so-obvious ones. And remember, the chances are 50/50 that the source of the problem lies with your partner. If you are extremely athletic or underweight, you may not have enough body fat. Recently, the medical community has determined that women whose fat falls below one-quarter of their total body weight have trouble conceiving because they often do not ovulate. This condition affects some world-class women athletes.

Plain stress can be another factor. Researchers at the Mind/Body Program for Infertility at New England Deaconess Hospital in Massachusetts found that one-third of previously infertile women became pregnant after they learned re-laxation techniques. For more information of herbal methods of relaxation, see "Stress" on page 52.

There are a number of herbs that increase fertility, such as vitex, Siberian ginseng, don quai from China and the aptly named motherwort. Numerous Chinese studies on don quai show that it helps the ovaries function better and helps to re-establish a normal cycle and fertility.

For many women, the problem is not becoming pregnant, but avoiding miscarriage once they are pregnant. Fertility experts say that women often miscarry before they even realize that they are pregnant. In Germany, quite a bit of research has been done on vitex. This herb has been found to increase levels of three hormones in pregnant women: progesterone, prolactin and luteinizing hormone (LH). All of these hormones work together to help a woman become pregnant, sustain pregnancy and promote the production of breast milk. These fertility-increasing herbs also decrease the likelihood of miscarriage. Another way to prevent miscarriage is to keep the uterus relaxed with wild yam and cramp bark.

There may also be a connection between early miscarriage and the immune system. Medical researchers at Methodist Hospital in Indiana discovered that the immune systems of almost half of the infertile women they examined were either too lax or too aggressive.

I've seen many cases where women who have built up their immunity with herbs have become pregnant. Lisa, for example, was unable to conceive for many years and also found that she was prone to colds and flus. She decided to build up her immunity against these viruses by taking herbs. Six months later, she was very happily surprised to find herself pregnant.

I know a number of other mothers who say that herbs helped them to get pregnant. While we cannot say for sure that herbs made the difference, it is my hunch that they did. Take Debra, for instance. I used to see her only once a year at a crafts fair where I sell aromatherapy products. She often bought a bottle of the Pregnant Belly Oil (see page 175) I make, but she always said that it was for a friend. Once, she mentioned that one of these years, she hoped to be buying a bottle for herself. When she asked me if I had ever heard of don quai helping infertility, I readily admitted that I had and even knew quite a few babies whose births were attributed to the herb. I did not see Debra again until a year later, and she was carrying her newborn. She proudly held him up, saying, "This is Evan, who is here thanks to herbs." Three years later, she was back with Evan, now a toddler, and little Sarah, another herbal-success baby.

Fertility Tea

1 teaspoon each don quai root, Siberian ginseng root and vitex berries
1 teaspoon each motherwort leaves, cramp bark and wild yam rhizome
1 quart water

🌿 Place herbs and water in a pot and simmer for 5 minutes. Turn off heat and steep for 20 minutes. Strain out herbs. Drink 2 cups a day. These herbs can also be taken in tincture form.

IRREGULAR MENSTRUATION

Menstruation usually follows ovulation like clockwork: 14 days after releasing an egg, a woman begins bleeding. If there is any variance in this cycle, it is most often during the time after menstruation. However, to be normal, your cycle need not be exactly 28 days long; it should only be fairly regular. It is also normal for the menstrual cycle to shorten and become irregular as you approach menopause.

A changeable cycle probably means a hormone imbalance. Ginseng, Siberian ginseng, motherwort, vitex, don quai and licorice can help. The Chinese have been using don quai to regulate menstruation since at least the sixth century B.C. Typically, don quai is taken during the two weeks before menstruation. Results of studies conducted in China led researchers to conclude that this herb enhances the utilization of oxygen in the liver and also that it contains small amounts of nutrients important to women: vitamins B_2, B_6 and E, pantothenic acid, choline and zinc. Since don quai can increase uterine bleeding, avoid it if you are pregnant or have heavy menstrual bleeding, endometriosis or uterine fibroids, unless a knowledgeable herb practitioner gives it to you as part of a formula.

Other herbs used in both Chinese and Western formulas to regulate a woman's cycle are motherwort, skullcap and ginger. They are especially useful to encourage menstruation that has been delayed by illness, stress or overexertion. Studies conducted in India showed that aloe vera juice, traditionally used there as a female tonic, also regulates menstruation. You can purchase this juice ready to drink in a natural food store.

Most of the women I know who have regulated their menstrual cycle with herbs—and there are dozens of them—do not tell very dramatic stories. They took the herbs and the herbs worked. Depending upon the situation and the severity of the problem, it took from one month to almost a year for these women to see results. Many of these women have told me that the effects of the herbs were not limited to normalizing their cycle—problems with PMS, especially the emotional ups and downs, also went away and the women experienced less cramping during menstruation.

Irregular menstrual cycles can also be a warning sign of more serious disorders, especially endometriosis and uterine fibroids and tumors. If your cycle is irregular, see your doctor to make sure these conditions do not exist. If they do, treat them first, then look to herbs to regulate your cycle.

Hormonal Tonic

1 teaspoon each vitex berries, don quai
*   root and licorice root*
½ teaspoon each motherwort leaves and
*   Siberian ginseng root*
1 quart water
＊ Put herbs and water in an uncovered pot and bring to a boil. Turn down heat and simmer for 5 minutes. Turn off heat, cover and steep for 30 minutes. Strain out herbs. Drink 1 cup once or twice daily from the time of menstrua-

tion until ovulation. If there is no menstruation at all, drink the tonic throughout the month.

MENOPAUSE

The word "menopause" means "monthly pause." Anthropologist Margaret Mead suggested that menopause be renamed PMZ, or "postmenopausal zeal!" For many women experiencing menopause, though, zeal is the last thing on their minds. As if the weight gain, skin and vaginal dryness, loss of muscle tone and hot flashes are not bad enough, it is also common to experience depression, lethargy, confusion and emotional withdrawal.

For centuries, the average age for menopause has been around 50. (Smoking cigarettes is the only factor known to cause menopause to start earlier, usually only by a couple of years.) But in recent decades, our life expectancy has lengthened so that today's woman can expect to live much longer after menopause. I'd like to help you make those years as enjoyable as possible.

All the problems associated with menopause are thought to be due to the erratic activity of the pituitary hormones LH (luteinizing hormone) and FSH (follicle-stimulating hormone) as they try to overcompensate for the declining levels of estrogen and progesterone. During menopause, FSH levels sometimes increase to as much as 20 times their original levels!

Physicians commonly prescribe estrogen replacement supplements for menopausal women. It is a scientific fact that estrogen increases the bones' ability to absorb calcium, reducing the risk of weak bones and osteoporosis. Estrogen also lowers your risk of heart disease and stroke, which is certainly no small matter, considering that heart disease is the leading killer of women over age 45. But studies show that estrogen supplements can increase the risk of breast and uterine cancer. This is making some doctors more conservative about dispensing prescriptions for estrogen, particularly to women who have a family history of reproductive-system cancer.

Many of these high-risk women are successfully using herbs instead of estrogen to treat their menopausal symptoms. Even women who are not at high risk for reproductive-system cancers find that herbs offer a positive solution to their menopausal woes. And for many women who do take estrogen, the herbs often allow them to take a lower dose.

Licorice, black cohosh, fenugreek, hops, don quai, vitex and ginseng can be used to treat many menopausal complaints, including hot flashes. In fact, black cohosh preparations, such as Cimicifuga-Pentakran, are commonly sold in European pharmacies to reduce the frequency and severity of hot flashes or to which is used to relieve hot flashes. After two months, the herbs lowered the women's luteinizing hormone levels. At least three different synergistic compounds that have this effect were found in black cohosh.

Robert Atkins, M.D., a well-known nutritional specialist, says that out of hundreds of his patients who complained of hot flashes, approximately 80 percent of them responded to ginseng.

Most of the rest of the women improved when vitamin E was taken with the herb. It takes most women two to six weeks before they begin to notice the difference, but once they become aware of it, most are amazed that a simple therapy like this one can make such a difference.

Gloria was pleased to be breezing through menopause with only a slight rise in temperature now and again, but then the "big one" hit. She was attending her niece's wedding when she suddenly began to feel uncomfortable. She began fanning her face, but in a minute found herself fleeing for the veranda where no one could see that she was flushed the color of a beet and that her lovely silk dress was soaked with sweat. The very next day, Gloria marched into a bookstore and headed for the health section. In her reading, she discovered that ginseng helps many women in her predicament and has quite a few other beneficial effects as well. She was especially pleased to read that this herb increases energy and mental power—two things she felt she could use a little more of.

So Gloria gave ginseng a try. At first, she noticed little difference except maybe a little more energy. She also had two more devastating hot flashes, but tried not to feel discouraged. Her perseverance paid off. After taking ginseng for a couple of months, she realized that she had not had even a mild hot flash for well over a month.

Gloria was thrilled, and she started a one-woman campaign to convince everyone she thought might benefit from this wonderful herb. Several of her friends tried it—soon, Bev and Jan were also symptom-free. Her friend Mary, however, was still having four to six hot flashes a day. So Gloria got out her books again and read about vitamin E. She told Mary to take this vitamin with the ginseng, and gradually Mary's hot flashes became less severe. They still have not completely gone away, but they have diminished enough to make Mary happy.

If you find that your menopausal symptoms include nervousness or irritability, a good herbal relaxant to choose is hops. Its estrogenlike effects were first discovered when female hops pickers noticed changes occurring in their menstrual cycles. It turned out that hops caused their estrogen levels to rise. For

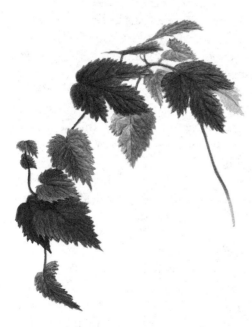

King Henry VIII of England forbade the use of hops, saying that this plant was a wicked weed that "would spoil the taste of the drink and endanger the people."

more information on relaxation herbs, see "Stress" on page 52.

In the course of her extensive field-work, Margaret Mead found that women in many non-Western cultures do not seem to experience menopausal symptoms. She could not determine why, but many theories have been posed, most focusing on diet, lifestyle and, of course, herbal medicines.

It seems that certain plants can increase estrogen during menopause—and not just the plants that we think of as herbs. In one British study, Gisela Wilcox, M.D., and associates gave 25 women who had gone through menopause foods and herbs that were supposed to increase estrogen. When these women ate red clover sprouts, flaxseeds and soy flour every day for two weeks, their estrogen levels rose and remained high. Once they stopped the special diet, the levels fell back down to their original postmenopausal level.

Alfalfa seeds and sprouts may produce a similar effect. These herbs have long been used as a folk cure to relieve hot flashes for women in New Mexico. The large amount of estrogenlike substances in soy and soy products is thought to be one reason that Japanese women experience so few menopausal symptoms. The plant source with the highest level of these substances is pomegranate seeds. This is followed by garden rhubarb stalks and pineapple. Even whole grains, nuts, seeds and avocados contain some estrogenlike compounds.

This is a book about herbs, but sometimes women find that herbs alone are not enough and that they also need to take vitamin E. Herbalists suspect that vitamin E enhances the functioning of some herbs. The use of vitamin E to treat menopausal symptoms is not new. In 1949, the British menopause researcher Hugh McLaren, M.D., who had found this vitamin extremely successful in fighting menopause, predicted that vitamin E would become the preferred menopause therapy, since he thought that estrogen therapy would prove to be carcinogenic. In a 1974 health survey conducted by *Prevention* magazine, 2,000 postmenopausal women mentioned how useful vitamin E was for them even though the survey questionnaire did not mention menopause. They reported that after taking vitamin E they experienced more energy, fewer leg cramps and hot flashes, and less vaginal dryness. One herb that contains vitamin E is don quai.

It seems that herbs not only can help you avoid menopausal complaints, but also should help prevent osteoporosis and heart disease. We do not know this for sure, however, so you should not rely solely on herbs. So far, mineral supplements and exercise have a more proven track record. A study conducted in New Zealand showed that postmenopausal women who took 1,000 milligrams of calcium a day were able to cut their bone loss in half. Equally as important is magnesium to help with calcium's assimilation. Another way to slow bone loss is with a half-hour session of weight-bearing exercises, or even exercising in a chair, three times a week. All postmenopausal women can take a hint from vegetarian women, who experience

less bone loss: Go easy on protein since high amounts block calcium absorption.

Some essential oils also mildly stimulate estrogenlike activity, and when used in massage oils they go right through the skin into the bloodstream. Of course, the massage itself is very relaxing. Fennel, anise, clary sage, cypress and, to some degree, basil can be made into a massage oil. Rose geranium, neroli and lavender are hormonal balancers that are traditionally used in European facial creams to reduce aging and wrinkles. Used in a rejuvenation cream applied inside the vagina, these oils can also counter vaginal dryness. I like to add vitamin E to this herbal cream. Studies conducted in 1949 by Dr. McLaren showed that using vitamin E this way can improve the strength and flexibility of the vaginal lining and help any abrasion that results from a dry vaginal lining to heal more quickly.

Estrogen is not the only hormone you should concern yourself with during menopause. While the emphasis during menopause has previously been on estrogen, progesterone has recently come to be considered equally important. This is probably why vitex helps so many women during menopause. Taking a hint from German herbalists, North American herbalists are now using vitex, usually combined with other menopause herbs, to treat such menopausal symptoms as hot flashes, dizziness, a dry vagina and depression.

While some sources claim that wild yam contains progesterone, this is not true, and much confusion has arisen as a result of the conflicting opinions. Women going through menopause often

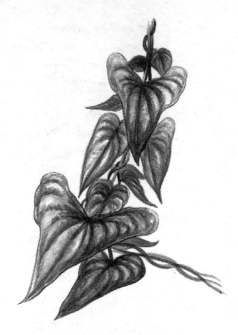

Once upon a time, wild yam was a survival food for the Polynesians—now it's available at most natural food stores.

ask me if taking a tincture of wild yam will provide a natural progesterone increase. I always say no. Although chemists use wild yam for starting compounds to synthesize progesterone, this can be done only in the laboratory. Many of the "natural progesterone" creams with wild yam that are popular for treating symptoms of menopause and PMS do contain a wild yam extract, but their active ingredient is usually the hormone progesterone (even though it does not always appear on the label). Like any hormone, this cream should be used only under the supervision of a professional health care practitioner. Although wild yam (or, more likely, soy bean) is used as a starting point to make progesterone pills and creams, many

women do not realize that by the time it is processed in the lab, it is no more herbal than estrogen pills and creams.

Strong adrenal glands and a healthy liver are also important during menopause. Your adrenal glands provide a backup system to supply female hormones that your ovaries are no longer producing and your liver helps to regulate hormones, making menopause easier. For more information on herbal support for the adrenal glands, see chapter 3.

Menopause Tincture
1 teaspoon black cohosh root
½ teaspoon each tinctures of vitex berry, ginseng root, red clover flower, licorice root, don quai root, motherwort leaf and fenugreek seed
🌿 Combine ingredients. This recipe can also be made into a tea using the same proportions of dried herbs and steeping them in 1 quart of boiling water. As a tea, however, this brew is too strong for most people's taste. Take 2 to 5 dropperfuls of tincture or 3 to 6 cups of tea a day.

Vaginal Rejuvenation Cream
2 ounces almond oil or vegetable oil
6 drops each rose geranium and lavender essential oils
1,500 International Units vitamin E oil (in liquid or capsule form)
1 drop neroli essential oil (expensive, so it's optional)
🌿 Combine ingredients. For the vitamin E, use either the liquid vitamin or pop open a couple of capsules and empty out the contents. Apply as needed inside the vagina.

MENSTRUAL CRAMPS

Menstrual cramps (or dysmenorrhea, as doctors call them) have long been an unrecognized women's ailment—unrecognized, that is, by everyone but the women suffering from them. As recently as the 1970s, 25 percent of U.S. doctors believed menstrual cramps to be psychosomatic—all in a woman's head. I find this astonishing, considering how many women experience cramps. Today, menstrual cramps are recognized as the single greatest cause of lost school and working hours among women— estimated at 140 million hours annually in the United States alone.

Most often, the pain is at least partly due to calcium that drops to low levels just before menstruation and to the increase in a hormonelike substance called prostaglandin 2 (PG2). Both are affected by another promoter of menstrual cramps—stress. Endometriosis, uterine infection and fibroids, a troublesome IUD and chronic constipation can all increase cramping. Even drinking alcohol or eating lots of eggs, meat and dairy foods can worsen menstrual cramps.

Some herbs can decrease PG2 levels and the resulting cramping without the side effects that sometimes result from the use of painkillers such as aspirin and ibuprofen. Among the most beneficial herbs are evening primrose, meadowsweet, feverfew, hops, ginger, cinnamon, cloves, thyme, garlic and flaxseed. Many of these can be used to flavor foods. Cereals containing flaxseed can be found in most grocery stores— just check the labels.

Start taking these herbs about a week before menstruation, since that is when PG2 levels begin to rise. It could be as long as three months before you see results. At the same time, avoid fried foods such as potato chips and corn chips, as well as crackers, baked goods and anything containing hydrogenated oils (this includes most store-bought crackers and baked goods) because they increase PG2.

Cramp bark, false unicorn root, motherwort and red raspberry have been used by herbalists for hundreds of years to ease uterine pain, reduce inflammation and stop cramps. They were all highly recommended for these purposes by the Eclectic physicians, nineteenth-century doctors who used several natural treatments, including herbs. The Eclectic physician John King, M.D., mentioned cramp bark's value as a uterine tonic in his American Family Physician in 1878, and it eventually found its way into the physician's main drug reference, the U.S. Pharmacopoeia. Dr. King called motherwort a "superior nervine and antispasmodic" and suggested it to relieve pelvic pain. So far, only studies using laboratory animals give scientific support, but herbalists who use these herbs know how successful they can be in stopping menstrual cramps.

Another Eclectic favorite for reducing cramps is a tincture of fresh oats. You will even find a little medicinal dose of this relaxant in your morning oatmeal. In addition to oat's other properties, it contains the muscle-relaxing minerals calcium and magnesium.

Simply relaxing can also cause menstrual cramps to subside. I know that this is often easier said than done, but do try to take some time out for yourself each month. If your schedule does not allow for this, you can at least take time for a relaxing massage or bath with an oil made with chamomile, lavender, marjoram, ginger and/or clary sage. Also try an herb tea or tincture. The sedative properties of wild yam, chamomile, hops, valerian, skullcap, ginger, oats, motherwort and California poppy have a relaxing effect on the uterus.

Menstrual Cramp Tea

1 teaspoon cramp bark
½ teaspoon each motherwort leaves, chamomile flowers, wild yam root, fresh oats, hops strobiles and skullcap leaves
¼ teaspoon ginger rhizome
1 quart water

Combine the herbs and water in an uncovered saucepan. Bring to a boil, then turn down heat and simmer for 5 minutes. Turn off heat, cover pan and let mixture steep for 20 minutes. Strain out herbs. Drink at least 1 cup to start, then drink freely, as needed.

Menstrual Cramp Oil

2 ounces Saint-John's-wort oil
8 drops each lavender, marjoram and chamomile essential oils

Combine ingredients. Apply as often as needed by rubbing over the lower abdomen. This formula is also excellent for lower back or shoulder pain, or any type of muscle cramps, even when you are not menstruating. You can buy Saint-John's-wort oil already made or make your own following the Body Oil recipe on page 19.

OVARIAN CYSTS

Ovarian cysts are fluid-filled sacs that develop on the ovary. If they are not malignant—and they seldom are— physicians do not bother to treat them, unless they become so large that they put pressure on nearby organs, become painful or impair circulation. To treat ovarian cysts, follow the suggestions for the treatment of breast cysts in "Fibro-cystic Breasts" on page 160. Try to find time to use the Castor Oil Pack and Sitz Bath on page 159.

A tincture, pills or tea of vitex will help balance your hormones. Red raspberry and motherwort are good toners for the uterine area. My friend Liz used the following formula when her gynecologist told her she had ovarian

Raspberries are always a tasty treat— whether eaten fresh or in jam—and the leaves may also ease morning sickness.

cysts. Although her cysts were benign, Liz was nervous because her grandmother had had uterine cancer. (Her formula also contained skullcap to help her anxiety.) The cysts disappeared in only a few weeks.

Ovarian Cyst Tincture

1 teaspoon each tinctures of burdock root, vitex berries, red raspberry leaves and motherwort leaves
½ teaspoon each tinctures of prickly ash bark and ginger rhizome
 Combine ingredients. Take half a dropperful 2 or 3 times a day.

PREGNANCY

Traditional Chinese have a delightful way of looking at childbirth. They say that the experience gives a woman a new life, one in which she can become healthier and more vigorous than before—providing she pays careful attention to her health. The Chinese traditionally recommend herbs to make sure that she does.

TONING THE UTERUS

For centuries, pregnant women in Europe were also told to take herbs. Those who drank raspberry tea throughout their pregnancy reported an easier labor. Scientists, however, have not shown much interest in investigating raspberry. In 1941, a study using animals found that raspberry leaves contain a "uterine relaxant principle," but this theory was never tested on people. Today, European doctors prescribe a number of raspberry preparations to

ease morning sickness and to prevent miscarriage.

In the old European herbals, lemon balm, a gentle, relaxing herb that aids digestion and alleviates nausea, was also recommended for pregnant women. Native Americans in the eastern United States used partridge berry; like raspberry, this small plant works as a uterine tonic to make pregnancy easier. Modern women who have tried these same herbs when they were pregnant agree with their sisters from past generations—these plants make labor easier and keep you healthier during pregnancy.

Oat straw and nettles provide trace nutrients—especially calcium—that are important for a pregnant woman and enhance the assimilation of these nutrients from other sources. Dandelion and nettle teas are even said to prevent the development of high blood pressure and water retention, which add up to a potentially dangerous condition during pregnancy known as eclampsia. (Since this condition is dangerous to both you and your baby, you must be treated by an obstetrician if you do develop it.)

MORNING SICKNESS

One of the most common complaints during pregnancy is morning sickness, a combination of nausea, headache and dizziness that is experienced by about half of pregnant women during their first few months of pregnancy. To relieve this problem, take ginger first thing in the morning and repeat at the first hint of nausea during the day. You can drink a ginger tea or take a couple of capsules. Even a few ginger-snap cookies or a large glass of ginger ale can help! You can also make a tasty morning-sickness reliever by combining ginger with lemon juice.

The causes of morning sickness are not clear, but there is thought to be a connection with liver functions. This is a logical conclusion when you consider that the liver is responsible for breaking down the excess hormones produced during pregnancy. Other herbs that work to reduce morning sickness are wild yam, false unicorn root and, of course, liver herbs such as burdock. For more on enhancing the liver's functioning, see chapter 7.

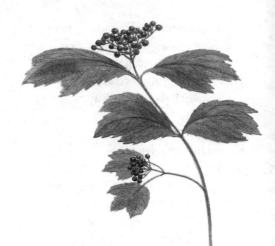

Cramp bark was listed in the *U.S. Pharmacopoeia* as a uterine tonic from 1882 to 1926.

PAIN DURING PREGNANCY

As a fetus grows, it puts pressure on places in your body not used to carrying so much weight. Wild yam, skullcap and chamomile are safe herbs to help you relax and to reduce any pain due to muscle problems. American spikenard, an herb related to ginseng, helps to reduce lower back pain, a common complaint of pregnant women. If sore breasts and water retention trouble you, a tea of wild yam and dandelion might relieve both.

MISCARRIAGE

If miscarriage threatens (clues include uterine cramping and spotting) or if you have had miscarriages before, there are herbs that can stop cramping and spotting. Prepare a tea or get a tincture of vitex, wild yam, false unicorn root and cramp bark. Vitex is important because it promotes progesterone production, and the other herbs are good because they stop uterine cramps. Then lie in

bed, in a place where you can relax completely, with your legs and hips elevated. Drink half a cup of tea or take half a dropperful of tincture about every 20 minutes for several hours or until the cramping or spotting stops. You should also contact your obstetrician or midwife.

A few times, I have found myself trying to calm nervous friends who thought they were losing their babies. All of these women took the above-mentioned herbs and later delivered healthy, full-term babies. Even though I have often seen such good results, these herbs are not guaranteed to prevent a miscarriage. I know other women who have not had such good luck with them. There are times when the reasons that the body has for discontinuing a pregnancy are too strong to overcome. But try not to despair—herbs can also help you strengthen your body and make it less likely that you will miscarry the next time.

Miscarriage Prevention Tea
*1 teaspoon each false unicorn root and
cramp bark*
*½ teaspoon each red raspberry leaves
and wild yam root*
3 cups water

Bring herbs and water to a boil in an uncovered pot. Turn down heat and simmer for 5 minutes. Turn off heat, cover and steep for another 20 minutes. Strain out herbs. Drink 2 cups every hour. These same herbs can also be taken as a tincture, which is more convenient when you are trying to stay off your feet. To make a tincture, purchase all 4 herbs as tinctures and combine them, using the same proportions as above. Similar formulas using these herbs can be purchased already prepared. Take half a dropperful every 20 minutes.

TENSION AND STRETCH MARKS PREVENTION
For years, I have made Pregnant Belly Oil, and I must have sold a thousand bottles by now, with not one report yet of stretch marks. I have been selling it at one craft show for so long that the grown-up children of women who used my oil years ago are now coming to buy bottles for themselves!

To prevent stretch marks, use a massage oil specially designed for the expanding skin of your growing belly. I like to add lavender and cocoa butter, since both have reputations for preventing stretch marks. Almost all pregnant women, who tend to be fussy about smells, like the fragrance of lavender. One year, I experimented by replacing lavender with jasmine, but the pregnant

women complained, saying, "But I liked it so much better when I used it for my first baby!" Now I stick with lavender.

Lavender is most fitting in an oil for pregnancy. A muscle relaxant, lavender flowers were traditionally heated and pounded into a poultice, then placed on the woman's lower back to ease tension and loosen tight muscles during childbirth. As one of the first things the baby smelled, lavender also became a bonding fragrance. European mothers made lavender pillows for their children to sleep with as a reminder that they would always be loved.

It would be nice to see lavender return to the birthing room. Poultices are messy to make and use, however, especially during birth, when a pregnant woman is likely to be changing positions. Since a women often appreciates massage during labor, the perfect solution is to use the lavender-scented belly oil as a massage oil.

Pregnant Belly Oil
*4 400–International Unit vitamin
E capsules*
*4 ounces almond (or any light
vegetable) oil*
*½ ounce cocoa butter (available in
drugstores)*
15 drops lavender essential oil

Pop open the vitamin E capsules and squirt contents into almond oil. Heat mixture in a saucepan over low heat. Add cocoa butter. After cocoa butter melts, remove mixture from heat and let cool. Add essential oil and stir to blend. Massage the oil on your belly— or get someone to do it for you—at least once a day, or as often as you like.

DELIVERY: BEFORE AND AFTER

Birth requires a tremendous amount of energy—I have even heard it compared to a 30-mile run. Some women will swear that it is more like twice that! If you choose to bring herbs to your birth, have someone there in charge of them; a woman in labor has better things to do than educate her labor crew on the use of herbs.

Many midwives and herbalists suggest taking very small amounts of black cohosh and blue cohosh during the last two weeks of pregnancy, because they believe that these herbs prepare the uterus for the final run by encouraging the light, early contractions women begin to feel weeks before labor begins. The two types of cohosh are also used to encourage a slow labor once serious contractions begin. Although it is suggested in some herb books that these herbs should be taken throughout pregnancy, this is definitely not a good idea. In other books, women are warned against using them at all because both herbs can affect blood pressure adversely. Many midwives and nurse-practitioners are familiar with the herbs that are discussed here; ask them to help you develop an herbal regimen that is right for you.

After delivery, drink lightly sweetened, warm tea. An excellent choice is a ginger tea, which you can buy at a natural food store or make by grating a teaspoonful of ginger and steeping it in a cup of boiling water. A tincture of shepherd's purse, cayenne or yarrow will slow postpartum bleeding. I know several nurse-midwives who carry shepherd's purse in their birthing kits and report that it provides great results. When a friend gave birth, I saw how effective cayenne can be as her bleeding stopped after she swallowed two capsules. A few days after the birth, start taking daily sitz baths in calendula, comfrey, chamomile and rosemary to ease any lingering discomfort and promote healing.

Massage the abdomen with the Pregnant Belly Oil (see page 175), which contains skin-toning herbs such as lavender. The uplifting fragrances of these herbs provides emotional balance for postpartum blues, which are thought to result from the sudden hormonal changes, especially the drop in progesterone (which increases to about 15 times its normal level during pregnancy!), following childbirth. A tea, a tincture or capsules of wild yam, vitex and motherwort can also help you through the slump.

Pregnancy Tea

½ teaspoon wild yam rhizome
¼ teaspoon ginger rhizome
5 cups water
2 teaspoons red raspberry leaves
1 teaspoon lemon balm leaves
½ teaspoon fresh oats
¼ teaspoon dandelion root
½ teaspoon peppermint leaves (optional)
2 ounces lemon juice (optional)
♨ Gently simmer wild yam and ginger in water in an uncovered pot for about 5 minutes. Turn off heat and stir in other herbs. Cover and steep for 20 minutes. Strain out herbs. Drink 1 to 4 cups a day, either warm or iced. For variety, add peppermint leaves to recipe or lemon juice to finished tea.

BREASTFEEDING

Breastfeeding provides your baby with natural defenses against disease, but is not always as natural for the mother as she might wish. If your milk comes slowly, try milk thistle, blessed thistle, nettles, vervain, vitex or the seeds of anise, dill, fenugreek, fennel and vitex. Then, when you are ready to wean your baby, drink a tea of sage or eat lentils flavored with sage to slow your milk flow.

Nursing Tea

1 quart boiling water
1 teaspoon each vitex berries and blessed thistle leaves
½ teaspoon each nettle leaves and vervain leaf (optional—it may be hard to find)
¼ teaspoon each fenugreek seed and anise seed
Pour boiling water over herbs and let steep for 20 minutes. Strain out herbs. Drink 1 to 3 cups daily.

PREMENSTRUAL SYNDROME (PMS)

The phrase "premenstrual syndrome" was coined only in the last decade. Although the problem is not new, it went almost unrecognized by the medical profession until the 1950s. Even after that, many doctors continued to scoff at the idea that physical and emotional changes occur before menstruation. Women who have experienced PMS— and this includes almost half of the women in their reproductive years— can tell you how real it is!

A complex problem, PMS is often divided into several different types. If you truly have PMS, the symptoms should disappear at the onset of menstruation, or very shortly afterward. If they do not, your problem may be hormonal but is probably not PMS.

Since PMS is a syndrome—that is, a collection of symptoms, not a single problem—the list of symptoms is rather long. One popular book on women's health describes 150 of them! Tension, lethargy, depression and irritability, along with food cravings, migraine headaches, weight gain, bloating, skin eruption, sore breasts, muscle cramps and nausea top the list. Several surveys show that PMS does not impair a woman's ability to function intelligently, although about 12 percent of women with PMS think that they perform below their normal level.

The problems associated with PMS are caused by a series of changes in your body's chemistry. PMS generally starts causing trouble three to eight days before menstruation. This is when your levels of progesterone, along with the minerals calcium and magnesium, begin to fall. At the same time, the hormonal substance prostaglandin 2 (PG2) increases. Women who experience PMS often also have too much of the hormone prolactin.

As if this is not enough to deal with, your immunity is also low just before menstruation. This makes you more susceptible to colds, flus, allergies, outbreaks of herpes and even flare-ups of rheumatoid arthritis. Stress, lack of exercise, poor nutrition, alcohol consumption, weight gain and poor tolerance of birth control pills all contribute to PMS. Scientists believe that the relief some women find by taking vitamin B$_6$ and progesterone supplements, using relaxation methods and engaging in regular aerobic exercise may be because all these alter the brain chemicals known as endorphins.

In a study of women who suffered from PMS conducted by researchers at Harvard University, symptoms were relieved when the women chanted or prayed for 10 to 20 minutes per day. Also, according to clinical studies reported in the early 1980s, vitamins B$_6$ and E combined with magnesium seem to lower prolactin and estrogen levels and to relieve certain PMS symptoms—breast pain, nervousness, nausea and uterine cramps—and prevent weight gain.

SORE, SWOLLEN BREASTS

Breast tenderness is a common symptom of PMS. It usually indicates that there is too much prolactin and possibly too much PG2. Two herbal treatments that have proved successful in reducing breast soreness are wild yam and evening primrose oil (which can be purchased only in capsule form). When researchers at the Premenstrual Syndrome Clinic in London, England, gave evening primrose oil to women with severe PMS, it was found that the symptoms, especially sore, swollen breasts, disappeared in more than half the women. This treatment even helped women who had previously tried other remedies with no success. If your breasts are sore because of cysts, see "Fibrocystic Breasts" on page 160.

DEPRESSION, HEADACHES, MUSCLE CRAMPING AND NERVOUSNESS

If you experience depression, irritability and mood swings from PMS, excessive prolactin may be to blame. One herb with an impressive track record in treating emotional changes due to PMS is vitex. Herbal sedatives such as valerian, passionflower, wild yam, motherwort and chamomile may also help. If you are lucky enough to have a garden, you will be happy to know a use for purslane. This weed contains omega-3 oils, which also help to relieve PMS symptoms. You can chop up purslane and eat it raw or add it to soups. I even pickle it!

You can also turn to aromatherapy to treat depression, headaches and nervousness. For an enjoyable aromatherapy blend, make a bath or massage oil with the essential oils of clary sage, lavender and rose geranium. Aromatherapists view all these antidepressant oils as hormone normalizers.

Previously, I discussed studies in which women with fibrocystic breasts stopped taking caffeine and related substances. In one of those studies, the women who had PMS experienced another benefit—their mood swings, anxiety and irritability disappeared! If it is too hard to eliminate coffee, tea and chocolate from your diet, try to do so for the two weeks before you menstruate and see if that makes a difference.

WATER RETENTION AND WEIGHT GAIN

Although you may gain only a few premenstrual pounds at the most, the sudden pressure, bloating and swollen breasts make it feel like much more. This weight gain is due mostly to water retention that occurs when calcium and magnesium levels begin to drop about a week before menstruation. Your problems will be greater if you ingest a lot of salt—it dramatically lowers your potassium level, causing you to gain weight and retain water.

Too much of the hormone prolactin may also be at fault, but taking vitex can balance hormone levels and may reduce fluid retention. Some sources recommend strong diuretic herbs to rid you of all that extra water. This makes sense until you consider that diuretics also flush out calcium, magnesium and potassium—all of which may already be low. A better approach is to avoid salty foods and stick to gentle diuretics that retain these minerals, such as asparagus, artichokes and dandelion root.

FOOD CRAVINGS, DIZZINESS AND FATIGUE

Blood sugar levels also take a dip just before menstruation, triggering fatigue, dizziness, appetite increase, headaches, fainting, mood swings and sometimes heart palpitations, especially if you are under stress. Both ginseng and Siberian ginseng help to stabilize blood sugar and alleviate depression and fatigue. In several different studies on PMS, evening primrose oil was shown to reduce many of these symptoms.

Women with PMS who like carbohydrates will be happy to learn that researchers at the Massachusetts Institute of Technology think that women should indulge these cravings. These scientists recommend a diet high in complex car-

bohydrates, such as potatoes and whole grains, to relieve depression, anger, anxiety, insomnia and mood swings. But, they say, you should avoid sweets.

Finally, wild yam and chamomile can be used to relieve the nausea, indigestion, tension and food allergies that can be intensified by PMS.

ACNE

In addition to all the PMS symptoms already mentioned, many women also develop acne just before menstruation. Take vitex to reduce the severity of this problem. You might also want to read chapter 17.

Premenstrual Tea
1 teaspoon each vitex berries and wild yam rhizome
½ teaspoon each burdock root, dandelion root, feverfew leaves and hops strobiles (the flowering parts)
1 quart water
Combine herbs and water in a pot and bring to a boil. Turn off heat and steep for at least 20 minutes. Strain out herbs. Drink at least 2 cups daily, as needed. This formula can also be taken as a tincture; there are many commercial formulas available for menstrual pain. To make your own tincture, use the same proportions as for this tea.

UTERINE FIBROIDS

Uterine fibroids—fibrous tissue growing inside or just outside the uterus—are fairly common, especially in women between the ages of 35 and 40. Some sources claim that almost half of all women in this age group have at least 1 fibroid, and that some have up to 100. Fibroids appear to be at least partially the result of genes, so be aware of your family history. Other risk factors include a high-fat diet, alcohol consumption, B-vitamin deficiency, stress and excess weight. But often, fibroids are due to too much of a potentially carcinogenic form of estrogen. While estrogen's ability to stimulate cell growth is great for skin and hair, it can be a major problem when it comes to uterine tissue.

Fibroids are easiest to treat when they are small, but they are also very hard to detect at this stage—tiny fibroids rarely produce any symptoms. Many women are not aware that they even have them. As fibroids grow larger, however, they cause menstrual bleeding to increase, and they become quite painful, especially during menstruation. Eventually, they can press on your surrounding organs, especially the bladder and kidneys, and this sometimes causes such severe symptoms that removal is the only option. Some surgeons, however, are able to remove only the fibroids and keep the uterus intact, but this does not solve the problem. About half of the women who keep their uteruses find that their fibroids grow back. Fibroids are responsible for about one-third of all hysterectomies.

Because fibroids normally shrink during menopause (although taking estrogen may reactivate them), some women choose to wait and see if the fibroids go away by themselves. If you do opt for a hysterectomy, talk to your surgeon about whether or not you should leave your uterus intact.

One way to prevent the return of fibroids—and often to avoid surgery in the first place—is to adopt a natural prevention and treatment plan using herbs. I do not know many women whose fibroids have been eliminated as a result of herbs, but I do know several whose fibroids shrank so much that the women could easily live with them.

Since fibroids are rarely life-threatening and generally grow slowly, you may have time to try herbs. You may also be able to speed things along by using other natural healing methods, especially acupuncture, in your therapy. I suggest seeking the help of a natural health care professional who has had success treating fibroids.

Vitex slows the growth of fibroids and even helps dissolve them by normalizing hormonal imbalances. As fibroids are dissolved, herbs such as prickly ash bark, ginger, cleavers, mullein and burdock assist the lymph and blood systems in eliminating the fibroid tissue. Regular use of castor oil packs and sitz baths also help to eliminate fibroids, probably by improving circulation. Castor oil packs should be used at least three times a week, 30 to 60 minutes a session; sitz baths should be taken as often as possible, every day if you can manage it.

While you are working on getting rid of your fibroids, you can also take herbs to relieve the symptoms. It is important to keep excessive bleeding, menstrual cramps and anemia controlled with the appropriate herbs because these problems will slow the healing process. Herbs that reduce bleeding and strengthen the uterus include red raspberry and motherwort. It is best to avoid herbs that stimulate menstrual bleeding, such as don quai, unless a knowledgeable herbalist includes them in a formula designed for you.

Uterine Fibroid Tea

1 teaspoon each burdock root, cramp bark, motherwort leaves and wild yam rhizome

½ teaspoon each prickly ash bark, cleavers leaves, mullein leaves and ginger rhizome

1 quart water

🌸 Combine herbs and water in a pot and bring to a boil. Lower heat and simmer for a few minutes. Turn off heat and let sit for about 20 minutes. Strain and drink at least 2 cups a day. This formula can also be taken as a tincture or pills, which can be more practical, since you may need to take it for several months.

VAGINAL INFECTIONS

Most women have had at least one bout with a vaginal yeast infection, and many women experience recurring infections. The incidence of these infections has more than doubled in the last 20 years. One reason that they are becoming more prevalent is the increased use of antibiotics, which kill off beneficial natural flora found in the vagina and allow more harmful bacteria and yeast to multiply.

Antibiotics are especially notorious in promoting vaginal yeast infections, which are caused by candida. A fungus that is a natural resident of the intestines and vagina, Candida creates a problem only when it overpopulates, causing a yeasty, irritating discharge that leads to swelling, itching and general discomfort. Opinion varies among gynecologists on whether yeast infections are transmitted between partners, but just to be safe, why not use herbs to treat both parties?

Trichomoniasis is another common vaginal infection. This infection, which is caused by the microorganism *Trichomonas vaginalis*, produces a thick, yellowish discharge, often resulting in swollen, inflamed genitals. Trichomoniasis is rarely serious, but can be harder to get rid of than a yeast infection. It also tends to be much more unpleasant, with more intense burning and itching.

In addition to these common infections, there are several other types of minor vaginal infections. If you are not sure what you have or how serious it is, you can find out by visiting your gynecologist, a health clinic or your local women's health center. If you suspect for any reason that you may have picked up a vaginal infection, even if you have no symptoms, it is a good idea to get checked.

One infection that you can have without experiencing any symptoms is chlamydia (men can get this too, but it is more common among women). If untreated, it can lead to sterility. You may not be familiar with this infection, since it was barely heard of a decade ago, but it now heads the list of sexually transmitted diseases with an estimated four million new infections occurring every year worldwide. Chlamydia can be passed on to a baby during childbirth and is one of the leading causes of blindness in the world.

Herbal remedies are effective in combatting trichomoniasis, yeast infections and chlamydia, which together cause about 90 percent of all vaginal infections. If you have any vaginal infection and you experience fever or pain, see a physician or go to a women's health clinic.

An herbal douche is one of the best ways to treat minor vaginal infections. I know that some gynecologists frown on douching because it can upset the vaginal balance or possibly spread infection into the uterus. Nevertheless, I've never heard of this being a problem. If you douche, do it right: Make sure that the spray is not too forceful by suspending the bag no higher than shoulder level. Also, remember to use a douche only to treat an occasional infection, not as a daily freshener.

By now, you must be wondering which herbs are best for douching. Various studies tell us that lavender, tea tree, garlic and berberine (found in goldenseal, barberry and Oregon grape root) kill harmful microorganisms, including yeast and trichomonads. One study showed that tea tree was especially good at ridding women of a variety of different vaginal infections. Slippery elm is soothing, and uva ursi is a disinfectant and astringent that dries the discharge caused by an infection.

Along with the herbs, yogurt is good in a douche because it reduces unwanted bacteria, especially yeast. It is also very soothing to irritated areas. Just be sure to use a live strain of Acidophilus (read the label on your yogurt to find out what kind it con-tains)—Bulgaris and S. thermophilus are ineffective.

Even eating yogurt helps. Studies have shown that eating eight ounces of yogurt a day for six months can significantly reduce vaginal infections.

Be sure you do not ignore even a simple vaginal infection. Untreated, it can spread into the uterus, fallopian tubes and ovaries and eventually work its way into the bloodstream. This can lead to pelvic inflammatory disease (PID), which can leave scar tissue in its wake. As of 1995, PID was one of the most common causes of infertility and tubal pregnancies in North American women. The National Institute of Child Health and Human Development reports that women who smoke, especially those who smoke ten or more cigarettes a day, are twice as likely to develop PID as those who don't.

Most cases of PID are the result of chlamydia, with the sexually transmitted disease gonorrhea a close second. Gonorrhea was on the wane in the 1970s, thanks to antibiotics, but has come back during the last decade because it has developed new, drug-resistant strains that the old antibiotics cannot kill. As new, stronger drugs are created, tougher strains of gonorrhea are appearing.

A woman's reproductive organs contain special immune cells designed to fight infection. If your system is rundown, your immunity may need a boost. As you would for any infection, use immune-stimulating, infection-fighting herbs such as echinacea. If you are dealing with recurring vaginal infections, the problem might also be linked to a hormonal imbalance. For example, too little progesterone can cause vaginal irritation and infection and thicken cervical secretions. To adjust your hormones, take vitex in pills or a tincture or as a tea. One teaspoon of vitex can also be added to the formula below. Reproductive toners like wild yam, red raspberry and nettles come in handy if you wish to strengthen the uterus. And, if you have not thought of it already, avoid tight or synthetic clothing that does not allow free circulation of air.

Douche for Vaginal Infections

3 drops each lavender and tea tree
  essential oils
3 cups warm water
2 heaping tablespoons yogurt
Combine ingredients in a douche bag. Slosh around to mix well. Use treatment once a day. If the problem doesn't clear up within 5 days, consult a professional health practitioner.

Women's Infection Tea

1 teaspoon each cramp bark,
  burdock root, echinacea root,
  Oregon grape root and vitex seeds
  (optional)
1 quart water
Combine herbs and water in a saucepan and bring to a boil. Boil for a few minutes, then turn down heat and simmer gently for 15 minutes. Turn off heat and steep for 20 minutes. Strain out herbs. Drink 3 to 4 cups a day. This formula can also be made into a tincture; take a dropperful 3 to 4 times a day.

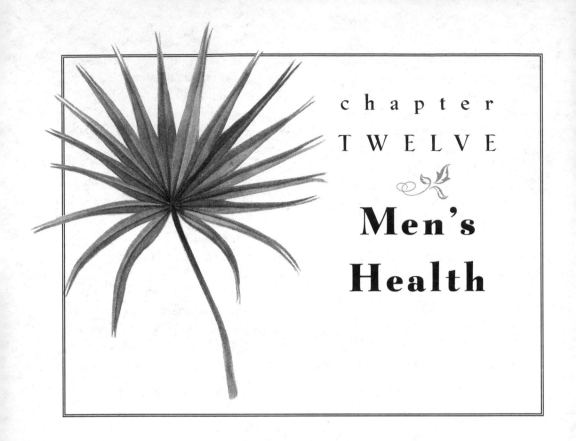

chapter
TWELVE

Men's
Health

Surprisingly little has been written about natural health care for men. This is really too bad, because nature has so much to offer men plagued by such physical problems as prostate inflammation, impotence and infertility.

Most of the physical problems unique to men are caused by imbalances in their hormone levels, especially in the level of testosterone. Produced in the testes and in the adrenal glands, testosterone develops a man's muscles, deepens his voice and makes him fertile. On the negative side, testosterone can also cause the prostate to enlarge, and high testosterone levels have been blamed for overaggressive behavior.

Of course, as a woman, I have not had any personal experience with the health problems that are specific to men, but I certainly know many men who have! And there is much evidence to show that numerous herbal treatments can effectively address these problems.

BALDNESS

It's not easy for a man to go bald. Hair—and lots of it—is an age-old symbol of virility. Many men think that they look better with a full head of hair than without. If you glance at any magazine, you are certain to find at least one magic formula for promoting hair growth. The truth is that there is no cure for baldness—the best such products can do is to slow the loss of any remaining hair.

Healthy hair grows in a cyclical pattern; a strand of hair grows for a while, then it falls out and its root takes a rest before sprouting again. Balding occurs when hair roots never "wake up" again! This is the case with "male pattern baldness," which is especially common when hair growth begins to slow, around age 50 or 60. It is the male hormone testosterone, helped along by certain genes, that encourages hair roots to shut down. Genetic researcher and dermatologist Mary Sawaya, M.D., headed a team from the University of Florida in Miami that discovered certain enzymes in balding scalps that double testosterone's potency and thus discourage hair growth. Because of this enzyme-testosterone connection, this harmless but distressing problem afflicts mostly men—and a lot of them. Over half of North American men are destined to go bald.

If you are concerned about keeping your locks, your best bet is first to feed the hair from within with a healthy diet and to improve your blood circulation. You should also try to keep your cholesterol level low. Ilona Schreck-Purola, M.D., of the University of Helsinki hospital in Finland, found that when cholesterol builds up on the scalp, it actually chokes out growing hair. For herbs that cut cholesterol and generally improve the functioning of the circulatory system, see chapter 4.

The best diet for your hair is the same as that for your general health. Be sure to get plenty of nutrients from fresh fruits and vegetables and whole grains and go easy on saturated fats. According to the American Academy of Dermatology, hair needs a steady supply of protein. Malnutrition and even heavy dieting can cause hair loss, but don't go overboard in planning a high-protein diet to save your head. Nutritional expert Carl Pheiffer of the Brain-Bio Institute in Princeton, New Jersey, found that although hair requires protein, it is actually more likely to fall out when your diet is more than 20 percent protein.

Although herbs will not bring hair back once it is gone (there is no wonder cure), a few herbs do seem to slow hair loss, especially aloe vera gel, nettle and rosemary. For centuries, both men and women have massaged rosemary in olive oil into their scalps to keep their hair healthy and lush. According to Wilma F. Bergfeld, M.D., of the Cleveland Clinic Foundation in Ohio, the massage itself serves an important function: It stimulates circulation and encourages hair roots to grow. Even today, French men are known to splash an old folk remedy of nettles extracted in apple cider vinegar on their heads. Also called stinging nettles, this wild weed actually stings a person when touched. Don't worry, though—it loses this characteristic when processed. Aloe vera not only is good for hair, but also serves as protection against sun and wind for a scalp that becomes exposed when hair begins to thin.

While it is difficult to know for sure that the herbs are helping, all the men I know who use them swear that they can tell the difference. When you use any hair-growth treatment, remember that the scalp is the most important area to address. Hair itself is dead. Certain types of hair conditioners can make it look a little thicker or smooth it down, but little else can be done. The scalp, however, is

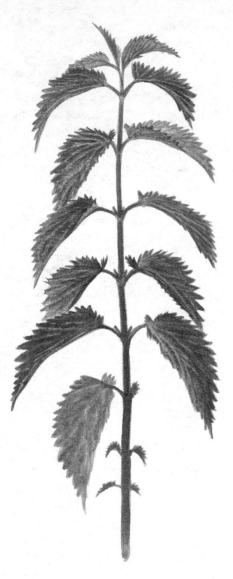

Strangely, one of the historical uses of stinging nettle was as cloth— during World War I, the Germans used it to stretch their cotton supply.

very much alive and can respond to herbal treatments.

Of course, testosterone, genes and poor circulation are not the only factors that cause men to lose their locks. Unlike

the man who sprouts it, the body considers hair one of its least important assets. It is one of the first things to go when a serious illness, nervous-system disease or advancing years demand their share of limited nutrients. Some drug treatments, especially ones for arthritis, gout, depression, high blood pressure and heart problems, can also shut down hair growth. So can radiation therapy and the various scalp problems that fall under the umbrella of dermatitis. If you think that any of these could be causing your baldness, choose herbs from the other chapters of this book that help treat the specific condition.

Rosemary Hair Oil
½ teaspoon rosemary essential oil
½ ounce jojoba oil (or castor oil)
◆ Combine ingredients. Dab a small amount on your fingertips and rub it into the scalp, using circular motions. Although this treatment will make your hair oily, use it twice a week and leave it on your hair at least a few hours before washing it off.

Hair Formula
1 cup aloe vera gel
4 tablespoons apple cider vinegar
1 tablespoon nettle tincture
½ teaspoon vitamin E oil
½ teaspoon rosemary essential oil
◆ Combine ingredients in a blender and process until smooth. Massage a small amount of the formula into your scalp every day and whenever you wash your hair. If you aren't able to find nettle tincture, make the recipe without it or see chapter 2 for instructions on how to make your own.

GENITAL RASH, INFECTIONS AND IRRITATIONS

For the most part, sexually transmitted diseases (STDs) are not a subject you are likely to hear discussed in casual conversation. These reproductive-system infections can cause all sorts of problems in your reproductive organs and eventually impair your general health. Today more North Americans are infected with sexually transmitted diseases than ever before. The U.S. Center for Disease Control in Atlanta estimates that there are a whopping 33,000 new cases every day; that's more than 12 million every year!

Before antibiotics came to be commonly used to keep them under control, gonorrhea and syphilis were the most widespread of these diseases. Others, including chlamydia and HIV, have now joined their ranks. Some of these newcomers are especially sneaky. Twenty-five percent of the men carrying chlamydia—now the most common of all STDs—have no symptoms at all. If there's any chance you've picked up a sexually transmitted disease, be sure to get checked by your doctor. Sexually transmitted diseases require professional help.

That doesn't mean, however, that herbs can't help. Take Bill, for example. After getting an irritating rash on his genitals, Bill decided that he would try herbs to cure it. He read one of the very few books on male herbs—*Male Herbalism*, written by my good friend Jim Green. In this book, Jim describes using herbs in an herbal soak. At first, Bill was taken aback by this suggestion, but Jim's argument for using herbs sounded convincing, so Bill figured "what the heck" and dunked his genitals into a strong herb tea twice a day. Afterward, he applied a skin-healing salve that contained tea tree and lavender essential oils. After about a week of doing this faithfully, the redness and irritation ceased. Bill continued the treatment for a few extra days, and just to be sure, he went to the local clinic for an exam. As he suspected, the tests showed nothing. The doctor, who was not much of an herbal advocate, shrugged and said he probably never had anything to begin with. This could be true, but you will never be able to convince Bill of that!

Herbal Genital Soak

2 cups boiling water
1 teaspoon each yarrow flowers, lavender
*   flowers and goldenseal rhizome*
*   (or Oregon grape root)*

Pour boiling water over herbs and let steep at least 20 minutes. Strain out herbs, and let cool to a comfortable temperature. Fill a large drinking glass half way with the "tea" and submerge the afflicted area. Soak twice daily, or as often as possible, for at least 5 minutes.

Oil for Genital Infection/Irritation

1/8 teaspoon each lavender and tea tree
*   essential oils*
1 ounce vegetable oil

Combine ingredients. If you cannot find a salve containing these essential oils like the one Bill used, you can easily make up this antiseptic oil. Apply to the infected or irritated area at least twice a day. (It works well even when the irritation is not caused by infection.)

The Oil for Genital Infection/Irritation also works well on most rashes and other irritations that occur on the genitals, including "jock itch," which is really a fungal infection. One way to cure and also prevent this is to keep the area dry. You can also apply the herbs as a dusting powder, which is much more drying than the oil. If this does not do the trick, try wearing loose-fitting pants that allow air to circulate.

To completely get rid of an infection, it may also be important to treat it internally. To do this, try taking immune system stimulants such as echinacea and pau d'arco, which seem to work especially well for skin infections. These herbs are particularly effective in treating genital infections. They can be taken as a tea or in pill form, although most men find a tincture most convenient. When you think the infection is gone, play it safe and get rechecked by a physician or a health practitioner in a clinic.

Dusting Powder for Fungal Infections

4 ounces cornstarch or powdered cosmetic clay (available at natural food stores)
½ teaspoon each lavender and tea tree essential oils

Place cornstarch in a plastic bag and add essential oils drop by drop, redistributing the cornstarch as you go to disperse the oils evenly. Break up any clumps with your fingers on the outside of the bag. Let sit for 2 days. Use a few times daily, and always after bathing or swimming. This powder works great on athlete's foot, too!

Infection-Fighting Extract

½ ounce each tinctures of echinacea root, goldenseal root, pau d'arco bark and Siberian ginseng root (optional)

Combine ingredients. Take half a dropperful 5 times daily during an active infection. You can purchase the individual tinctures in a natural food store or choose a similar formula that is already blended.

GENITAL WARTS

Like other warts, genital warts are caused by a virus—the human papillomavirus (HPV), to be exact. A different breed from the common skin wart, genital warts usually grow in raised, bumpy clumps that resemble a cauliflower. At first, they're difficult to detect, but a vinegar wash makes them more obvious. If you suspect that you have warts, soak a cloth with a mixture of one-quarter vinegar and three-quarters water and apply it to the affected area. After two minutes, genital warts usually turn white on top. But don't take any chances with your health. Have a health professional examine any questionable bumps, even tiny ones, to know for sure.

If you have genital warts, you're not alone. Between the start of the "sexual revolution" in the 1960s and the late 1980s, reported occurrences of these warts increased tenfold. By 1990, one million cases a year were being reported in the United States alone. Concern over genital warts, which are transmitted sexually, is well-founded. It is surprising how many men (and women) are unaware of the consequences they present for women—genital warts put women at higher risk for cervical cancer.

There is some inconclusive evidence that these warts also increase the risk of male cancers—especially if left untreated.

A person who has genital warts should always seek medical attention. Herbs, however, can be used for at least part of the treatment. The essential oils of thuja and tea tree help eliminate genital warts. Since these oils are quite potent—and they have to be to conquer warts—use them carefully. Dilute them in vegetable oil—or castor oil, which is a folk remedy for removing warts—then apply them directly to the wart.

I learned about the effectiveness of castor oil in a roundabout way. Many people are curious about old remedies, so I did not think much about it when a man casually asked me to list some traditional wart remedies. I told him about several curious folklore methods, which included keeping a cotton ball saturated with castor oil on the warts and even swearing at them! At the time, I had no idea that he had personal reasons for asking his question, or that the warts he was concerned about were not typical skin warts, but genital warts. A few weeks later, the same man thanked me profusely. The castor oil had gotten rid of his warts. I was happy to have helped him, but also surprised that castor oil alone had worked so well. Since then, I have used it with the essential oils to make them more effective.

Jerry is another example of someone who eliminated genital warts. He had these warts once before he was married, so when he noticed the tiny bumps emerging on his genitals, he suspected right away that they were a recurrence of the infection. Of course, Jerry wanted to get rid of them as soon as possible—he did not want to give them to his wife! Figuring he had nothing to lose by trying an herbal treatment for a few days, he put together a wart oil formula almost identical to the one below. For the first two days, it looked like there was no change, but by the third day, Jerry was convinced that the warts were smaller. He stuck with the treatment for two weeks, and they disappeared completely.

Wart Oil

½ ounce castor oil
¼ teaspoon each thuja and tea tree
    essential oils
800 International Units vitamin E oil

🔊 Combine ingredients. (The vitamin E, added to facilitate healing, can be obtained by opening two 400–International Unit capsules.) First, protect the skin around the wart with some salve, leaving the wart itself exposed. Carefully apply the mixture with a glass rod applicator or a cotton swab 2 to 4 times a day. Apply it only to the wart itself—thuja oil is extremely strong and this formula can burn sensitive skin.

Getting rid of warts is one thing, but that still doesn't eliminate the virus that causes them in the first place. The first time Jerry had warts, his dermatologist explained that they would be removed, but that there was no way to prevent a recurrence. You can, however, increase your immunity with herbs, which will help keep this virus from taking hold. If necessary, you may also need to improve your diet. Not wanting to get the warts again, Jerry did just this. He cleaned up his diet and periodically takes echinacea and other immunity-enhancing herbs to put the virus permanently to rest.

Herbal treatments will not make everyone's genital warts disappear. Roger, for instance, diligently used the Wart Oil for over a week, and although the warts stopped growing larger, they did not get any smaller. He decided to have them removed by a dermatologist. If you don't see results in a week or so, go see a doctor. The caustic solution often used by dermatologists to burn off warts is actually a derivative of a substance found in an herb called mayapple. This plant is poisonous and therefore inappropriate for home use, so be sure to leave its use to a professional.

IMPOTENCE

Because most men find it difficult to speak about their problems, especially sexual dysfunctions, there is little discussion about impotence, which is more common than you might think. The truth is that impotence affects about ten million men in the United States alone. By age 65, a quarter of North American men are impotent. *The Merck Manual,* a referral book for doctors, kindly informs us that "aging is not an inevitable cause of impotence, even into the seventies and eighties." This is especially encouraging, considering that a lowered testosterone level—a marker of advancing years—is often the source of the problem.

Until recently, the cause of most impotence was often dismissed as being in the mind. While some specialists still estimate that up to 80 percent of men's sexual dysfunction is linked to their emotions or to unresolved psychological issues, modern research makes such clear-cut distinctions less obvious. Emotions do play a role—we know that testosterone levels can drop from fatigue, depression, overwork, stress and insufficient sleep—but poor circulation and nerve damage also take their toll and can lead to impotence.

Impotence is sometimes caused by prescription drugs, especially some sedative, tranquilizer, ulcer and high blood pressure medications—the very prescriptions an older man is likely to take. When possible, avoid the drug's side effects by using herbs to treat the conditions that these drugs fight. It is not just pharmaceutical drugs that are to blame for impotence; many recreational drugs, including heroin, amphetamines, "downers" (like Quaaludes) and alcohol, also reduce performance. While cocaine and amphetamines do stimulate the nerves that control ejaculation, these drugs can be self-defeating since they also block another set of nerves that control and sustain sexual interest. The result is short-lived performance with little gratification.

About a quarter of impotent men have too much of a pituitary hormone called prolactin. Stress increases prolactin, but the stressed-out man who figures he will relax with a beer should know that the hops in beer slightly increases prolactin, as well as increasing estrogen. This in turn makes testosterone levels drop. In fact, hops may be part of the reason why heavy beer drinkers often experience hormonal shifts and develop enlarged bellies and breasts. A report in the *New England Journal of Medicine* noted that marijuana use also increases prolactin and lowers testosterone.

Not many men talk openly about their impotence, but because I'm an herbalist, I have had men confide to me that they are looking for a natural solution to this problem. They usually start the conversation with some other topic, but I soon get the hint. I encourage them to investigate herbal ways to deal with impotence. While herbs are not always successful by themselves, they are often helpful when combined with other holistic therapies such as acupuncture, massage and relaxation techniques. Of course, having a compassionate partner is always very helpful.

The first step to conquering impotence is to explore natural remedies for relaxation. Unlike many pharmaceutical relaxants, valerian, skullcap, California poppy, kava and fresh oats ease both physical and emotional stress without decreasing sexual desire or interfering with performance. Some herbalists even consider oats and kava to be mild sexual enhancers. In addition, oats, and possibly damiana and valerian, help counter depression, which can be a cause of impotence. When researchers at the San Francisco Institute for Advanced Study of Human Sexuality gave a blend of fresh oats, nettle leaves and seaweed to men who were experiencing sexual problems, it took only two months for the men's libido and performance to improve and their sensation to increase. California poppy,

damiana, kava and oats are all best used as tinctures. Seaweed can be added to your diet. Aromatherapy techniques for relaxation (see page 281) will also help you to relax and thus to perform better.

What about trying an aphrodisiac? Do they really exist? There certainly are enough stories and folk tales about them. If there are true aphrodisiacs, it is very likely that they can help some cases of impotence. I have heard of all sorts of foods and, of course, herbs that are reputed to be aphrodisiacs; some of them are mentioned in this section. For information about some traditional aphrodisiac fragrances for men and women, such as rose, jasmine, ylang-ylang and patchouli, see Stimulant for Fatigue on page 293.

You might also try addressing the specific causes of impotence: poor circulation, poor functioning of nerves that play a major role in sexual activity, and low testosterone levels.

IMPROVING CIRCULATION

It may seem that "hardening of the arteries" (atherosclerosis) and related circulation problems—the same problems that lead to heart disease and stroke—would have little to do with impotence. But poor circulation is a common cause of impotence because it prevents blood vessels from expanding and filling with blood. Studies reported in the British medical journal *Lancet* confirm that when damaged or weak blood vessels cannot function properly, neither can the man! Adult-onset diabetes—a disorder that impedes circulation and injures nerves—exacerbates atherosclerosis and is blamed for nearly half the cases of impotence. (Impotence gets even worse when someone with diabetes lets blood sugar levels get out of control, putting extra stress on the body.)

Circulation problems that impair sexual function, even those resulting from diabetes, can be treated with herbs. Ginkgo strengthens blood vessels that are just under the skin's surface, improves their ability to dilate and helps provide a sufficient blood flow. It does all this without increasing blood pressure. Studies conducted on ginkgo in 1991 showed that this herb contains a compound that improves poor circulation and helps most men under 70 years old who have erectile problems. In most of the studies, it was found that ginkgo takes less than two months to improve sexual functioning, and many researchers suggest continuing treatments for another four months. For more tips on maintaining good circulation with herbs such as ginger, see chapter 4.

TONING THE NERVES

The African herb yohimbe has been proven to improve a man's staying power, although it doesn't fit most people's idea of a true aphrodisiac. For one thing, yohimbe usually doesn't increase sexual excitement, although some men interpret its stimulating effect that way. It does improve the operation of the nerves that promote desire while dampening those that stimulate ejaculation (this is just the opposite action of cocaine). This translates to prolonged and increased pleasure. But before you

rush out to buy some, remember that it is men with sexual dysfunction problems who notice the benefits the most. Men without sexual dysfunctions tend to experience either a mild stimulating effect or no change at all.

Yohimbe's action takes about 30 minutes to take effect and then continues for a couple of hours. During one of my classes, one man agreed that yohimbe was effective for sexual dysfunction and then admitted that he knew this because he had used it himself. He did not offer any details about his situation, but did say that he took it every morning, just before going to work. Presuming that he was a faithful husband, I suggested that he might try taking it in the evening instead. He came early to the next class just to thank me for that suggestion, and said that the herb was helping much more now.

If yohimbe is so great, you may be asking, how come doctors don't recommend it? The answer is that they do! Yohimbe contains the compound yohimbine, a major ingredient in several prescription drugs for impotence. This compound has an impressive track record, but you will be able to get it only with a prescription. A number of studies have shown that yohimbine helps impotence caused by poor circulation, emotional problems or diabetes—all of which are primary causes of sexual dysfunction. In one study of impotent men, researchers at Queen's University in Ontario, Canada, discovered that it helped almost half the participants. Of those who took a placebo (dummy pill), only half as many experienced a change. The researchers who conducted this study declared yohimbine a "safe treatment for psychogenic impotence that seems to be as effective as sex and marital therapy"— a pretty strong statement! Both yohimbe and its extract, yohimbine, often take a couple of months to produce lasting results.

No problems have been reported from using the herb, but the concentrate yohimbine occasionally increases heartbeat, raises blood pressure or increases irritability, depression, nervousness or dizziness—certainly none of which inspire passion. To be safe, if you have high blood pressure or diabetes, use yohimbe only under the care of a professional. Also, don't take it with diet aids, commercial nasal decongestants that contain ephedrine, or with cheese, red wine or liver, since combining any of these with yohimbine sometimes causes side effects, such as headaches.

INCREASING TESTOSTERONE

If any herbs really do inspire passion, the most likely ones are those that increase testosterone—raising your testosterone levels will raise your libido. For thousands of years, Chinese folklore has claimed that ginseng (which translates as "man root") improves not only virility, but also stamina and longevity (both sexual and general). This is one reason that Chinese herbalists still recommend it for many men over 40.

Another possible sexual healer is a Chinese herb called fo-ti in North America, which is considered an aphrodisiac and longevity herb. The Chinese, who call this creeping vine *ho shou wu*,

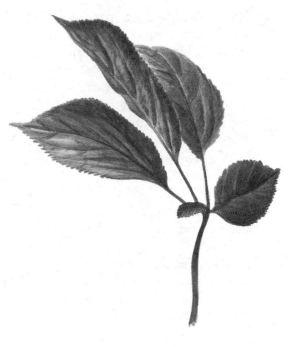

Because of overharvesting, American ginseng is now an endangered species.

ascribe many amazing properties to it. According to folklore, a 50-year-old fo-ti root is said to turn gray hair dark again, and a 150-year-old root will cause teeth to grow back in the elderly! While I assume that these stories are rather exaggerated, practitioners of Chinese medicine have long used this root to counter the effects of aging and to treat impotence.

Three Central and South American herbs are also rumored to be aphrodisiacs: muira puama, damiana and sarsaparilla. Brazilian herbalists use the wood of muira puama, appropriately nicknamed "potency wood," as a male tonic and stimulant. German researchers have found that it may indeed have aphrodisiac-like effects, possibly by affecting men's hormones. Back in 1874, the native Mexican herb damiana was sold in the United States as a tonic "to improve the sexual ability of the enfeebled and aged." It is still made into a popular alcoholic drink in Mexico, where it is widely recognized as an aphrodisiac. Tablets of sarsaparilla are sold throughout Mexico and South America to improve virility and sexual stamina in both men and women, although there have been no scientific tests to show that it is effective.

When considering male health, remember that general health has a strong impact on a man's sexual health. A healthy liver is especially vital to maintaining a good balance of male hormones. Any serious liver problem, such as cirrhosis caused by heavy alcohol consumption, can be responsible for impotence.

Many male alcoholics eventually become impotent as a result of liver damage. Indications that a drinker's testosterone is on the wane include the development of enlarged breasts, a reduction of the frequency with which he needs to shave and a diminishing of his sex drive. Herbs like milk thistle and probably shizandra help rebuild the liver if it has not been damaged too severely. For herbs to heal and maintain your liver, see chapter 7, and for more advice on enhancing testosterone, see "Infertility" on page 195.

A friend of mine made an interesting herbal discovery somewhat by accident. Matt had already successfully used herbs to treat a digestive problem. Now approaching 50, Matt went in for a phys-ical and complained about a minor urinary problem as well as a decrease in libido. His physician told him that they needed to "watch" his prostate and that there was not much he could offer right now to increase libido. Matt figured that he could at least use some preventive herbal medicine for his prostate. He started taking ginseng and saw palmetto to help his prostate and also to increase his stamina when he worked out at the gym twice a week.

As Matt had no idea that herbs could increase libido, he was quite surprised when he realized that his herbal treatment was not only helping these two conditions, but also improving his sexual stamina. He asked me if I had ever heard of such a thing. I said that I certainly had, and suggested that he read up on some other herbs, such as yohimbe and damiana. He did his homework and added these herbs to his herbal regimen. Much later, I ran into him and his wife, Sue, at a party. We were discussing herbs anyway, so I boldly asked, "Did your new herbal formula work?" Matt turned bright red and I instantly regretted asking the question, but then I saw Sue wink. Enough said.

Impotence Tincture

½ ounce each tinctures of ginseng root, ginkgo leaves, yohimbe bark, fresh oats and damiana leaves (if available)

◆ Combine ingredients. Take 30 drops of tincture 3 or 4 times a day for at least 2 months. (Oats and damiana are usually most effective in tincture form. The fall-harvested ginkgo can be taken as a tincture or in pill form.)

INFERTILITY

Many men who want to be fathers but find that they are infertile have told me that they feel a deep sadness at not being able to father children. Fertility and virility are often thought of as being synonymous, and few men want to have their virility questioned. Maybe this is why I hear many men automatically assume that their wives are responsible for the couple's infertility problems. In fact, in about half the cases of infertility, the root of the problem lies with the man.

Over the last few decades, medical experts have seen a dramatic drop in men's sperm counts. Some scientists worry about the possibility of even greater fertility declines in future generations. One chilling theory posed by some European researchers is that the rising rates of infertility result from overexposure to estrogen that starts even before the child is born. It is true that high levels of estrogenlike substances, which lower the male hormone testosterone, are found in birth control pills, pesticides and many meat and dairy products—a good argument for eating organically grown foods! Water sources are also polluted by estrogen-type detergents; biologists have even found male fish in such water behaving like females because of a dramatic shift in the balance of their hormones.

A sufficient quantity of testosterone is necessary to manufacture healthy sperm in sufficient quantities to make a man fertile. Herbs do not offer a surefire cure for infertility, but they do work some of the time. They are most successful when the infertility is a result of out-of-whack hormones or weak sperm, rather then when infertility is due to structural problems such as a blocked sperm duct.

So far, ginseng is the only herb recognized by science to stimulate testosterone production. The Chinese tell folk tales about men in their nineties fathering children after taking ginseng. As far as we know, these are only stories, but if any herb can maintain a man's fertility, ginseng seems the most likely candidate. In fact, its powers in this regard caught a couple of men I know by surprise. Both of these fellows started taking ginseng, along with other herbs such as shizandra and saw palmetto, to build up their physical stamina. After many years to the contrary, they were extremely surprised when their wives announced that they were pregnant!

It is probable that other herbs also stimulate testosterone production. Researchers are just beginning to investigate the Chinese herb fo-ti as a treatment for infertility. Other possibilities include two relative newcomers to the North American market: the African herb pygeum and the Indian herb ashwaganda. Pygeum is a tall evergreen tree, also called African bitter almond, whose bark has been used by the Zulus and other African tribes and now also by European doctors. The root of ashwaganda is an ancient Indian sexual tonic for the treatment of infertility. Practitioners of Ayurvedic medicine view this herb in much the same way the Chinese view ginseng; according to Ayurvedic medicine, ashwaganda also "strengthens" sperm.

When a man suspects infertility, one of the first things a physician checks is whether there is a sufficient amount of sperm to do the job. Although it takes only one sperm to fertilize an egg, it takes many to accomplish the task—fertility experts call this a "team effort." The Chinese have used fo-ti for centuries to increase the sperm count. A 1989 study showed that the common kitchen herb ginger stimulated hormone production and increased the sperm count in animals. Although no studies have been done on humans as yet, researchers believe that this herb has the same effect on men. In fact, you get a medicinal dose every time you flavor food with ginger.

And while you are at it, try adding pumpkin seeds to your meals. Endocrinologist Ali A. Abbasi, M.D., formerly of the Allen Park Veterans Administration Hospital in Maryland, found that zinc deficiency causes the sperm count to plunge, but adding zinc to the diet increases the count. Pumpkin seeds, a popular folk remedy for infertility, are especially rich in zinc. They are easy to take; buy them already shelled and eat them by the handful, or grind them and add them to your morning cereal.

Aromatherapists also report improvements in fertility for men who use rose essential oil—an expensive but wonderfully fragrant treatment. It has been speculated that rose essential oil, which has an age-old reputation as an aphrodisiac for both men and women, increases the sperm count. Emotional or physical stress can easily make conception more difficult, but this fragrance also relaxes the body and mind. If you think that stress may be a contributing factor to your infertility, try using the rose essential oil along with some of the sedative herbs suggested in "Stress" on page 52 and the relaxing aromas discussed in chapter sixteen.

The testes and seminal vesicles also need to be in top health to produce and house sperm. One herb that protects them from damage is pygeum, which is discussed on page 195 as a testosterone stimulator.

It is also a good idea for men who want to reverse their infertility to take plenty of red raspberry leaves. Usually considered a woman's reproductive tonic, raspberry seems to be equally helpful for men. Ask animal breeders; they will tell you that raspberry leaves are added to feed to increase male fertility.

Experience with animals also provides another hint for treating human male fertility: oats, which are fed to racehorses to keep them healthy and fertile. As oats are best when harvested during their fresh, milky stage, your best bet is to use a tincture. You may also derive some benefit by eating oatmeal. (It seems that the old saw about men sowing their wild oats has some basis in fact.)

Some plants encourage estrogen production and thus discourage male fertility. According to Robert C. Kolodny, M.D., reporting in the New England Journal of Medicine in 1974, regular use of marijuana lowers testosterone levels and also decreases sperm production. Sage is also suspect; while I know of no problem with moderate consumption, if you are trying to conceive, avoid seasoning your food with lots of sage. In the fourth century B.C., the Greek healer

Theophrastus called garden sage an "excellent article for excessive desire"—to limit it, that is.

And just in case you have unusual dietary tastes, go easy on the date pits; Arab women used to place ground pits in their men's food before they departed on camel caravans to help keep them faithful! However, do not worry about the dates themselves; estrogenlike compounds are found only in the pits.

Finally, tobacco and coffee consumption also seem to cause fertility problems, probably because they impair circulation. If impotence is a cause of infertility, see "Impotence" on page 190.

Fertility Formula

1 ounce tincture of panax ginseng root
½ ounce each tinctures of fresh oats, ashwaganda leaves (if available) and raspberry leaves
☙ Combine ingredients. Take 1 dropperful twice a day.

Aromatherapy Fertility Oil

5 drops rose essential oil
1 ounce vegetable oil
☙ Combine ingredients. Massage into the lower abdomen and inner thigh once a day. Be sure to use only pure rose essential oil, preferably Bulgarian or Turkish rose attar.

MALE MENOPAUSE

Although men don't have hormonal cycles as obvious as those of women, researchers speculate that there may be male cycles as well. Certainly, men experience an annual cycle; a man's testosterone levels rise in the fall and drop in the spring. Studies from Syracuse University in New York, Wittenberg University in Ohio and Georgia State University show that it isn't only seasonal changes that affect a man's hormones. Emotional events also have an effect—both love and war sharply increase testosterone levels. A man's hormone level also increases after a success, such as earning a degree or winning an athletic prize, and even during everyday speech.

Experiencing hormone changes as one grows older is not limited to women; recent research indicates that men undergo similar changes. Many of the symptoms of male menopause are surprisingly similar to those experienced by women during menopause—irritability, anxiousness, fatigue, hot flashes, night sweats and decreased libido. British research indicates that a substance called sex hormone binding globulin (or SHBG), which increases with age, makes the tissues in a man's body resistant to testosterone. So even if a man has a fairly high testosterone level, the hormone's action will be diminished.

What to do when male menopause hits? The treatment is similar to the one suggested for women. Strengthen your adrenal glands so that they can take over the responsibility of producing sufficient male hormones, and tone your liver to help it properly detoxify hormones circulating in your blood.

The same herbs used to increase physical stamina—Siberian ginseng, shizandra, licorice and ginseng—are some of the best choices to help you get through male menopause. You can try making the Male Change Formula, or you can use ginseng by itself. This herb is available in several forms, including the whole plant or root, or as tea, tincture, semi-solid extract (which is stirred into hot water) or various pills. One way to use the whole root is to soak it in a jar of water and bite off a small amount every morning. Kept in the refrigerator, a root will last about two weeks.

Male Change Formula

1 ounce tincture of ginseng root
½ ounce each Siberian ginseng root,
    shizandra seed and licorice root
🌿 Combine ingredients. Take half a dropperful once or twice a day.

PROSTATE ENLARGEMENT

Many men will be surprised to learn that herbs can help correct prostate enlargement. Also known as benign prostatic hyperplasia (BPH), this is the most common problem with the prostate. In fact, it is so common that roughly half of North American men between the ages of 40 and 60 are plagued by it. Standard medical opinion points to only two solutions—surgery or hormone therapy—but neither is appealing.

In 1990, an estimated $3 billion was spent on prostate surgery in the United States alone. But after about five years, most men find, to their dismay, that the surgery needs to be repeated. Hormone therapy, which uses drug treatments to inhibit the hormones testosterone and prolactin, also carries undesirable side effects, including possible impotence.

Before we discuss the helpful herbs, let's first consider the prostate. This small gland, which is located next to the bladder, is made of muscle, gland and connective tissue. The thin fluid that it secretes helps carry sperm down the urethra, the same tube that transports urine from the bladder. Since the urethra passes right through the prostate, when the prostate enlarges, it pinches the tube and causes urine retention. This also creates an urge to urinate more often since the bladder never fully empties. The uncomfortable result can be an inability to void, false starts, dribbling and burning pain.

Since there are usually no symptoms in the early stages, it is easy to understand why so many men let prostate problems go untreated at first. They don't even know something is wrong until the urethra is blocked and the problem can no longer be ignored!

The severity of symptoms doesn't necessarily tell you the extent of enlargement, but a doctor's examination will. You need to be examined by a doctor because problems such as an obstruction in the urinary tube, a bacterial infection and bladder or prostate cancer need to be ruled out. If a survey by the Prostate Cancer Education Council is any indication, most men are not well-informed about the health of their prostates. Studies conducted by the council show that most men don't have regular physicals and that of those who do, less than half have their prostate checked.

The most common cause of prostate enlargement is changes in hormone levels. As a man ages, his testosterone levels begin to fall. At the same time, his levels of the "female" hormones prolactin, estrogen, LH and FSH rise. This dramatic hormonal shift results in many body changes, such as weight gain, changes in fat distribution and a decrease in muscle strength. Even the testosterone itself changes. An especially potent form of testosterone called dihydrotestosterone (DHT) begins to dominate. Unfortunately, DHT can cause prostate cells to multiply excessively; four to six times the normal amount of DHT is found in most enlarged prostates. While DHT increases with age, a number of environmental pollutants (the chemicals dioxin, polyhalogenated biphenyls, and hexachlorobenzene) also make this hormone accumulate in the prostate.

The Agency for Health Care Policy and Research in the United States has recently concluded that "watchful waiting" with regard to an enlarged prostate is better than surgery or drug therapy. There is also another avenue to explore: herbs. North American doctors, less schooled in the use of herbs than their European and Asian counterparts, are just beginning to pay attention to the exciting research on herbs that can be used to correct prostate problems. I know plenty of men who have been helped by using herbs. For most of these men, herbal therapy was a last-ditch effort to avoid surgery after nothing else they tried worked.

Jesse is a good example. Like most men, he did not have prostate problems until he was in his sixties. He had looked forward to his retirement for a long time but hadn't counted on the pain and other uncomfortable symptoms of an enlarged prostate. His physician sent him to a urologist at the well-known medical center at the University of California at Los Angeles. Jesse tried to focus on sailing and his hobbies and put off thinking about the inevitable prostate surgery, but eventually the symptoms were just too much to live with.

Jesse wasn't really an "herbal convert," but he figured it couldn't hurt to try herbs. After only a few weeks of using an herbal formula similar to the one recommended below, he felt better, but he thought it was probably his imagination since nothing had helped his condition over the last year. Still, he stuck with it, and after a couple of months, the problems seemed to disappear.

His next trip to the urologist confirmed that this was true. The astonished doctor reported that the prostate was much smaller and declared that in his many years of practice he had never seen a prostate reduce in size without surgery or hormonal drugs. He even asked Jesse for the formula! Both Jesse and the urologist, unaware of ongoing research in Europe, thought that they might be on the brink of discovering new therapies to save millions of men from surgery or hormonal drug treatments.

Prostate-Reducing Tincture

1 ounce tincture of saw palmetto berries
½ ounce each tinctures of nettle root,
* sarsaparilla root, wild yam root,*
* echinacea root and pipsissewa or*
* uva ursi leaves*

Combine ingredients. Take half a dropperful 3 times a day. For a maintenance dose, take once a day.

This research has been going on for many years, especially on saw palmetto. Compounds in this herb have demonstrated a remarkable ability to inhibit DHT, the hormone that causes prostate inflammation. Saw palmetto does not change the level of testosterone or other hormones in the blood, but it does stop tissues, especially those in the prostate, from utilizing it. In fact, this herb is about 25 times stronger than cyproterone, a once-common prostate anti-inflammation and cancer drug now considered too toxic for noncancerous conditions.

Clinical trials on saw palmetto have been performed in France. W. Vahlensieck, M.D., and his associate researchers found that saw palmetto greatly reduced symptoms associated with prostate enlargement—including pain and incontinence—within three months.

In Germany, 11 separate studies on saw palmetto, involving a total of 500 men, were conducted over a period of a few years. When the results for men over 60 years old were pooled, it was shown that the men who took this herb had less than half as many symptoms as those who did not. The other good news is that almost no side effects were reported.

The bad news is that saw palmetto's soapy, bitter taste is not pleasant; the best way to take this herb is to dilute the tincture in a small amount of water and chug it down.

Unfortunately, herbs have difficulty finding their way into mainstream medicine in North America. It is unlikely that anything but the standard prescription drugs suggested for prostate treatment will be available here in the near future.

Alternative over-the-counter products for prostate enlargement, including saw palmetto and amino acids, were banned by the Food and Drug Administration (the U.S. governmental agency that determines which medicines—drugs or otherwise—and foods can legally be sold in the United States) in 1990 because this condition is not considered suitable for self-treatment. You can still buy saw palmetto, but the label will not dare mention anything about using it for the prostate. In Germany, however, the use of saw palmetto is approved by the health authorities and is so well-established among doctors that pharmacies sell an over-the-counter suppository containing saw palmetto and the immune stimulant echinacea, so men can self-treat prostate irritation and inflammation.

Another medicinal plant that is effective for the treatment of this condition is pygeum. In France, this herb is found in over 75 percent of all doctors' prescriptions for enlarged prostate. Doctors there report that the herb reduces symptoms in at least half of the men who try it, and it does so in less than six weeks. Pygeum, which has been under scientific investigation since the 1960s, has been used to treat thousands of men. Researchers say that it seems as effective as the pharmaceutical drugs commonly suggested for enlarged prostate. They even recommend it as a suitable replacement for such drugs.

Usually, pygeum causes swelling and uncontrollable urination to disappear fairly soon, and there are almost never side effects. Only a rare case of upset digestion has been reported. In one study on pygeum involving dozens of men who took the herb for two months, the herb improved all of their symptoms, including difficult urination, uncontrollable urination at night and problems with residual urine. It also decreased the size of the prostate.

Pygeum helps all but the most serious cases. Many researchers who have conducted studies on this herb suggest that pygeum is most effective when used at the first signs of prostate problems. Even the men who do opt for surgery find that they have fewer related problems and that their circulation improves when they take pygeum afterward. It appears that this herb decreases prolactin production and also reduces the detrimental effects of testosterone. Pygeum is currently available only as a tincture or in pill form, and is often combined with saw palmetto. The suggested dose recommended by researchers is two 100- or 200-milligram capsules a day.

Nettle leaves have long been known as an excellent diuretic and are used to stop the urine retention that often accompanies prostate inflammation. The roots of the nettle are what have drawn the attention of scientists. After conducting a study of this root at the Department of Phytotherapy in Paris, French researchers declared that the nettle root appears to be a useful therapy for milder cases of prostate inflammation and a good alternative to surgery. Men with mild prostate enlargement who took nettle root found that their symptoms disappeared after only three weeks.

These researchers added that nettle root, saw palmetto berry and pumpkin seed all help prostate problems, possibly because they contain abundant amounts of b-sitosterol, a hormonelike substance known to reduce prostate inflammation. Other researchers have proposed that the reason nettle is so effective might be that it reduces the amount of testosterone circulating in the blood or that it inhibits the enzyme responsible for making testosterone. In another study, men given both pygeum and nettle root had their prostate problems eliminated.

The French studies mentioned above and several others conducted in Germany have led German health authorities to declare nettle root an appropriate and effective treatment for the early stages of prostate inflammation. It can be taken in any form, including a tea.

Gamma linoleic acid (GLA), which is found in evening primrose, borage and black currant seed oils, also helps relieve prostate inflammation. You can encourage GLA production in your body by eating a handful of pumpkin seeds or by taking one or two teaspoons of flaxseed oil every day.

Pumpkin seeds, a Ukrainian folk remedy for prostate inflammation, also contain an unusual amino acid called cucurbitin. Modern European pharmacies sell a popular enlarged prostate remedy called Curbicin that combines pumpkin seeds with saw palmetto. In 1991, A. Hasler, Ph.D., conducted a study in which he gave Curbicin to men suffering from enlarged prostates. Within three months, their urinary flow problems greatly improved, with almost no side effects.

Good circulation is imperative for good health, and a sedentary lifestyle, especially one that involves sitting in chairs for long periods of time, has been accused of contributing to prostate problems. Stone root, Saint-John's-wort, prickly ash and horse chestnut, a popular European treatment for enlarged prostate, all improve circulation. An herbal sitz bath (a warm bath in which you sit in water up to your waist) with rosemary is also good for pelvic circulation. An anti-inflammatory oil made of Saint-John's-wort and the essential oils of rosemary and lavender can also be applied behind the scrotum to increase circulation, reduce inflammation and relax muscles.

Anti-Inflammatory Prostate Oil

⅛ teaspoon each lavender and rosemary
    essential oils
4 drops Roman chamomile essential oil
    (optional)
2 ounces Saint-John's-wort oil
❧ Combine ingredients. Rub on the skin under the scrotum once or twice a day.

Studies conducted by the American Urological Association have shown that it is common for cholesterol to build up in enlarged prostates, often to a level 80 percent higher than normal. So a second front in the war against prostate inflammation begins with the fight against cholesterol. Both GLA and pygeum specifically reduce the accumulation of cholesterol in the prostate. See chapter 4 for ways to use other cholesterol-fighting herbs.

Several other herbs can also come in handy for treating prostate problems. When the urine flow is constricted, see chapter 8 for ways to use wild yam root to relax and open the passage and to reduce pain.

Herbalists also successfully use hydrangea and joe-pye weed, sometimes with uva ursi, pipsissewa, yarrow and/or horsetail, to clear up the urinary tract infections that often accompany prostate problems. Echinacea is an excellent choice to improve immunity and

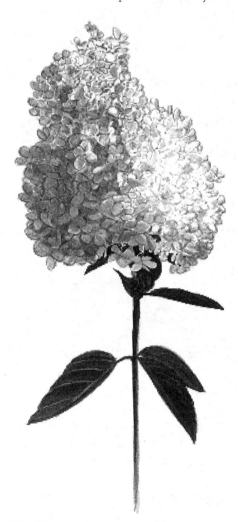

The Native Americans called hydrangea "seven barks" because the stems are covered with many thin layers of different colored bark.

fend off infections. For more advice on treating a urinary tract infection, see chapter 8.

Once the size of the prostate is reduced, you may need to continue taking herbs (at a reduced level) to keep symptoms at bay. When symptoms began to recur, Jesse (who was mentioned earlier) found out he needed to take his formula every few months; after about a year, he discovered that he no longer needed the herbs. Al, who successfully used herbs to control his prostate growth, tried to discontinue them several times. About two months after stopping the herbs, he kept having flare-ups, so he decided to keep taking a small dose on a regular basis. Considering that the likely alternative is surgery or hormone therapy, he does not mind that he may need to continue taking them for the rest of his life.

SWOLLEN TESTICLES

Swollen testicles is a painful and potentially serious condition that requires a physician's care, unless it is obviously a temporary situation—perhaps caused by a spider bite, a minor blow to the area or restrictive clothing. Even then, this condition can be serious enough for a doctor's care if the testicles swell a lot, become extremely painful or stay swollen for several days. If this condition is accompanied by chills, fever or vomiting, do not try to self-treat it—go see your doctor. Lumps or "knots" inside the testicles also need to be checked out by a physician. A more chronic condition can be caused by an infection or by

⚘ THE MAN ROOT

Ginseng is often referred to as the "man's herb," and indeed its name is translated from the Chinese as "man root." Despite the name, however, ginseng is good for women as well as men.

There is a great deal of confusion over ginseng. Chinese and American ginseng are quite similar. In fact, the United States ships great quantities of its ginseng to the Orient. American ginseng is often less expensive than the Chinese variety and just as suitable, but it is best to buy cultivated ginseng, which is grown on farms, instead of the wild collected roots—ginseng is being overharvested and is becoming endangered. Try to seek out organic ginseng; because this plant is a valuable crop that is prone to disease, pesticides are used on much of the commercial ginseng.

Siberian ginseng is an entirely different plant—it is actually a prickly bush, while ginseng is a small forest herb with one main stalk. Siberian ginseng's name was coined because it shares some, but not all, of ginseng's properties. To avoid confusion, herbalists often refer to Siberian ginseng as eleuthro (which is short for its botanical name, *Eleutherococcus senticosus*).

structural problems in the testicles, an enlarged prostate, a sexually transmitted disease, mumps or an inflamed urinary tract. A chronic case sometimes leads to infertility.

For a case that you feel confident self-treating or for more chronic conditions—*after* you have seen a doctor—use herbs such as lavender or chamomile to reduce the swelling and pain. These herbs also help fight the infections that sometimes accompany swollen testicles. Doctors usually recommend wearing an athletic supporter to ease the stress on the area, and sitting in a hot bath.

In her book *Herbs and Aromatherapy for the Reproductive System,* herbalist Jeanne Rose tells of a man whose swollen testicles were due to an infection. For a week, he took the antibiotics prescribed by his doctor, but there was little change. The doctor then recommended that he sit in a very hot bath for an hour, two or three times a day. The next week, the ailing man sought the advice of an herbal-

ist, who suggested that he turn this into an herbal bath by adding a strong tea of comfrey, echinacea and mullein. He also started taking a mixture of the infection-fighting herbs echinacea and goldenseal, along with ginseng and yellow dock. He saw definite improvement almost right away, and the pain and swelling noticeably diminished in a couple days. Five days after starting the herbs, he was finally able to walk without pain.

If bathing this much is not practical, you can soak once a day and gently rub on an oil a few times daily. The Oil for Genital Infection/Irritation (see page 187) is a good one to use, especially if an infection is present.

Testicle Bath
1 quart water
¼ cup each comfrey and mullein leaves
⅛ cup chamomile flowers
Bring water to a boil and pour it over the herbs. Let steep at least 15 minutes. Strain and pour into your bath.

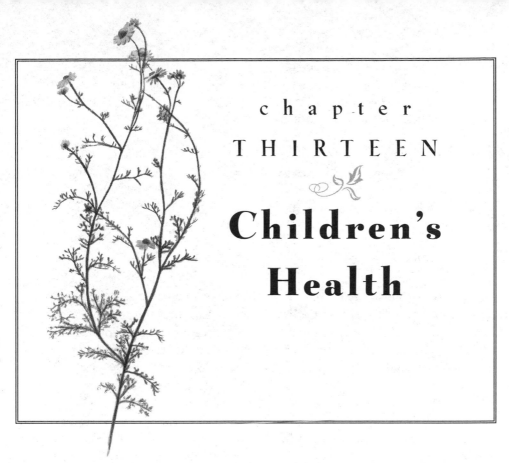

E ven the healthiest child occasionally comes down with sniffles,
an earache or a fever. If you are
a parent, your family medicine cabinet
is probably already well stocked with
cough syrup, children's pain relievers
and other assorted children's medicines.
However, many health care professionals
are beginning to wonder if drugs are
overprescribed and whether their short-
term beneficial results are not out-
weighed by long-term hazards.

Antibiotics are among the medicines
under question. The U.S. Public Health
Service has issued new guidelines for
physicians treating children with an
excess of middle-ear fluid, essentially
cautioning doctors to hold off on
prescribing antibiotics. According to

government statistics, in 85 percent of
children this condition clears up on its
own within six months; nevertheless,
87 percent of doctor's office visits for
ear problems result in a drug being
prescribed.

In one Australian study, children
who were given antibiotics to treat their
sore throats actually stayed ill longer and
experienced more severe symptoms than
those who were not given the drugs.
Robert Mendelsohn, M.D., pediatrician
and author of *How to Raise a Healthy
Child,* challenged his colleagues when he
stated, "The vast majority of childhood
illnesses do not require medical attention
and when they receive it needlessly, the
treatment given may do more harm than
good." What can you, as a responsible

parent, do when faced with the choice between overmedicating and not doing enough? The answer is simple: Turn to herbal remedies. If the illness is treatable at home with over-the-counter drugs, herbs most likely offer a better alternative. If your doctor prescribes drugs, be sure he isn't doing so "just in case" or simply to make you feel the visit was worthwhile.

Perhaps you have thought about using herbs for your children's health problems, but you've resisted this alternative because you were not sure which herbs to use or even how to use them. Plenty of herb books provide information on treatments for adults, but say nothing about children. In fact, there are numerous herbal remedies that are not only safe for kids, but also easy to use. And many of the same herbs can be used for different conditions. This means that you only need to buy (or grow!) a few herbs to treat many of your child's illnesses. You can be sure that the remedies in this chapter have been kid-tested for effectiveness and gentleness.

It is not always easy to persuade children to take medicine—even good herbal medicine—so I have tried to make all the remedies in this chapter pleasant-tasting and easy to administer. Otherwise, children may later turn their nose up at anything that even hints at being herbal. If you take the right approach, you may be surprised how a sick child takes to natural remedies without much resistance at all. In time, you may hear your child asking for Peter Rabbit's Tea (see page 235) to settle an upset stomach or Soothing Cough Syrup (see page 233) to ease a sore throat.

Because a child's gag reflex is so strong, many kids simply won't swallow pills. Babies can take herb tea in a bottle, or a nursing mother can take the herbs herself and thus dose her baby through her milk. If your child does not like tea, you may have better luck with a tincture or an herbal body oil.

For the finicky child, you can disguise many herbal remedies as "normal" food. After all, the herbal pharmacy includes many fruits and vegetables that have medicinal properties. Herbalists even count juices and oatmeal among their remedies! Teas sweetened with fruit juice can be transformed into fizzy drinks or frozen into enticing popsicles. (*Note:* Don't use honey as a sweetener for children under two years of age— there is a microorganism in honey, which is otherwise quite innocent, that sometimes makes them ill. Alternatives include barley and fruit-based sweeteners.)

Sometimes a little parental creativity is more effective than the tastiest sweeteners. One of my students, Jennifer, found that her two young children did not want anything to do with herbs. When either one complained of feeling ill, Jennifer would say, "I'll get the herbal remedies," and the child always quickly responded, "No, no, I'm not sick now, Mommy!" Jennifer's solution was to make the remedies more tasty and give them cute names so that they would be more appealing to children. She even wrote her children a story about a Grandma Bunny who dispensed healing herbs to the local animal population. Because of Jennifer's patience and imagination, five-year-old Jessa has become

✿ CLARK'S RULE FOR CHILDREN'S REMEDIES

Children's bodies are especially receptive to herbs and, since their bodies are smaller than adults', it takes only a small dose to bounce them back into good health. Many of the formulas given in the other chapters of this book can be used to treat children as well as adults, but you must remember to reduce the dosage accordingly. When treating children, calculate dosages using Clark's Rule, a standard formula for prescribing pediatric doses. This rule, in which the average adult is assumed to weigh 150 pounds, allows you to convert adult formulas to suit your child's weight. This means that if the suggested dosage for an adult is one cup of herb tea and your child weighs 50 pounds,

you would give him or her one-third of a cup. Likewise, 30 drops of tincture to treat a sick adult would be reduced to 10 drops for the same child. A 15-pound baby would get only one-tenth of a cup of tea, or 3 drops of tincture. Because I have chosen remedies that I know to be safe, this rule can be applied to all the formulas provided in this book. Remember, though, that Clark's Rule cannot be applied to all herbal remedies; some are simply too potent to give to any child, no matter how small the dose.

Note: The formulas throughout this chapter are suitable for a child whose weight is between 36 and 65 pounds. If, for example, the recommended dose is a half cup of tea, the dosage for children who do not fall into this weight range would be as follows:

WEIGHT	DOSAGE
Up to 5 pounds	$\frac{1}{16}$ cup (or 1 tablespoon)
5 to 15 pounds	$\frac{1}{8}$ cup (or 2 tablespoons)
16 to 35 pounds	$\frac{1}{4}$ cup (or 4 tablespoons)
66 to 80 pounds	$\frac{3}{4}$ cup
81 to 110 pounds	1 cup

quite an advocate of herbalism. She carries a bottle of garlic in glycerin almost
everywhere—even when she is not sick.
This concoction, which is used to ward
off most types of infections and to prevent coughs, earaches and stomach flu,
is so special to Jessa that she once placed
her bottle among the family's holiday
decorations.

ASTHMA

Asthma is a respiratory ailment in which
the throat and lungs constrict, making it
difficult for a person to breathe. In its
mildest form, this condition, which
manifests itself as recurring attacks, is
uncomfortable; at its worst, it can be
life-threatening. Most people with
asthma are constantly battling congestion in their lungs. Asthma can occur in
anyone, but it is most prevalent during
childhood and early adulthood. According to the U.S. Center for Disease Control and Prevention in Atlanta, the
division of the U.S. Public Health Services that investigates and tries to control
the incidence of various diseases, the
asthma rate in children increased almost
40 percent from 1980 to 1990.

Many things can trigger an asthma
attack, including exhaustion, stress, lung
infection and even cold air, but exposure
to allergic substances, such as dust and
smoke, tops the list. Although attacks are
usually brief, they are still frightening for
child and parent alike.

Modern medicine offers children
with asthma little more than temporary
relief for their symptoms. The right
herbs, however, not only help these children to catch their breath, but also re-

⚘ NUTRITIONAL SUPPLEMENTS FOR CHILDREN

When choosing nutritional supplements for children, avoid the
isolated nutrients and the "mega"
vitamins found in formulas made
for adults. Look for vitamins and
minerals designed especially for
children, and avoid those sweetened with sugar to make them
chewable.

For children with asthma,
200 milligrams of vitamin C (for
a 50-pound child) is recommended as an antihistamine. To
support their adrenal glands,
children with asthma can also
take pantothenic acid 1 ½ hours
before exercising. Other vitamins
recommended for children with
asthma include magnesium and
the B-complex vitamins, particularly B_6, which have been shown
in various studies to reduce the
severity of asthma attacks. When
treating constipation, diarrhea, or
intestinal parasites, or after giving
your child antibiotics, give her
acidophilus, a natural culture
that encourages the growth and
health of the natural intestinal
bacteria that help to digest foods
and break down important nutrients. This culture can be found
in various foods, such as some
yogurts, or can be given as a supplement.

duce attacks by strengthening their lungs and their immune systems. You will find mullein and elecampane—which herbalists have found to be exceptionally tonic and healing to the lungs—in almost every commercially available herbal formula for asthma. These herbs also arrest or eliminate symptoms such as wheezing and shortness of breath by opening the constricted bronchial passages.

Other herbs also act as antihistamines to open air passages and relieve wheezing. (Histamines are substances released in the body that produce swelling and constrict bronchial passages.) These herbs include some familiar and tasty children's favorites, such as anise, ginger, peppermint and chamomile. German studies have shown that chamomile may slow allergic reactions, such as those that trigger asthma attacks, by increasing the adrenal glands' production of cortisone, which reduces lung inflammation and makes breathing easier. Motherwort and passionflower, which are commonly used by Italian physicians to treat asthma, not only decrease the severity of lung spasms but also reduce anxiety, thus lessening the chance of an attack. Lemon verbena tea—a flavorful drink that almost any child will appreciate—is commonly given to South American children to reduce their wheezing. If your child suffers from asthma, you too may want to try a tea made with these herbs, but you may also want to keep a tincture of these same herbs on hand for times when making tea is inconvenient. Many herbal asthma formulas are available in natural food stores.

Breathe-Easy Tea

1 quart boiling water
1 teaspoon each chamomile flowers,
    echinacea root, mullein leaves and
    passionflower leaves
½ teaspoon each elecampane root and
    lemon verbena leaves (if available)

Pour boiling water over the herbs in a saucepan and steep for 10 to 15 minutes. Strain out herbs. For a 50-pound child, give a half cup of tea at least once a day as a preventive, or a few times a day when breathing becomes strained or when emotional conditions may lead to an attack. If you use a tincture of these herbs, give ¼ dropperful (15 drops) to replace each half-cup of tea. Store extra tea in the refrigerator.

According to studies reported at a doctors' conference in Florence, Italy, in 1986, ginkgo reduces the susceptibility of children to various allergic substances and thus greatly decreases the frequency of asthma attacks. The researchers found that ginkgo keeps the bronchial passages in the lungs from constricting. In traditional Chinese medicine, ginkgo throat spray is used in much the same way as the modern asthmatic inhaler. Ginkgo, which can be found at most natural food stores in both pill and tincture form, is an effective and easy-to-use herb.

Ginkgo Throat Spray

1 teaspoon tincture of ginkgo leaves
5 drops chamomile essential oil (optional)
¼ cup water

Combine ingredients and store the mixture in a sprayer bottle. Shake well before using. Use as needed to keep airways clear.

For thousands of years, another Chinese herb, ma huang, has been used to dilate bronchial passages and stop asthma symptoms for hours. Ma huang, which is also known as Chinese ephedra, is a potent herbal antihistamine. It also stimulates the adrenal glands and the nervous system and misuse of this herb has caused several deaths, so you *must* discuss its use with a doctor knowledgeable about herbs before giving it to your child—it can be particularly detrimental for a child who has a weak heart or is run-down. A gentler approach comes from onions, which contain a newly discovered compound that reduces the severity of asthma attacks. In one German study of a group of people with asthma, about half the subjects experienced much less severe attacks when they drank onion juice every day. Your child will most likely refuse to drink onion juice, so you could try adding onions to his meals.

Many of these herbs can be combined into effective asthma remedies, but it is also important to give your child herbs that build up the immune system, such as echinacea and chamomile. This may seem contradictory, since allergies are the result of an overactive immune system—that is, the system treats harmless foreign substances as objects to be destroyed, and in the process harms rather than protects the body—but these "immune-boosting" herbs also "balance" the immune system so it can better realize when substances are harmful and when they are not. Allergic reactions, such as those that trigger attacks in many people with asthma, often indicate that an individual is suffering from prob-

lems with her immune system. Children with difficult-to-treat asthma cases often benefit from taking a Chinese formula of magnolia, rehmannia and don quai. In one Chinese study, these herbs allowed several people of various ages who suffered from severe asthma to stop taking the powerful steroid drugs that they were given to fight their asthma. Other people with asthma were able to reduce the amount of their drugs.

Chinese Asthma Tea

1 teaspoon each magnolia flowers and rehmannia root
½ teaspoon don quai root
3 cups water

❧ Combine ingredients in a saucepan and bring to a boil. Turn down heat and simmer for 20 minutes. Turn off heat and steep for 20 minutes. Give 1 cup daily. Store extra tea in the refrigerator. These herbs can be special-ordered though a natural food store or bought from a mail-order Chinese herb source.

Herbs alone can work wonders in helping your child, and a few additional measures will contribute to the success of these remedies. Since asthma is associated with allergies, keep the air your child breathes as clean as possible. Air filters help to eliminate many common airborne allergens: pollen, mites, mold, animal dander and dust. Check that your air-conditioning and heating-system filters are not recycling dust through your home. You might also remove feather pillows and comforters from your child's bed, and wash his toys to see if either of these measures makes a difference. In addition, avoid giving your child foods to which people with asthma tend to be sensitive, especially fruit dried with sulfites (additives used to help vegetables keep their color) or foods containing the flavor-enhancer MSG (monosodium glutamate), which is used in some Chinese restaurants and in many processed foods. Studies show that one way to prevent asthma in the first place is by breastfeeding your baby; breastfeeding is known to help build up the natural immunities that prevent children from developing allergies.

I met eight-year-old Heather and her mother, Lori, soon after Heather started suffering asthma attacks. A doctor had advised stripping the child's room of everything, including the carpet and most of her toys, to turn it into a sterile, hospital-like ward. As is the case with many people with asthma, stress played a key role in Heather's condition, and Lori was worried that removing her daughter's special curtains and favorite toys might prove really upsetting. Indeed, as we talked about it, Heather could barely contain her tears. As a compromise, they worked together to redecorate Heather's room and make it less allergenic and easier to keep clean. Most of the stuffed animals took a "carnival ride" in the washing machine, while others vacationed in another part of the house.

They then began herbal treatments, focusing on substances that could fend off asthma. When Lori heard that I was writing about asthma, she wanted me to assure other parents who are dealing with asthmatic children for the first time that it can get better. Heather no longer has asthma attacks, and Lori credits herbs, especially those that bolster the immune system, such as echinacea, for improving her daughter's condition. As an added benefit, Heather does not come down with as many colds and flus as she once did. There was even a day at school when Heather picked up a pet rat, once a sure trigger for her asthma; her eyes reddened, but she did not start wheezing.

Janet, a registered nurse, uses both medical and herbal approaches to treat her son Ryan's asthma. Janet and her husband, Dan, say that the best prevention for seven-year-old Ryan's asthma attacks is a lavender chest rub just before he goes to sleep. The lavender does double duty: As a muscle relaxant, it keeps chest muscles and bronchial passages from constricting; as a mind relaxer, it reduces the stress that might trigger an attack. If the child tends to become congested while sleeping, an antihistamine such as chamomile can be used in conjunction with the lavender.

Lavender Chest Rub

8 drops lavender essential oil
2 drops chamomile essential oil (optional)
¼ cup olive (or other vegetable) oil
🍂 Combine ingredients. Rub on chest as needed, especially before bedtime. If you wish to add chamomile as an antihistamine, replace 2 drops of the lavender essential oil with 2 drops of chamomile essential oil.

An alternative to the chest rub is an herbal steam that uses these same essential oils. Add two drops of lavender essential oil to a humidifier (check the instructions to make sure yours will not clog or otherwise be damaged by essential oils) in your child's room or have your child inhale the steam from a pan of water containing four drops of lavender essential oil. For more information, see Herbal Steam on page 232.

Janet and Dan tried a lavender steam with Ryan but he did not like putting his head over the hot steam. In exploring other ways to administer this herb, they eventually discovered that if they put him in a hot bath containing a few drops of lavender essential oil at the first signs of a serious attack, Ryan breathed easily for at least an hour. Dan says that it is amazing how dramatically the herbal bath works in halting even the worst attacks—a great relief, since Ryan's asthma is so bad that he has ended up in the hospital a few times, once in intensive care. Since the herbal treatments began, there have been no hospital visits, and Janet and Dan have been able to reduce Ryan's medication.

Unlike teas and pills, the ginkgo spray, chest rub, steam and hot lavender bath can be safely used even after the child begins to wheeze. To play it safe, have your child sniff the oils before you use the chest rub, steam or bath for the first time—some asthma sufferers are sensitive to any fragrance.

BABY SKIN CARE AND DIAPER RASH

A bad case of diaper rash can turn even the most loving, cooing baby into an irritable complainer. According to surveys from Loyola University, over 75 percent of newborns get diaper rash within the first few months after birth. This condition is caused by a combination of fac-tors, the most common of which are bacteria and detergent residues that are not completely rinsed out of diapers. These are not the only factors, though—a rash can even arise from super-clean diapers rubbing against your baby's sensitive skin. You can prevent diaper rash by changing your baby's diapers more frequently and increasing air circulation, first by using diaper covers that do not seal in moisture, then by allowing your child some time without a diaper.

Some of the products that promise to moisturize, soften and cleanse a baby's skin can also contribute to diaper rash. Most baby oils and salves sold in drugstores are made with mineral (petroleum) oil, which is a good machinery lubricant but is questionable for anyone's skin care, especially a baby's. Commercial powders are also suspect. Most of them contain additives, coloring, preservatives, artificial scents and compounds that increase water repellency and enhance the powder's ability to pour evenly and without clumping—these are extras that your baby's skin does not need.

Some ingredients in commercial powders, such as zinc stearate, do not harm skin, but can be harmful if inhaled. Poison centers regularly get reports about children who suffer coughing fits, labored breathing, insufficient blood oxygen and vomiting after inhaling baby powder. Even talcum powder, which is favored by parents because of its smoothness, can lead to trouble. If inhaled, its tiny sharp molecules can injure lungs, and it sometimes contains traces of arsenic (which is poisonous) or asbestos (which is carcinogenic).

Good alternatives to chemical-laden commercial products include baby salves and powders made with chamomile, calendula, comfrey and lavender. These herbs soothe, heal and protect a baby's sensitive skin. Herbal salves also contain beeswax, oil and lanolin, which provide a barrier against moisture and thus keep rashes from recurring. Baby powder made with cornstarch absorbs moisture and also reduces chafing. You can purchase herbal baby salves and powders in natural food stores, or you can make your own.

Fragrant Baby Powder
½ pound cornstarch
¼ teaspoon lavender essential oil
Place cornstarch in a self-sealing plastic bag and add the essential oil drop by drop. Tightly close the bag and shake it to distribute the oil, breaking up any clumps through the bag. Let stand 4 days to distribute the essential oil. Use with every diaper change, or as needed. Potato starch or arrowroot powder can be used instead of cornstarch. Some herbalists use white clay, also called China clay, but this substance tends to clump when wet. Spice or salt shakers with large perforations in their lids make good powder containers.

My friend Bob launched his herbal career with a homemade diaper rash salve. I first met Bob in the early 1970s at a crafts fair where I was selling herbal products. He said that he had made an herbal salve to heal his son Sierra's diaper rash, and when he told his friends about it, the requests poured in. After his second son, Sage, was born, Bob named his product for the two boys and began selling "Sierra Sage" salve to stores. He later expanded his herb business to include cough syrup for children. Today, he owns a large herb business.

Diaper Rash Salve
1 cup Baby Flower Oil (see page 214)
½ ounce beeswax
½ teaspoon lanolin (optional)
5 400–International Unit vitamin E capsules
2 1,000–International Unit Vitamin A (with added Vitamin D) capsules
Heat the Baby Flower Oil just enough so that you can melt the beeswax and lanolin in it. Pop the vitamin capsules with a pin and squeeze their contents into the oil. Stir well. While the mixture is still hot and liquid, pour it into widemouthed jars and let cool. (You can also use the refillable tubes sold in backpacking supply stores.) Apply with every diaper change, or as needed. Be aware, though, that lanolin causes a reaction on some people's skin. If you wish, you can test your baby beforehand by rubbing a tiny amount of pure lanolin on her skin. This salve can be used to treat abrasions anywhere on the body and to combat diaper rash.

Infant bathing may be one case where less is actually more. According to Loyola University researchers, the average one-month-old baby is bathed four times each week and shampooed three times in the same period. Most babies need only an occasional bath in warm water with no soap or shampoo, unless you are treating a condition such as cradle cap. Following a bath, a gentle rubdown with a quality baby oil (preferably herbal) helps to replace lost skin oils. Mother Nature can also help you to protect your newborn's skin. The *vernix caseosa*, a whitish protective coating that covers the skin after birth, can have long-term beneficial properties: Natural childbirth advocates believe that if this coating is rubbed into the child's skin instead of being washed off (as is the practice at most hospitals), the child's chances of developing skin problems in the future will be reduced.

Baby Flower Oil

½ cup each lavender flowers, calendula flowers and elder flowers
3 cups almond (or vegetable) oil

Chop dried herbs and place them in a clean glass jar. Cover herbs with almond oil and stir to remove air bubbles. Put the oil in a warm place (near a radiator or in the sun) for 2 to 3 days, then strain out herbs. If necessary, strain again using a coffee filter or fine strainer to remove the tiniest particles. Store in a cool place. Use as frequently as needed for skin treatment and massage.

Herbs can also be used to heal cradle cap, a thick, yellowish, crusty rash that forms on the scalp and sometimes the face of newborns. This rash is caused partly by an overproduction of oil. The standard medical treatment is cortisone cream, but most pediatricians would rather not use such strong steroids on babies. Instead, wash the scalp with a gentle baby shampoo to reduce excess oils, and treat daily with antiseptic and skin-healing lavender, tea tree and aloe vera.

Cradle Cap Remedy

¼ cup aloe vera
3 drops each lavender and tea tree essential oils

Combine ingredients in a bottle and shake well to blend. Apply directly onto the skin a few times daily.

BEDWETTING

Typically, a child is between two and seven years old before he can make it through the night without having to empty his bladder. Although bedwetting can be exacerbated by psychological problems or emotional stress, it generally involves poor muscle control or crossed signals in the communication between the nervous system and the brain. It tends to disappear as the child grows older, but for some parents, the wait can seem endless. In any case, most child psychologists agree that reprimanding a child who wets the bed does more harm than good.

Fortunately, bedwetting can often be remedied with an herbal tincture. Studies have shown that Saint-John's-wort and oats help the nervous system to control the bladder. Likewise, corn silk and plantain leaf (which is used in many Chinese herbal formulas to treat urinary problems) have been shown to improve the urinary tract muscles that control the bladder. Be patient; it may take several weeks before you see results, but this formula usually works! Do not give your child any liquids, including herb tea, for three hours before bedtime, since this can encourage bedwetting. If your child seems to be overly tense or anxious, or if he gets upset about wetting the bed, some Calming Tea (see page 237) will help relax him. Since these herbs lose much of their potency when dried, use a tincture that has been prepared from fresh plants.

My friend Mary was surprised when her 11-year-old son, Bobby, started wetting the bed—a problem he had never had before. As you can imagine, Bobby was terribly embarrassed, and he was eager to try any concoction his mother came up with, as long as there was any chance it might help. Mary had made her own Saint-John's-wort tincture and had purchased a tincture of fresh oats, but she was unable to find a corn silk tincture. I suggested that she buy some fresh, organically grown corn (corn not grown organically generally has pesticides clinging to the silk) and make her own tincture. Meanwhile, Mary started Bobby on the Saint-John's-wort and oats tincture. At first, he still wet the bed every night, but after a week, he awoke to a dry bed. The newly finished corn silk tincture was added, and there continued to be fewer and fewer bedwetting episodes. After about a month of taking the tincture, Bobby completely stopped wetting his bed. Mary continued the treatment for a few more days, just to be sure. Bobby has had a dry bed ever since.

Dry Bed Tincture
Equal parts tinctures of Saint-John's-wort tops, fresh oat berries, corn silk and plantain leaves

Combine tinctures in a bottle. For a 50-pound child, give 15 drops (¼ dropperful) 3 times a day. Before or after meals is an easy time to remember.

Another bedwetting treatment is aloe vera juice. Researchers in Russia found that almost all the children in their study not only stopped wetting their beds when they were given aloe, but also became noticeably less irritable. The few who continued to wet the bed did so much less frequently. Mix aloe juice with an equal amount of the child's favorite fruit juice. But don't overdo it—I suggest one-half to one cup a day.

Bedwetting is occasionally caused by a bladder infection. If this is the cause, your child will probably complain of discomfort and burning while urinating. If you suspect that your child may have an infection, have your pediatrician examine him so that a kidney infection or other serious disorder can be ruled out. For more information, see chapter 8, and don't forget to adjust the proportions according to Clark's Rule (see page 207).

CHILDHOOD DISEASES

The primary childhood diseases— measles, German measles, mumps and chickenpox —are caused by viruses. Most of us are affected by them only once in our lives—after the first exposure, the body recognizes the virus and usually builds up a lifelong immunity to it. Until recently, most people encountered all four viruses as children (which is why the illnesses are called childhood diseases). Today, vaccines are used to foster a person's immunity without his ever having to experience the illness, but even vaccinated children occasionally come down with one of these illnesses. In fact, according to the *Merck Manual,* the incidence of German measles has been increasing since 1988, and most children who have contracted this disease during this time have been vaccinated. The symptoms of these diseases, as well as minor adverse reactions to the vaccinations, can be fought using herbs. If your child experiences breathing problems, a rash, persistent fever or crying, or appears unusually inattentive after being vaccinated, this could be because of a reaction to the vaccine. You should contact your pediatrician immediately.

Measles start off with itchy pink spots on the face that spread to the rest of the body. The child will probably also have a cough, high fever, sensitive eyes and a runny nose. German measles, also called rubella, is less contagious and usually less severe, with fewer spots and a low fever, if any. The child's glands will swell, but this swelling is rarely accompanied by a sore throat. Chickenpox causes only a moderate fever, but results in itchy spots that scab over, headaches, and an occasional sore throat. Mumps produces a moderate fever and noticeable swollen glands on the neck. It rarely occurs in children under two years old, and at least 25 percent of cases are so mild that they go unnoticed.

Most likely, your doctor will recommend the same treatment for all these childhood diseases: bed rest. You can, however, lessen your child's symptoms and make her more comfortable with an herbal remedy. A child suffering from any of these illnesses always seems to get well much more quickly and to have a relatively light case if he drinks a tea of

catnip, lemon balm, burdock and the Chinese herb bupleurum. Catnip lowers a fever and reduces the eruptions of measles and chickenpox. Long before viruses were found to be the root of these diseases and vaccines were developed to fight viruses, the Chinese treated these illnesses with burdock and bupleurum in an effort to enhance immunity and liver function. Laboratory studies have shown that burdock and bupleurum destroy the measles virus. The virus responsible for chickenpox is inhibited by antiviral agents in lemon balm and by bergamot essential oil. Lemon balm also destroys the mumps virus. Lemon and

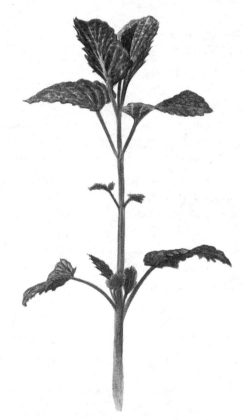

Sweet-smelling lemon balm is a common ingredient in potpourris.

yarrow reduce the fever that generally accompanies these diseases, and mullein encourages the drainage of swollen glands.

Childhood Diseases Tea
1 teaspoon burdock root
½ teaspoon bupleurum root (optional)
1 quart water
1 teaspoon each catnip leaves, lemon
   balm leaves, mullein leaves and
   elder flowers
½ teaspoon each yarrow flowers and
   peppermint leaves (for taste)

🍃 Combine burdock, bupleurum and water in a saucepan and simmer for 5 minutes. Turn off heat, add other herbs and steep for 15 minutes. Strain out herbs. Give as much as the child will drink—at least 2 cups daily for a 50-pound child. If your child does not like the taste of this tea, mix it with fruit juice to make it more palatable. Store extra tea in the refrigerator.

If your child comes down with one of these diseases, her appetite and ability to hold down food will probably be reduced. However, if she can tolerate food, the sickness can be treated through the addition of certain herbs to her meals. A small amount of burdock can be prepared as a vegetable, Japanese-style. The Chinese recommend saffron and coriander leaves (known as cilantro in Mexican and Oriental cooking) to encourage sweating in eruptive skin diseases like chickenpox and measles. If your child has one of these diseases, it is also a good idea to sponge off her skin with an herbal wash or to apply wet compresses. These treatments reduce the itching, speed healing of the sores and reduce possible spread of the infection. Use a strong "tea" of burdock, calendula and lemon balm for the wash or compresses.

Eruptive Skin Wash
2 teaspoons each burdock root, calendula
   flowers and lemon balm leaves
6 drops bergamot essential oil (for
   chickenpox only)
3 cups water

🍃 Place burdock root and water in a saucepan and simmer uncovered for about 5 minutes. Remove from heat and add remaining herbs. Cover pan and steep for 10 minutes. Strain out herbs. Add essential oil and stir well to distribute evenly. Sponge gently over skin eruptions, or make a compress by soaking soft cloths in this wash. Wring out the cloth and apply on afflicted skin.

For mumps, drain the glands and reduce the pain and swelling with the neck compress suggested for swollen glands (see page 232). A child with mumps will also benefit by taking a tincture that encourages lymph drainage. If ear or other infections are also present, follow the instructions given in this chapter to combat these problems.

Mumps Tincture
Equal parts calendula flowers, barberry
   and mullein leaf (if available)

🍃 For a 50-pound child, give 10 drops 3 times a day. Take this along with the Childhood Diseases Tea. Because this formula is not very tasty, it is best given as a tincture with a small amount of water or fruit juice.

BOLSTERING IMMUNITY

All children are exposed to numerous illnesses at school and day care, but some kids seem to have sniffles or stomach upsets almost constantly, while others suffer only an occasional bout of a cold or flu. Resistance to illness is determined by many factors; diet, heredity and stress are all relevant, but the strength of the immune system is likely the most important consideration. The best kind of herbal medicine (like the best modern medicine) is not treating your child once he falls sick, but preventing him from getting sick in the first place.

When I began writing this chapter, I asked for herbal success stories from parents. Over and over I heard stories similar to the one that Joan told me about her baby Nathaniel: "Except for an earache, which I treated herbally, he hasn't been sick yet. I think this is because of the immune herbs I give him at the first sign of any problem." Marsha's son is 11, so I figured he had had more chances to get sick, but she said, "Well, Zaya has never really been sick. Maybe that is because since he was little, I have given him herbs like echinacea to boost his immune system."

Repeated illnesses are a sign that a child's immunity needs to be bolstered with herbs such as echinacea, chamomile and shizandra. In one Russian study, more than 200 young children were given an herbal combination based on echinacea; these kids had fewer colds and fewer days of fever than children who had not taken herbs. Chamomile, used traditionally in Germany and also heavily researched there, has been proven to increase resistance to disease. A study done in the Russian town of Chirchik showed that children given shizandra proved more resistant than other children to a serious flu epidemic that swept through town. Echinacea, chamomile and shizandra can be given as a tea, pills or a tincture. You can purchase these herbs at a natural food store.

Immune Booster Tea

2 cups water
1 teaspoon echinacea root
½ teaspoon each chamomile flowers, shizandra berries (if available) and peppermint leaves (for taste)

Boil water and pour it over the herbs. Steep for 15 minutes, then strain out herbs. At first signs of illness, give 1 cup daily for every 50 pounds of body weight. As a preventive measure—for instance, when your child is about to start school or go on a long trip—give him 1 cup daily for a week. Store extra tea in the refrigerator.

COLDS AND FLU

In my herb class, Don, a single father, told of his success giving his six-year-old daughter, Libby, a tea of equal parts elder, peppermint and hyssop. (See Fever Tea on page 226; this formula not only reduces a fever, but also fights colds and flu and helps to relieve the congestion that often accompanies these sicknesses.) Don uses this flavorful formula, which he found in an herb book, to fend off sniffles. Whenever Libby wakes up with a slight rattle in her throat—a warning sign Don has learned to recognize—he gives her a cup of this tea. If there is any sign of fever, he adds yarrow. For three years in a row, she was not sick once, even though plenty of her classmates had runny noses and coughs. In fact, since she never has any sick days, Don occasionally takes her out of school just so they can do something fun together. This last year, Libby, who is now nine years old, finally did get a little cold, but that's okay—researchers believe that an occasional cold may be a good thing because it stimulates natural immunity.

Jennifer, whom I mentioned earlier in this chapter, also gave her two young children, Jessa and Bohdi, herbs before ever attending an herb class. Her husband, Andrew, once had a bad case of bronchitis that a friend treated by placing ginger compresses on his chest. Remarkably, the bronchitis cleared up in a few days. So when Andrew's children come down with colds or flus, he does not hesitate to use herbs. One of his favorite herbs is ginger. To treat his kids' congestion, Andrew stirs two table-spoons of ginger powder into a hot bath. This is a lot of ginger, but it does the trick almost every time. He and Jennifer say that their kids rarely have runny noses, colds or flus. You can overdo it, though, as Jennifer and Andrew once did when Jessa was sick. They prepared a ginger bath for Jessa, and a few seconds after getting into the tub Jessa said, "Hot, hot," and they realized that she was complaining not about the temperature, but about the tingly-hot sensation produced by too much ginger in her bath.

Even though antibiotics continue to be prescribed for colds and flu, it is well known that these drugs have no effect on viruses. They only help to prevent bacterial infections from developing. Evidence indicates that the overuse of antibiotics decreases their effectiveness when a true emergency arises, and may even lessen one's natural immunity in the long run. Use of antibiotics also encourages the development of strains of infectious microorganisms that are resistant to them—because the microorganisms adapt to the drugs and become stronger—and drug developers are forced to create stronger and stronger drugs.

So what can you do to protect your child from secondary infections developing once a cold or flu sets in? There are many natural antibiotic herbs that work much differently to destroy microorganisms than their drug counterparts. These herbs do not compromise the immune system, as pharmaceutical antibiotics can—they make the body healthier. One of the most popular of these natural antibiotics is garlic, which is mentioned often in this chapter, and for good reason. Garlic fights the microorganisms responsible for many types of infection. You can administer garlic in any form your child will take. First, try adding it to your kid's meals. If your child resists, try giving her garlic supplements (there are many types available) or use the Garlic Vinegar on page 231.

Another well-known herbal antibiotic is goldenseal, although I often replace it with barberry or Oregon grape root, which grows wild where I live and is not an endangered plant like goldenseal. Oregon grape root tastes slightly better than goldenseal, so most children prefer it. They also like the name. No matter how many times I correct them, children almost always think that this formula contains Oregon "grapefruit." I also use licorice, the antiviral value of which was reported in two journals in 1980, and echinacea, which was shown in a 1978 German study to fight against and protect from infection. These herbs deter or halt viral infections by making the virus inactive, slowing its reproduction and preventing it from breaking down cell walls.

Children's Antibiotic Formula

2 cups water
½ teaspoon each echinacea root, licorice root and barberry bark (or Oregon grape root)

🌿 Place water and herbs in a saucepan. Simmer for 2 minutes, then remove from heat and steep for about 20 minutes. Strain out herbs. For a 50-pound child, give 1 cup of tea or half a dropperful (30 drops) of tincture daily. To improve the flavor, the tea can be mixed with an equal amount of juice. In fact, homemade apple and grape juice, unlike bottled juices, contain strong antiviral agents that fight colds and flu.

CONSTIPATION

Constipation is very common among children, which is not surprising, considering the foods that many children love. Lots of white bread, peanut butter, cheese and sweets all lead to constipation. So can bouts of worry or fear. And the young couch potato who forgoes exercise to spend hours in front of a television or computer tends to suffer more from constipation than an active child.

Laxatives suggested for constipated adults, even herbal ones, are generally too strong—in both taste and action—for children. To treat a constipated child, turn to a gentle combination of licorice and apple juice, with either fennel or ginger to relieve intestinal gas.

Laxative Juice

1 cup boiling water
½ teaspoon licorice root
¼ teaspoon ginger rhizome (or fennel seeds)
¼ cup each apple and prune juice (optional)

🌿 Pour boiling water over herbs and steep for 10 minutes. Strain out herbs, then add juices. If your child balks at the taste of prunes, use only apple juice. For a 50-pound child, give ¼ cup every 2 hours until a change for the better becomes apparent.

and make sure that the child's morning schedule is not too hectic. If these measures do not produce enough results, add half a teaspoon of ground psyllium seed to your child's favorite juice each morning or serve her Slippery Elm Gruel before bed. If your child continues to be constipated despite these treatments, be sure to see your pediatrician.

Psyllium Juice

½ teaspoon ground psyllium seed
½ cup warm fruit juice or vegetable juice
Mix ground psyllium into juice and stir. For a 50-pound child, give entire amount every morning as long as needed.

Slippery Elm Gruel

1 tablespoon slippery elm powder
¾ cup cold water
1 teaspoon lemon juice (optional)
Combine powder and water in a saucepan and heat until warm, stirring the mixture to prevent clumping. Add lemon juice for flavor, if you wish. You can also sweeten the gruel with your child's favorite herbal or fruit-based sweetener. Have your child drink the entire amount (for every 50 pounds of body weight) before it cools—as gruel cools down, it thickens, and the thicker it gets, the more likely your child is to push it away.

Willow, an herbalist who uses Slippery Elm Gruel, says that as a working mother, she appreciates how fast-acting and effective it is. Willow was surprised that her daughter even liked it, but when Jenny was quite young she asked for some of the extra-thick gruel that

While the aroma of catnip is a great attraction for cats, it is also an effective insect repellent.

Another easy-to-dispense laxative is elderberry jam. If these remedies are not successful, an enema with catnip tea does the trick when all else fails.

If constipation is a common condition for your child, be sure to treat the causes of this problem as well as the symptoms. If you are not serving these items already, switch to high-fiber, whole-grain breakfast cereals or oatmeal,

Willow was drinking to treat her own constipation. Jenny drank the entire cup; it turned out that she was having the same problem!

DIARRHEA

Most healthy children occasionally suffer bouts of diarrhea; generally, these bouts last only a day, if that. Diarrhea may be due to having eaten too fast or too much, or may be the result of a pesky flu. Even overexcitement can occasionally result in loose bowels. With minor cases (for instance, those that last only a day), it is sometimes better to let nature run its course. Diarrhea is one way in which the body eliminates unwanted visitors, such as an intestinal flu virus or badly digested food.

Even when diarrhea is severe or lasts longer than a day, it is rarely a sign for alarm, since it can be quickly relieved with herbs. A tea of catnip, cinnamon, peppermint, slippery elm and raspberry or blackberry leaves usually stops diarrhea. Or you can use a tincture of blackberry root, an old backwoods favorite for curing diarrhea. Garlic also helps to rid the body of flu and other viruses that can cause diarrhea.

Diarrhea Tea
3 cups water
1 teaspoon catnip leaves
½ teaspoon each raspberry or blackberry leaves, slippery elm bark and peppermint leaves
½ teaspoon cinnamon bark powder
🌿 Combine ingredients and water in a saucepan. Bring mixture to a simmer, then remove it from heat. Steep for 15 minutes, then strain out herbs. For a 50-pound child, give 1 cup every half-hour until the symptoms go away.

Blackberries alone are a great diarrhea remedy for small children, as they are not as potent as the blackberry root. (Do not include the blackberry seeds—they act as a bulk laxative.) If your child is reluctant to take herbal remedies, you can easily disguise a diarrhea remedy as food. Simply combine blackberries, cinnamon and bananas into a delicious smoothie. Or sprinkle cinnamon on oatmeal or rice porridge with bananas.

Blackberry Smoothie
½ cup blackberry juice (or jam)
1 banana
½ teaspoon cinnamon bark
🌿 Blend ingredients and serve. Sweeten to taste if needed. Have the child drink as desired.

Rice Porridge
½ cup rice
2 cups water
¼ teaspoon powdered Oregon grape root
½ teaspoon cinnamon
🌿 Place rice and water in a saucepan and simmer for 30 minutes or until very soft. Using a blender, mix the cooked rice with the herbs. The porridge will become watery. Serve child-size portions, with bananas or a spoonful of blackberry jam, if you wish. The cinnamon can be mixed in or sprinkled on top.

The easy-to-make Slippery Elm Gruel on page 221 also works for diarrhea. (Although this may seem odd, herbalists have found that it helps stop constipation because it adds bulk and that it counters diarrhea because it is very absorbent.) Porridge, gruel and bananas not only treat diarrhea, but also replace the nutrients so easily lost with diarrhea. In fact, rice porridge is traditionally fed to children with diarrhea in many parts of the world. Remember also to give your child lots of fluids—children, especially tiny ones, can quickly become dehydrated when suffering from diarrhea.

In most cases, diarrhea can easily be treated at home, but do not let the situation get out of hand. If the problem continues for more than two days or if it keeps recurring, check your child's diet for foods that do not agree with him, intestinal parasites or an unresolved emotional trauma. If there is a fever, which may indicate the presence of infection, or other symptoms, consult your pediatrician before continuing home treatment.

EARACHES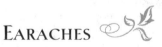

Middle-ear infection is one of the most common and troublesome childhood health problems. It is often a baby's first significant illness, but it is not always easy to spot until the child becomes irritable from the pain, develops a high fever or begins tugging at his ear. Chronic infections and the fear of hearing impairment can lead to a near-endless stream of visits to the doctor. Ear pain results in about one-third of

all pediatrician visits for children under six years old.

The eustachian tubes, which run from the ears to the throat, maintain air pressure in and drain fluids from the middle ear, but also provide an easy route for throat infections to travel to the ears. Because these tubes are so small in a child, swelling from infection or allergy inhibits drainage and compounds the problem. To treat this condition, pediatricians generally prescribe antibiotics. Eventually, if chronic ear infections persist, a doctor will insert small draining tubes into the child's ears.

There is, however, a more natural solution that I have seen work dozens of times, often with children already scheduled to have the tubes inserted: An oil of mullein flower and garlic dropped into the ear will reduce inflammation, stop pain and kill bacterial infections. Garlic also attacks fungal infections, such as "swimmer's ear," that usually occur in the outer ear. Fungal infections are generally less serious than bacterial infections, but they do cause lots of itching. (Some commercially available ear oils also include Saint-John's-wort and calendula to decrease inflammation.)

Years ago, when I was living in the high desert of New Mexico, a local naturopath asked if I knew where to get mullein oil. His ten-year-old daughter Kim's ear was so hot and swollen that she could not hear, and he had already tried all the other natural remedies that were available. This was before anyone sold herbal ear drops. Fortunately, I lived near a wild mullein patch and had just made some oil. During the next two days, we watched as the oil dramatically reduced the redness and swelling of Kim's ear. After a few days, a sprouted bean, the cause of all the trouble, popped out of her ear. (Kim assured us that she had no idea how it got there!) Kim's father continued to administer the mullein for a few days, until all signs of infection had disappeared.

Herbal ear drops are now sold in natural food stores. Or if you can properly identify mullein, you can make your own. Glycerin is included for a few reasons: It is the only natural product I know that cuts earwax buildup (a problem often compounded by infection); it helps to keep the drops in the ear (because it is slightly sticky); and it is an excellent preservative.

Mullein and Garlic Ear Drops

1 ounce Homemade Mullein Oil (see below)
1 ounce Garlic Vinegar (see page 231)
1 teaspoon glycerin
❧ Combine ingredients and stir well. After making sure that the ear drops are warm enough not to cause any discomfort, place 2 drops in each ear. Then, gently rub around the outside of the ear to work the drops in.

Homemade Mullein Oil

Fresh mullein flowers
Olive oil to cover
❧ To make your own mullein oil, you will need a source of fresh flowers to pick. (Be sure to properly identify any herb you pick yourself. Fortunately, once you are familiar with it, mullein's tall taper of yellow flowers is easy to spot.) Place—but do not pack—flowers in a clean glass jar. Cover with just enough olive oil to submerge all the flowers. Stir the flowers to release any air bubbles. Place in a warm location, such as the top of a refrigerator or in the sun, for about 3 days. Then, pour it through a fine strainer. Put 2 drops in each ear a few times daily during an infection, or once a day as a preventive measure. Stored in a cool place, this oil should last for 2 years.

Even if only one ear seems to be infected, treat both of them—these herbs will also help to protect the well ear from the infection. Be careful not to touch the dropper to the infected ear first because this can lead to the infection being transferred. If your child has recurring infections, herbal remedies can help diminish their frequency and severity, but to cure them you must find and solve the source of the problem. Food allergies may be a cause, so you may want to ask your doctor about testing.

Ear drops are not appropriate for serious ear problems—for instance, if the eardrum is perforated or something is lodged inside the ear. Although Kim's father used ear drops for her lodged bean, remember that he is a qualified professional; if you have reason to believe that your child's earache is due to a perforated eardrum, a lodged object or a fever, consult a pediatrician immediately.

In cases of minor irritation, place a compress or poultice over the ear or rub an antiseptic massage oil around the outside of the ear.

Antiseptic Ear Rub
¼ teaspoon each lavender and tea tree
    essential oils
1 tablespoon olive oil
Combine the oils and store the mixture in a clean glass bottle. Lay the child down comfortably on her side and rub the oil around the outside of her ear. Use this treatment a few times daily during an infection.

Onion Ear Poultice
½ onion, chopped
¼ cup water
Heat ingredients in a pan and bring to a simmer, then turn off heat. Wrap simmered onion in several layers of cheesecloth and apply this poultice over the ear, leaving it there for at least 5 minutes. The onion can be reheated and reapplied several times. Do this as many times as needed to ease the pain. This old-fashioned technique is a little messy, but useful when it is the only remedy on hand.

If your child's ear begins to hurt after he has been swimming or bathing, there may be water trapped in the ear— and this condition can be just as painful as an ear infection. To evaporate the water and ease the inflammation and resulting pain, place a drop or two of an anti-inflammatory tincture, such as mullein flower, Saint-John's-wort or chamomile, in the ear. The alcohol in the tincture will dry up the excess water in the ear, and the herb will reduce the swelling and the pain.

FEVER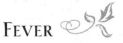

Fevers account for about one-third of all visits to pediatricians. Most fevers are due to a simple cold or flu, but do not be too quick to reduce your child's temperature. According to David Lang, M.D., chief of pediatrics at the University of Maryland School of Medicine, "The body is wiser than we; we shouldn't interfere with normal body responses to illness just because we can." Many pediatricians recommend staying calm and forcing a fever down only if the thermometer reaches 103°F (102° for toddlers or 101° for babies), or if the child becomes too uncomfortable or exhausted.

Although a child's rising temperature can be scary, a child's fever, unlike that of an adult, is not always a true indication of the severity of the problem. According to the National Institutes of Health, a government agency based in Rockville, Maryland, a parent's biggest concern is that a high fever will produce seizures, but these are uncommon— they are estimated to occur in only 4 percent of the children who experience a very high fever—and rarely occur in children over five years old. They are caused not by the severity of the fever, but by how quickly it rises. Any high fever in an infant warrants a call to a pediatrician, who will tell you whether the fever is cause for concern.

When you do need to reduce your child's temperature, serve a tea of elder and yarrow (with peppermint added for flavor). This blend also relieves the sinus and lung congestion that so often accompanies colds and flus. The skin may feel hotter temporarily as these herbs increase circulation, but the child will soon begin to sweat and her fever should break. Do not be surprised if her temperature rises again in the evening; it often does. If this happens, give your child more tea. If you use a tincture of these herbs instead of tea, dilute it in hot water to make an instant tea and have the child drink it hot. If you cannot get the child to drink tea, cool the tea and apply it as a cold wash to her skin (this is not nearly as effective, however, as having the child drink it).

Fever Tea

2 cups water

½ teaspoon each elder flowers, yarrow flowers, peppermint leaves and hyssop leaves (if fever is accompanied by a cold, flu or cough)

🌿 Pour boiling water over herbs, steep for 10 minutes, then strain out herbs. Give your child as much hot tea as she will drink. This tea can be mixed with an equal amount of fruit juice or lemon water, which also helps to reduce a fever.

One advantage to using herbs to reduce fever is that you probably do not have to worry about Reye's Syndrome, an often deadly illness that can occur from simply giving a child with the flu some aspirin to bring down her fever. There are no reports of Reye's Syndrome developing from the use of herbs that contain natural aspirins (salicylates), such as willow and meadowsweet.

A feverish child needs to drink plenty of liquids to keep from becoming dehydrated. Ginger ale is a good bet. Even today, I remember how much I enjoyed ginger ale when I was sick as a kid! Besides reducing fever, ginger fights the germs that cause a cold or flu, and helps relieve such cold and flu symptoms as a queasy stomach and congestion. It also helps eliminate toxins produced in the body during a cold or flu. You can buy a healthy version of ginger ale from the natural food store, or you can make your own.

Natural Ginger Ale

1 teaspoon thinly sliced fresh ginger rhizome (or ½ teaspoon ginger powder)

1 teaspoon red raspberry leaves

3 cups water

1 cup carbonated water

1 lemon slice

🌿 Combine herbs and plain water in a saucepan and bring to a boil. Turn down the heat and simmer for 5 minutes. Remove from heat and steep for 10 minutes. Strain out herbs. Add carbonated water and lemon just before serving.

FOOD ALLERGIES

Allergies occur when an unchecked immune system misidentifies and attacks innocent substances in the body. Children's allergies can be the result of many factors, and it is far better to correct the cause of the problem than simply to relieve the symptoms (for instance, a stuffy nose or upset stomach). In the case of food allergies, the cause is most likely undigested proteins, such as those found in milk, eggs, some processed foods and even wheat. The more a child eats foods to which he is allergic, the worse the allergy usually becomes. Unfortunately, the very foods that children like the most are often the ones to which they are allergic.

A food allergy can produce many symptoms. The most common are digestive disturbances such as upset stomach, constipation and diarrhea. But sinus congestion, hives, headaches, earaches and bedwetting—seemingly unrelated problems—can also be caused by allergies. While stress and fatigue both encourage allergic reactions, they can also be symptoms of allergic reactions. Others include "growing pains" and even some learning and attention deficit disorders (see "Hyperactivity" on page 229), although conventional physicians generally do not accept that these problems might be caused by food allergies.

One survey of English children who suffered frequent headaches showed that most experienced fewer and less severe headaches when they stopped eating certain foods, particularly eggs, dairy products and wheat. Researchers at Georgetown University believe that food allergies are also responsible for many children's ear problems. Most of the children they studied with chronic ear infections also had food allergies. The allergies usually cleared up when the offending foods were eliminated from the children's diets, and the ear problems returned when the children started eating these foods again.

The first step is to remove the foods that cause the allergic reaction. There is a blood test, available through many holisitically and nutritionally oriented physicians, that checks sensitivities to 96 commonly eaten foods. You can also try to figure out the culprits yourself. Eliminate questionable foods from your child's diet, then add them back one at a time while watching for adverse reactions. Symptoms may reappear in a few hours, but allergic reactions to food may be delayed for several hours or even until the next day. For this reason, you should wait a day or two after reintroducing each food item into the diet. It is easy to see why food allergies often go undetected; it is difficult to imagine that yesterday's ice cream is causing today's headache.

If you're a nursing mom, try changing your diet. The La Leche League, a national organization that advocates breastfeeding, recommends that nursing mothers who are seeking to reduce a baby's digestive problems start by avoiding chocolate, hot spices, peanuts, sugar and foods such as cabbage, which are high in sulfur.

You can also reduce the likelihood of your child having future allergic reactions by giving him herbs that balance the immune sytem, decrease inflammation and soothe indigestion. Chamomile and marshmallow perform all three of these roles, peppermint and ginger aid digestion and decrease inflammation, and echinacea provides the immune system with discretion in dealing with foreign substances. You will probably not see the effects of these herbs immedi-ately, since it usually takes time to correct food allergies, but they are safe for long-term use.

Allergy Tea

2 cups water
½ teaspoon each echinacea root and
    marshmallow root
1 teaspoon chamomile flowers
½ teaspoon peppermint leaf
¼ teaspoon ginger rhizome

Combine water and echinacea and marshmallow roots in a saucepan and simmer for about 5 minutes. Turn off heat and add remaining ingredients. Steep for 15 minutes, then strain out herbs. For a 50-pound child, give 1 to 2 cups daily. These herbs can also be used as tinc-tures; for a 50-pound child, give ½ to 1 dropperful (30–60 drops) daily.

Hives, the rashlike skin bumps that can drive kids crazy with itching, are another symptom of food allergy. To stop the itching, sponge the child's skin with a warm herbal wash. If that does not provide enough relief, apply an herbal poultice. Even children who normally object to having a poultice smeared on their skin often accept anything that relieves the discomfort of hives. When these herbs are not available, try a hot bath or shower.

Hives Skin Wash

1 cup boiling water
1 teaspoon each calendula flowers,
    chamomile flowers, echinacea root,
    elder flowers and yarrow flowers
3 tablespoons baking soda

Pour boiling water over herbs and steep for 15 minutes, then strain out herbs. Stir in baking soda. Apply to irritated skin with a soft cloth or a sponge until itching is reduced.

Hives Skin Poultice

¼ cup Hives Skin Wash
3 tablespoons bentonite clay
1 tablespoon slippery elm bark powder

Stir all ingredients into a paste. Let set 5 minutes to thicken. Apply to irritated skin with fingers or a tongue depressor. Let dry on skin and do not remove for at least 30 minutes. Wash off.

My friend's son Ethin complained of headaches so often that I suspected that he had food allergies. Whenever I heard him say he had a headache, I asked him what he had eaten a few hours earlier. Before long, that question made him smile sheepishly because the answer was always the same: ice cream, candy or other sweets.

When he was ten years old, Ethin once spent the night at my house after a holiday meal. He had just fallen asleep when he awoke with an unbearably itchy rash on his arms and chest that was quickly turning into raised welts and spreading all over his body. It was too late to do anything about the particular foods that caused this reaction, but I knew that herbs could stop the itching. Ethin took a cool shower (showing just how uncomfortable he must have been!), then I spread the skin paste on his hives. The itching did not stop right away, so I had to distract him from scratching off the medicine, but he slowly began to relax as the itching subsided. I gave him some Calming Tea (see page 237), and he was finally able to drift off to sleep. By morning, all traces of the hives were gone.

You should be aware that hives and rashes that appear shortly after ingesting a substance to which you are allergic can mark the beginning stages of a serious medical emergency. If a child's allergic reaction progresses rapidly to what looks like a total body response—with redness and difficulty breathing—get medical help immediately. Don't try to treat this kind of thing yourself.

HYPERACTIVITY

So far, no one has been able to pinpoint the cause of hyperactivity, or Attention Deficit Disorder (ADD). Current research points to physical rather than psychological causes, possibly problems with brain chemistry and a connection to prenatal trauma. For reasons unknown, ADD affects ten times more boys than girls. But

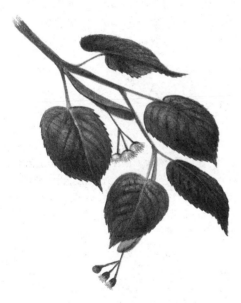

In the French countryside, a tea made of linden flowers is traditionally given to children to calm them down in the afternoons.

ADD can be treated—I have seen a number of hyperactive children dramatically change behavior when their parents instituted a comprehensive program that included herbs, a change in diet, avoiding potential allergic substances and counseling, usually for the whole family. Pediatrician and allergist Ben Feingold, M.D., found that hyperactive children improved when synthetic food colorings, milk, chocolate, sugar and certain preservatives were eliminated from their diets.

As any parent with a hyperactive child knows, a child who suffers from this condition can be quite a handful. It might not be so bad if these children were simply lively, but they are easily distracted, unable to concentrate, have a tendency to act impulsively and become aggressive without apparent reason. Parents may hesitate to take their hyperactive child anywhere, and teachers constantly struggle to get the child to concentrate. Such children are routinely given drugs such as methylphenidate, which can have serious long-term effects, including a drugged, docile state, appetite and weight loss, insomnia and an irregular heartbeat.

Natural treatments for hyperactivity are much more popular in Europe than they are in North America. The Germans have treated hyperactive children with valerian since the 1970s. In one German study, more than 100 hyperactive children experienced improved learning skills, muscle coordination and reaction time after only a few weeks of taking valerian. They were also less anxious, less aggressive, less restless and less fearful. Even more amazing, over 25 percent of these children recovered completely. Because valerian has an unpleasant taste, you should administer valerian-based formulas in tincture form. Another European remedy for hyperactivity is catnip, which contains compounds similar to those in valerian. Linden flower tea is a traditional afternoon drink given to French country children to settle them down. Linden is not widely available as a tincture, but it is sold in natural food stores and even in many grocery stores as a French or an English herb tea.

Hyperactivity Tincture

1 teaspoon tincture of valerian rhizome
½ teaspoon each tinctures of catnip leaves and passionflower leaves
¼ teaspoon each tinctures of peppermint leaves and linden flowers (if available)

Combine ingredients. For a 50-pound child, give half a dropperful several times a day.

When children at the London Children's Hyperactive Clinic took evening primrose oil, they were much less hyperactive, and two-thirds of them experienced fewer nightmares. Evening primrose oil is better known for successfully treating premenstrual syndrome (PMS), but the clinic has found a possible link between hyperactivity and PMS, and even alcoholism—problems that many hyperactive children eventually develop and that seem to run in their families. Researchers believe that this connection is due to an overproduction of certain hormonelike substances in the body called prostaglandins, which are reduced by evening primrose oil. This oil

is sold in natural food stores only in capsules; to adjust the recommended dosage on the package for your child, use Clark's Rule (see page 207).

While herbal treatments can reduce hyperactivity, children benefit most when dietary changes are also part of their program. Both the New York Institute for Child Development and Princeton's Brain-Bio Center are investigating the relationship of food and food additives, such as nitrates and food dyes, to children's behavioral and learning imbalances. Over half the hyperactive children treated at the Pain and Stress Therapy Center in San Antonio, Texas, began to function more normally when sugar and caffeine (which is present in colas and other soft drinks) were removed from their diets and they were given nutritional supplements such as magnesium and vitamins C and the B-complex, especially B_6.

INTESTINAL PARASITES

Although not a frequent topic of discussion, intestinal parasites are a common cause of digestive disturbances in children. Intestinal invaders such as pinworms are easily passed from one person to another through careless hygiene. Pinworms are the most common parasite in children living in temperate climates, which includes most of the United States. These worms can cause anal itching, but they often produce no symptoms at all; many people are therefore unaware of them and never treat them. Today, another parasite, giardia, is becoming more and more common, not only near rivers and lakes in North America, but also in many day-care centers! Giardia is believed to interfere with the digestion of fats; it manifests itself in diarrhea, cramps, belching and weight loss.

A number of culinary herbs can be used to kill intestinal parasites. Ginger has long been used in eastern Africa for this purpose. Researchers discovered that all 42 components in ginger essential oil kill roundworms, among other parasites. Some of these compounds were more effective than the commonly prescribed drug piperazine citrate. Various studies show that thyme and summer savory destroy hookworms and roundworms, and that rosemary, chamomile, elecampane and gentian kill many types of intestinal worms and also decrease intestinal inflammation.

Intestinal Parasite Tea

½ teaspoon chamomile flowers
½ teaspoon each elecampane root,
    ginger rhizome, rosemary leaves and
    thyme leaves
3 cups water
✍ Combine herbs and water in a saucepan. Bring to a boil, then turn off heat and steep for at least 30 minutes. Strain out herbs. For a 50-pound child, give at least 1 cup per day until parasites are gone (you may have to take your child to the doctor to be sure).

One of the best herbal preventive measures and treatments for the whole family, including pets, is garlic. It deters all sorts of intestinal problems, including pinworms, giardia and even intestinal

flu. If your kids will not eat garlic in any form, you can cut a garlic clove in half and rub it on the soles of their feet. This may sound like some sort of agricultural ritual, but it is actually a valid way of taking garlic. Although it is less effective than eating it, in this way garlic is absorbed through the skin and enters the bloodstream. Try it yourself (when you are not going to a dinner party), and you will taste garlic on your breath in less than 30 minutes.

Garlic Vinegar

4 garlic heads, divided into individual
    cloves
1 pint apple cider vinegar
1 tablespoon honey or glycerin (optional)
✍ Using a blender, blend the unpeeled garlic cloves and vinegar thoroughly. Transfer the mixture to a covered container and let sit at room temperature for at least 2 weeks. Strain and discard the garlic. If you wish to sweeten the vinegar, add honey, glycerin or the sweetener of your choice. (Remember that honey should not be given to children under 2 years old.) To treat parasites for a 50-pound child, give at least 3 teaspoons daily. You can also use this formula now and then as a preventive measure. This versatile preparation is good to have around to treat many different conditions. Stored in a cool place, it will keep for many years.

Although herbs are effective in destroying intestinal parasites, they need to be combined with fibrous, raw vegetables to help move things out of the intestine (carrots are a good choice—they contain a compound that kills worms)

In fact, parasites often take up residence when a poor diet has weakened the digestive process. You should also avoid giving your child foods that worms thrive on: starchy products, sugar and milk products. After three days, flush everything out with the Laxative Juice and Psyllium Juice suggested for constipation (see pages 220 and 221). To deter reinfestation, repeat the treatment in a week and again after another week.

To improve intestinal health, look for ways you can improve your child's diet, especially by reducing sweets and starchy foods. Since constipation impairs intestinal health and tone, if your child has been subject to this condition, use the children's remedies suggested for constipation in this chapter.

SORE THROAT, CONGESTION AND SWOLLEN GLANDS

When your child complains of a sore throat, cough or stuffy nose—whether due to tonsillitis, laryngitis, a cold or flu—herbal remedies can come to the rescue. Steaming with herbs or applying a vapor balm brings pain relief, fights infection, and relieves sinus and lung congestion. A sore throat can be treated with an herbal cough syrup, and swollen neck glands can be reduced if wrapped with a neck compress.

Perhaps you have noticed how much easier it is to breathe in a warm, steamy shower when your lungs or sinuses are congested. This is because the steam itself opens constricted air passages. To relieve a sore throat, combat infection

and reduce sinus and lung congestion, you can have your child steam with essential oils of eucalyptus, tea tree or the children's favorite, lavender. These same essential oils can also be added to a bath or put into a commercial humidifier (first make sure they won't harm your machine). When steaming is impractical—say, while traveling—use one of the herbal nasal inhalers sold in natural food stores, or place one drop of essential oil on a cloth, cover your child's nose and have her inhale.

Herbal Steam
1 quart water
3 drops eucalyptus, tea tree or lavender essential oil

❧ Heat water in a pot until it boils. Remove from heat. Add essential oil. Place child's face over the steaming pot, put a towel over the back of the child's head and tuck the ends around the pan to create a mini-sauna. *Caution:* Make sure that the steam is not too hot—it should be comfortable for the child. And make sure she keeps her eyes closed so that the essential oils do not sting. Some children think steaming is fun, but others will object. If so, it may help to eliminate the towel. What is important is to have the child breathe the steam twice a day, or as needed.

Covering your child's chest and throat with a vapor rub of these same herbs is another way to reduce congestion, fight infection and increase blood circulation in the chest area. If you read the label on any commercial vapor balm, you will notice that it contains components of many antiseptic essential oils, including thymol (from thyme), menthol (from mint) and eucalyptol (from eucalyptus). You can buy a commercial balm that contains these essential oils at the natural food store, or you can make your own. Once you apply the Vapor Rub, you can increase its warmth and action by laying a warm piece of flannel on your child's chest.

Vapor Rub

1/4 teaspoon eucalyptus essential oil
1/8 teaspoon each peppermint and thyme essential oils
1/4 cup olive oil

🐾 Combine ingredients in a glass bottle. Shake well. Gently massage onto chest and throat.

A sore throat can also be soothed with preparations of licorice and slippery elm. To stop your child's coughing, add anise, peppermint or eucalyptus to these treatments. As useful as coughing is to breaking up congestion, it can interfere with breathing or sleeping and can irritate the throat. The herbs discussed above are thought to work by suppressing the brain's cough reflex. As an added benefit, they are also antihistamines (which relieve sinus and lung congestion). Two more herbs, rose hips and lemon grass, provide the "anti-infection" vitamins C and A, respectively.

These herbs can be taken as tea, but cough syrup or lozenges will work better to soothe your child's sore or ticklish throat, since they coat the throat. You can purchase herbal cough syrups and lozenges at natural food stores and most drugstores. Or you can make your own herbal cough syrup.

Soothing Cough Syrup

1 tablespoon each licorice root, mullein leaves, thyme leaves, rose hips, slippery elm bark and lemongrass leaves
1 quart water
1/4 – 1/2 cup rice syrup or fruit syrup (or honey, for children who are at least 2 years old)

🐾 Bring herbs and water to a boil in a large uncovered saucepan. Remove from heat, cover and let steep for 30 minutes. Strain out herbs. Return to heat and simmer, then turn off heat. While still warm, stir in syrup or honey. Let cool. Give a suffering child 1 tablespoon, as needed. Store in the refrigerator.

Inspired by the Chinese honeyed licorice, I have developed a recipe for soft Honeyed Licorice Sticks that children can suck on. These are so good that you will need to remind your child that the licorice stick is medicine and not candy; limit him or her to an inch or two a day.

Honeyed Licorice Sticks

1/2 cup water
2 pieces of licorice root, about 5 inches long (available at natural food store)
1 tablespoon honey
1 teaspoon lemon extract or 5 drops lemon essential oil (optional)

🐾 Place water, licorice and honey in a saucepan and bring to a boil. Turn down heat and simmer 5 minutes. Remove from heat and add the extract or essential oil, if desired, and let sit 5 minutes. Strain out sticks and let cool. Store in refrigerator. Note: Remember not to give honey to children under 2 years old.

You can also do what Don does for his nine-year-old daughter, Libby. After taking a number of my classes, he learned how to make all sorts of elaborate herbal concoctions. However, when he or Libby comes down with a sore throat, he sticks to his tried-and-true method: sage tea. He learned of this treatment during his vagabond days traveling across the United States. A man offered to drive him to Don's next location, and Don's throat was so sore that he could barely manage a "thank you." The stranger told Don that a tea of common garden sage would soothe his throat. It worked so well that Don never forgot this simple remedy. Because this tea is fairly bitter, he sweetens it with a little honey before giving it to Libby; she readily drinks it, knowing that her sore throat will soon be gone. You probably already have some sage in your kitchen spice rack.

Sage Tea

1 cup boiling water
1 teaspoon garden sage leaves
¼ teaspoon honey (optional)
🌿 Pour boiling water over leaves and steep for 15 minutes. Sweeten with honey to taste (remember not to give honey to children under 2 years of age). For a 50-pound child, give at least half a cup (if she wants more, that's perfectly okay).

Although incidences of whooping cough, an infectious illness marked by a spasmodic, convulsive cough often followed by a noisy intake of breath, have greatly decreased with the advent of a vaccination against it, some children still contract this bacterial disease. According to the *Merck Manual,* the United States began seeing more cases of whooping cough in the 1980s, and in the early 1990s an epidemic of whooping cough spread through parts of the Pacific Northwest, hitting children who had been fully vaccinated as well as those who had not been. The *Manual* also says that the disease is rarely serious in children over two years old, but the characteristic high-pitched, "whooplike" cough is enough to worry any parent. For whooping cough, follow the treatments suggested for coughs in general. Be sure to use the Vapor Rub (see page 233), since thyme has long been considered an effective treatment for whooping cough.

STOMACHACHE, COLIC AND NAUSEA 🌿

Stomachaches are probably the most common health problem for children; fortunately, they are usually one of the easiest to treat. However, if indigestion is a recurring theme with your child, investigate the cause. The problem may be obvious (for instance, the child may have binged on candy) or more elusive. Other possibilities to consider include bacterial infection, parasites, poor diet—including an excess of refined foods—and food allergies.

Colic, which cramps the intestines and makes babies cranky and irritable, is often attributed to an immature digestive system. But since colic often disappears when the baby's diet (or a breastfeeding mother's diet) is changed, some doctors suspect that food allergies also play a part.

Lemon balm, catnip, caraway, fennel, dill and chamomile resolve most digestive upsets. These gentle and tasty herbs soothe stomachache and gas pains. Kids readily drink chamomile tea when reminded that Peter Rabbit's mom gave it to him after he ate too much, too quickly, while in Mr. McGregor's garden. For centuries, Indian and Lebanese mothers have given their babies dill, and Chinese mothers have traditionally used fennel to ease colic and gas. Nineteenth-century European children were given a syrup of these seeds that was called Gripe Water. Another nineteenth-century indigestion treatment, which is still sold in Europe today, contains fennel, chamomile, caraway, coriander and orange peel.

In a study conducted in Israel, researchers gave infants bottles of chamomile, fennel and lemon balm sweetened with licorice to see if it would really relieve their colic. As any mom who knows her herbs could have predicted, more than half the babies stopped crying and fussing soon after drinking the tea, while most of the infants given plain water continued to fret. The scientists who conducted the study believe that this tea relieves muscle spasms in the digestive tract, which are caused when a baby swallows air while feeding.

In the beginning, I mentioned the creative stories my friend Jennifer told her children to get them to take herbal remedies. In one of these, Grandma Bunny gives her grandkids a tummy tea of fennel, catnip and chamomile. A com-

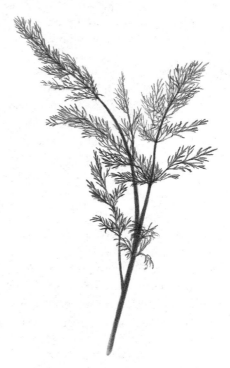

Dill pickles make a tasty snack, but the herb is also effective for lulling small children to sleep.

bination of chamomile, peppermint and red clover is another favorite. If your child likes basil on pasta or cinnamon on oatmeal, you are in luck. Like most culinary herbs, these help to improve digestion.

Peter Rabbit's Tea
2 cups boiling water
1 teaspoon each chamomile flowers and
lemon balm leaves
½ teaspoon each catnip leaves and fennel
or dill seeds

Pour boiling water over herbs and steep for 10 minutes. Strain out herbs and allow to cool. Have your ailing child sip this tea as needed. Sometimes as little as ¼ cup spells relief.

This tea is a wonderful multi-purpose treatment that can be used to address digestion problems as well as the stress and anxiety that can cause these problems. For colic, give your baby Peter Rabbit's Tea, diluted with an equal amount of water in a bottle, before or after eating. Most babies will need only ⅛ to ¼ cup of the diluted tea. You can also try the Tummy Rub Oil suggested below.

Do not overlook the possibility of emotional stress as a source of any digestive problem. Just like adults, children easily transfer unresolved problems and stress into physical ailments such as an upset stomach or bowel irregularities. Most parents know this, but they do not always realize that situations that may seem trivial to them can be quite disturbing for a child. A tea of lemon balm, chamomile, catnip and dill (see Peter Rabbit's Tea on page 235) soothes frayed nerves and anxiety. Because children with indigestion are often cranky, they sometimes refuse to drink even a tasty herbal tea. If this is the case with your child, try an herbal bath or tummy massage, which are soothing and help to eliminate gas pains. You can use essential oils such as lemongrass, orange and chamomile, which have calming fragrances, in either the bath or massage oil.

Child's Indigestion Bath
2 drops lemongrass essential oil
1 drop each orange and chamomile
   essential oils
Add essential oils directly to bath water. Stir to distribute on water's surface before child gets into the tub.

Tummy Rub Oil
6 drops lemongrass essential oil
1 drop each chamomile and fennel
   essential oils
2 ounces vegetable oil
Mix ingredients together. Rub on every hour, or as needed. (In this formula, I've used lemongrass instead of lemon balm, which is very expensive but is also very effective.)

Nausea is another digestion-related problem. Children are especially prone to becoming nauseated while in a moving vehicle, probably because their inner ear structure is so small that the irregular swaying back and forth disturbs the fluid-filled canals in the middle ear. The ear tells the brain that the body is moving, but the eyes say that it isn't. This conflict of information confuses the brain and causes dizziness and nausea. That's why activities like reading or playing lap games while traveling can prompt motion sickness more easily than looking out the window. In fact, a simple solution for "travel nausea" is to watch the landscape go by. This convinces the eyes that the inner ear is correct: The body is moving.

Nausea responds to a simple tea of peppermint, or even sucking on a peppermint candy. Peppermint often prevents vomiting, although not in the case of food poisoning or when the stomach really needs to be evacuated.

Peppermint Tea for Nausea
1 cup boiling water
1 teaspoon peppermint leaves
Pour boiling water over leaves and let sit for about 5 minutes. Strain out herbs and serve at least half a cup. If you

can't find fresh peppermint leaves, you can use commercial peppermint tea bags or even peppermint candy instead.

Another tasty herb that settles the stomach of a nauseated child is ginger. A good way to give a child ginger is by having him drink ginger ale or eat candied ginger, both of which are easy to carry in a car or boat. Sliced, crystallized ginger is sold in the Chinese food section of many grocery stores. If your child feels too ill to eat anything, try the Tummy Rub Oil on page 236.

STRESS, HEADACHES AND INSOMNIA

Children are subject to stress as much as adults are, perhaps even more so; situations that wouldn't faze an adult often push a child over the edge. We tend not to think of children as being tense, so it may come as a surprise that about 20 percent of North American children suffer from serious tension headaches or migraines. Tension is thought to cause the majority of children's headaches and insomnia.

Most parents expect children to be nervous before recitals or tests at school, overexcited about trips or filled with dread when going to the dentist. For some children, though, these emotional states are overwhelming. If nervousness or anxiety seem to come out of nowhere or if your child continually reacts inappropriately for his age, chances are that you have already sought professional help. But if you do not know where to turn, ask your child's school counselor or the local public health facility for resources.

A bit of quiet time and a comforting talk with a trusted adult or some "quality time" with a favorite stuffed animal or pet is often all that a child needs to overcome a stressful moment. A calming cup of tea can also help, and the best choice of herbs for that tea are relaxants such as chamomile, catnip and lemon balm, which soothe pain, nervousness, tension and headaches and even put an over-stimulated, cranky child to sleep. A cup or two of the same tea will also calm the frayed nerves of a worn-out parent!

At a Christmas party I went to one year, I met Maryanne, a spry 85-year-old German emigré with plenty of interesting stories to tell. She told me how she was introduced to herbs at an early age. Each night, Maryanne's mother would give each of her nine children a cup of chamomile tea before bed to calm them down. When the family emigrated—first to Russia, where Maryanne was born, then to the United States, where they settled in Montana—the tradition of an evening cup of chamomile was continued. To this day, Maryanne still drinks chamomile tea when she wants to relax.

Calming Tea
½ teaspoon each catnip leaves, chamomile flowers, passionflower leaves and lemon balm leaves
¼ teaspoon peppermint leaves
2 cups water

Place herbs and water in a saucepan and bring to a simmer. Remove from heat; steep for 15 minutes and strain out herbs. Give this tea freely, as needed.

European children of past centuries were given herb-stuffed "dilly" pillows to send them off to dreamland—these pillows work just as well on modern children and even knock out many adults. Heads begin to nod from simply smelling hops, lavender and dill, while chamomile and thyme help prevent nightmares. If you think this is too simple to be true, just try it yourself. Even I was at first amazed at how well it works. Scientific research in the field of aromatherapy shows that the smell of hops encourages sleep and that lavender is sedating.

Dilly Pillow

5-inch by 10-inch piece of cloth
Equal parts lavender flowers, hops strobiles, chamomile flowers and dill seeds

Fold the cloth in half (so that it measures 5 inches by 5 inches) and sew the edges, leaving an inch open. Combine the herbs and stuff them into the pillow, then sew the edge closed. Slip this pillow inside the child's pillowcase, and she will soon drift off to sleep.

A warm bath or a massage can also relax a child. Most children enjoy the emotionally relaxing fragrances of lavender, chamomile and marjoram, which you can combine with one drop of ylang-ylang. Don't hesitate to give your child a massage. You don't need to know any fancy techniques; gentle, circular motions can be most effective. Remember, though, that children can be very ticklish!

Relaxing Children's Massage Oil

3 drops lavender essential oil
2 drops orange essential oil
1 drop chamomile essential oil
1 drop ylang-ylang essential oil (optional)
2 ounces almond oil (or any light vegetable oil)

Combine ingredients. Use for massage as needed.

Relaxing Bath

2 drops lavender essential oil
1 drop each orange and chamomile essential oils
1 drop ylang-ylang essential oil (optional)

Add oils directly to bath and stir to distribute.

To relieve a headache, place a cool lavender compress on the forehead or over the eyes. Some children also like a warm or cool compress on the back of the neck. You can also serve your child Calming Tea and, if needed, give him a relaxing bath. Remember, though, that while the herbal treatments are good for temporary relief, it is also important to address underlying physiological or psychological problems.

Recurring headaches are a common symptom of allergies, especially to food, and as with any health problem, it is essential to combat the cause as well as to relieve the symptoms. (If food allergies are present, follow the suggestions given in "Food Allergies" on page 226.) If your child suffers from persistent and recurring headaches, or if his headache was caused by a blow to the head or accompanied by a high fever, have the child examined by a doctor to rule out some less obvious disorder.

Headache Compress
8 drops lavender essential oil
1 cup water
Soft cloth

Add essential oil to water and soak a soft cloth in the mixture. Wring excess water from the cloth, then fold and apply it directly over the eyes or forehead or to the back of the neck.

SUGAR BLUES

You will not find sugar blues listed in any medical books, and recent research has offered conflicting evidence about the link between sugar consumption and a child's moodiness. Still, many parents and teachers often complain that too many sweets make children irritable. In a study in which children were fed an amount of sugar equal to that in two frosted cupcakes, the young subjects felt weak and shaky afterward and found it difficult to concentrate or to remain in their seats. The children also responded differently to sugar than adults do. Like adults, their blood sugar levels increased, but unlike adults, their adrenaline levels also increased—an average of ten times higher than normal. No wonder they got the nervous jitters!

If you give an adult-size portion of sugar to a child, the effect is much stronger than it would be on an adult. Clark's Rule (see page 207) can be ap-

plied to colas and sweets as well as to doses of medicine. I'll do the math for you. Let's say your family goes out for ice cream cones and everyone gets a double-decker. According to Clark's Rule, for your 75-pound fifth-grader, eating this cone will be the equivalent of your eating 4 scoops; for your 25-pound tyke, it will be like eating 12 scoops. And sugar is not the only problem. Most parents wouldn't think of giving their child coffee, but colas and other carbonated soft drinks are loaded with caffeine (as well as sugar). For a child, one can of a caffeinated soft drink is equal to an entire cup of coffee for an adult. You can also figure in the eight teaspoons of sugar in the typical 12-ounce can of soda!

Sweet-tasting herbs such as licorice, hibiscus, rose hips and stevia provide a healthy alternative and can replace at least some sweets. Unlike sugar, they will not affect a child's blood sugar level in the slightest. In its native Paraguay, stevia, which is even sweeter than sugar, is used to keep blood sugar levels stable. Peppermint and spearmint are all-time children's favorites. Children also tend to like the sweet and fruity taste of herbs like lemongrass and lemon balm, and the spiciness of cinnamon, ginger and anise. Sarsaparilla and wintergreen taste like root beer. According to studies from the University of Michigan, parents can help curtail the development of a sweet tooth by not dispensing sweetened foods to begin with. Children under two years old are attracted to sweets, but as they grow older, their desire for sugar is based on how much they had as infants.

Herbal Root Beer

2 teaspoons sarsaparilla root
1 teaspoon each licorice root, wintergreen
*   leaves and stevia leaves (optional)*
½ teaspoon cinnamon bark
2 cups water
1 quart carbonated water

🌿 Simmer herbs in the plain water in an uncovered pan for 10 minutes, then remove from heat. Cover the pan and let cool. Strain out herbs, add carbonated water and serve. For variety, you can use flavored carbonated water. Because stevia is sometimes hard to find, it is optional.

Kid's Herbal Punch

2 cups boiling water
1 teaspoon each hibiscus flowers, lemon
*   grass leaves and rose hips*
½ teaspoon spearmint leaves

🌿 Pour boiling water over herbs and steep for 10 minutes. Strain out herbs and let cool. This punch is tasty when mixed with apple juice.

Although this is not exactly an herbal success story, it did impress upon me the importance of offering children herbal alternatives to sweets, such as the herbal root beer described above. When I was employed as a teaching assistant for second-graders, I worked with "problem" children. I needed to be especially patient with Renée, whose attention span lasted only a couple of minutes, and Malcolm, who simply could not stay in his seat, no matter what I did or said. It was only after I posed an addition problem to Renee, using the foods she ate, that I realized her diet was based on

sugar: a doughnut and sweetened juice for breakfast (if anything at all); Twinkies for lunch; cookies, soda pop and a hot dog with ketchup after school; and cake or cookies for dinner. That started me wondering about Malcolm's diet. When quizzed, he admitted that he shunned everything but sweets. He was so difficult to discipline, his mother said, that she always gave up and allowed him to have whatever he wanted. I was, of course, unable to instill changes at home, but when a school breakfast and lunch program was instituted, I noticed a dramatic change not only in Malcolm and Renée but also in other children in the classroom. Almost overnight, their concentration improved. (My job also improved; I was able to focus more on education and less on discipline.)

TEETHING PAIN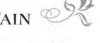

Because a baby's first four front teeth are so sharp, they tend to appear without much fanfare (when the baby is about six months old). The arrival of flat molars a month or two later is a different story. If your baby experiences pains from teething, give her a bottle of Calming Tea (see page 237) diluted with an equal amount of water, then rub the baby's gums with a clove teething oil. Your child will probably also enjoy a hard teething biscuit to gnaw on—try a mini-bagel. If teething is accompanied by a fever, also give a bottle of Fever Tea (see page 226), diluted with an equal amount of water.

Be sure to dilute the clove essential oil first or you may end up with a wailing baby who is screaming more from the treatment than from the teething pain! One time when I was buying groceries, I saw a woman with a fretting baby open a bottle of clove bud essential oil that she had just bought. "Oh no," I thought, anticipating her next move. Before I could reach her to warn her of the consequences, she had slathered her baby's gums with the essential oil. Of course, the baby began to scream.

Joan signed up for my six-month herbal apprenticeship program but missed the first weekend with one of the best excuses I have heard—she was in labor. Joan arrived at our next class with three-week-old Nathaniel, so it was no surprise that for the special project I had assigned her she chose to create an herbal kit for babies. One herbal recipe that came in especially handy was her Gummy Rub, which, like my Teething Oil, contains clove essential oil diluted in vegetable oil. Joan was surprised to see the dramatic change in her happy, mild baby when he started teething. But, of course, she was prepared. After the first application, it took only a few minutes for Nathaniel to calm down.

Teething Oil

4 drops clove bud essential oil
1 tablespoon vegetable oil
Combine ingredients. Try this out on your own gums first and adjust formula accordingly, keeping in mind that a baby's gums are much more sensitive than yours.

THRUSH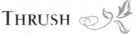

Thrush is a yeast infection that appears as creamy, white patches inside the mouth. It is especially common in babies and young children, and is often accompanied by a fever and poor digestion. Like most yeast infections, it is exacerbated if your child is given antibiotics. Studies from Germany, Russia, England and Hungary show that many essential oils, especially those of clove, tea tree and lavender, inhibit *Candida albicans*, the yeast that causes this infection. These essential oils can be diluted in any vegetable oil in your kitchen, such as olive or safflower. According to research on chamomile conducted in Hungary in 1976 and studies reported in the *Journal of General Microbiology* in 1988, the potent antifungal compounds in garlic and chamomile also combat this bacterium. To help fight thrush, try incorporating these foods into your child's diet.

My herb student Rosemary became concerned when her infant daughter Cerridwyn became unusually cranky and fitful. This concern increased when the baby developed a serious case of diarrhea with lots of intestinal gas. Until this time, Rosemary had treated her daughter's few disorders with simple herbs, but on this occasion all her natural remedies only worked temporarily. Despite all Rosemary's best efforts, Cerridwyn's mouth was soon so raw and painful that she could barely nurse and was becoming dehydrated. Rosemary took the baby to the pediatrician, who said that Cerridwyn was probably just suffering from the flu, which would disappear in a few days. This proved not to be the case, and the problem just got worse every day.

Rosemary guessed that Cerridwyn's illness might be thrush and could therefore be treated with herbs after all. Confirming her guess, a few of the typical white spots that indicate thrush finally became noticeable in Cerridwyn's mouth. Rosemary knew that lavender and tea tree essential oils destroyed Candida, but she also knew that they were too strong to use undiluted in the baby's mouth. She mixed the essential oils in some vegetable oil and gently swabbed the inside of Cerridwyn's mouth with the mixture. Since Candida often spreads to a nursing mother's nipples, Rosemary also treated herself so that she and Cerridwyn would not continue to pass the illness back and forth. For the first time in two weeks, improvement was almost immediate. In another week's time, Cerridwyn was again a happy, healthy baby.

Thrush Oil
8 drops each lavender and tea tree essential oils
2 tablespoons vegetable oil

Combine ingredients. Gently apply oil to inside of child's mouth with a cotton swab or a clean finger. A nursing mother whose child is suffering from thrush should apply this oil to her nipples so that she and her baby do not pass the illness back and forth.

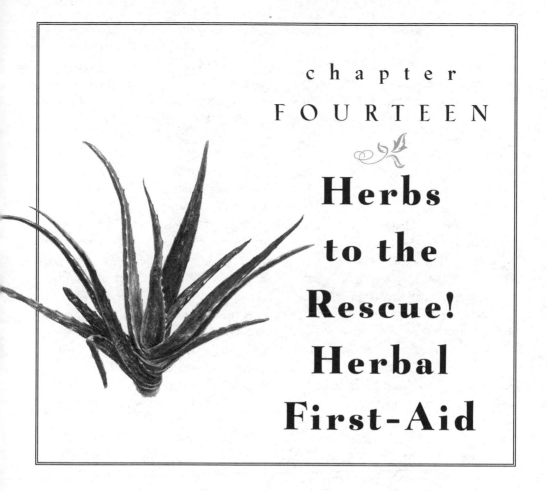

Herbs to the Rescue! Herbal First-Aid

Think of your medicine cabinet as an arsenal full of weapons that you can use to combat a variety of physical ailments. Most likely, the heavy artillery in this arsenal consists of brand-name drugs. I once had a medicine cabinet like that, but 25 years ago, I threw everything—every pill, drop and ointment—into the trash. I then re-created my medicine cabinet from scratch, replacing almost all the brand-name products with herbal remedies.

Why did I turn away from the latest advances of pharmaceutical science and go back to age-old herbal remedies? Although I was familiar with herbs—I'd been cooking with them for years—it had not occurred to me that they could replace all the drugs in my medicine cabinet. One day I picked up an old herb book, and as I read I became aware that my herb garden held more than culinary delights; it contained an entire pharmacopoeia.

Soon thereafter I came down with a flu. I recall thumbing through that old herb book, simply because it happened to be lying beside my bed, and realizing that some of the herbs listed for my condition were growing right outside my door! I stumbled out to the garden to pick my medicine. I can't remember exactly what that first remedy was, perhaps a mullein and yarrow tea, but I do recall my amazement at how well it worked. My second experiment, a concoction for bruises, was equally successful. I decided that the time was right to overhaul my medicine cabinet.

Ironically, the pharmaceutical companies have also begun to catch on. A few years ago, they discovered aloe vera, and now it's hard to find a lotion or baby wipe that doesn't advertise the curative powers of this succulent from the lily family.

You too can adopt a more natural approach to first-aid. This chapter will help you decide what you need to keep on hand and how to use it. But you must be sure that you know when herbs are a reasonable alternative to conventional medicines and when they are not.

Using herbs, you can take care of the same small emergencies that you already treat at home—the minor burns, cuts, scrapes, bruises and sprains that are a part of daily life. Of course, any serious or unusual injuries should send you scurrying for immediate medical attention. If a trip to the doctor is required, stabilize the condition as best you can with herbal remedies, then keep your patient as calm and comfortable as possible. Whenever you have any doubts that you can deal adequately with an emergency, choose the safe route—seek professional advice.

A natural medicine chest should get you through nearly every small emergency that you can reasonably and safely deal with on your own. But its effectiveness depends on your mental preparedness—no matter how many good herbs and gauze pads you have, there's no substitute for knowledge and practice, which will make you completely ready when you face an actual emergency. Once you are standing there with a burned or bleeding finger, it becomes impractical to start paging through an herbal guide, even this one. If you familiarize yourself with the uses of alternative remedies, you'll be prepared for any minor emergency. I recommend taking a first-aid course through the Red Cross, reading the American Medical Association's *Handbook of First-Aid and Emergency Care* and viewing the *Emergency Action* video produced by the American Lung Association. These will make you a better judge of which situations you can take care of by yourself and which ones need a doctor's care.

Of course, it is important not only to know the herbs, but to be able to use them properly—using them incorrectly can do more harm than good. When I was first studying herbs, I decided I should try all the natural remedies that I was learning about before suggesting them to anyone else. I had never seen a recipe for a mustard plaster, so I didn't know that the mustard was supposed to be cut with flour to prevent the plaster from overheating. I assumed that the intense heat I felt was part of the therapy (the "no pain, no gain" philosophy). Finally, with my back well-burned, I frantically peeled off the plaster. This experience taught me two things. The first was that I should never again approach first-aid without being fully informed about what I was doing; the second was that aloe vera sure does heal a burn.

STOCKING YOUR HERBAL FIRST-AID KIT

If you are intrigued by herbal first-aid but simply don't know where to begin, start slowly by stocking your medicine chest with a dozen or so basic, versatile herbs and herbal products that can be used to treat minor injuries. As you begin to feel more comfortable with treatments of this kind, and as your knowledge of herbs grows, you will find yourself turning to herbs first in most first-aid situations. Eventually, you may find yourself preparing your own herbal products and maybe even growing or collecting your own medicinals.

Choose items that best suit the needs of your family. Most of the things you will need can be purchased at a natural food store. Or, if you prefer, you can make your own herbal remedies—just follow the recipes provided in this book. You'll find yourself using salves, compresses, poultices, teas and tinctures (all of which are discussed in detail in chapter 2). Add a few bandages, a pair of tweezers and the usual first-aid paraphernalia, and you'll be all set. I keep my home medicine chest filled with herbal items, an herbal first-aid kit under the seat of my car and a travel bag of herbal remedies ready to pack in a suitcase or backpack. (For first-aid on the go, your supplies should fit neatly into a child's lunch box or a small fanny pack.)

The herbs suggested for first-aid are safe and effective, and generally cause few of the side effects normally associated with pharmaceutical drugs. As with any medicine, though, you should keep these remedies out of the reach of young children, who often eat anything that comes within their reach.

BITES, STINGS AND SPLINTERS

Does the high-pitched whine of a mosquito zeroing in on a patch of exposed skin discourage your next venture past the screen door? Fear not. While nature provides an array of bugs to pester you, she also supplies herbs to stop the itching and swelling of those bugs' bites and stings. There are even natural insect repellents to make flying and crawling pests keep their distance.

Minor bites from mosquitoes and other insects respond quickly to an herbal oil. There are many herbs that stop itching and reduce swelling, but my favorite is lavender, which not only smells great, but also reduces the risk of infection. Since it's neither practical nor comfortable to rub lavender flowers on a bite, use the Insect Bite Oil.

Insect Bite Oil
1 teaspoon lavender essential oil
1 tablespoon vegetable oil
Combine essential oil and vegetable oil and dab mixture directly on bite as needed. Store in a bottle with a tight lid. A glass container is best, but if you prefer a lighter, plastic container, choose one made of oil-resistant plastic (you can find these in camping goods stores). Make sure to keep the Insect Bite Oil away from your eyes.

For the more severe stings and bites of bees, wasps, ticks and spiders, combine lavender with echinacea and bentonite clay into a poultice. The clay pulls the poisonous material from the bite or sting to the skin's surface and keeps it from spreading. Echinacea dramatically lessens any allergic response that might occur. In fact, your patients may feel so good once the poultice is applied that you'll need to remind them to restrict activity for at least 20 minutes to prevent the poisons from circulating through the bloodstream. Lavender stops itching and reduces swelling.

Bite and Sting Poultice
1 tablespoon echinacea root tincture
1 tablespoon distilled water
⅛ teaspoon lavender essential oil
1 tablespoon bentonite clay
Combine the tincture, water and lavender essential oil. Add this mixture to the clay, stirring slowly as the liquid is absorbed. The resulting paste should be tacky enough to adhere to the skin. Apply directly to bite as needed. Store this remedy in a container with a tight-fitting lid, so that the mixture will not dry out. If it does dry out, stir in enough distilled water to turn it back into a paste.

I've put clay poultices on more bites and stings than I can count. Much of this experience comes from the week I spend each summer doing first-aid at a dance camp on a lake in the foothills of the Sierra Nevada mountain range in northern California. Unfortunately, people aren't the only ones attracted to the lake; it also draws "meat bees," pesky wasps that bite or sting with very little provocation. My patients often step on these bees, then tell me in great detail how badly they react to such stings and bites, even as I'm applying the poultice. It doesn't take them too long to realize that their feet have not puffed up like balloons or turned bright red, as they were expecting, and that the pain is gone. Honeybee stings, some spider bites and even scorpion stings (the scorpions there don't have a very strong poison—it won't kill you, but it will produce a nasty sting) all respond quickly to the Bite and Sting Poultice.

You must remember, though, that applying a poultice is only the first step in treating the bites and stings that might cause an allergic reaction. Give anyone who is susceptible to these reactions half a teaspoon of echinacea tincture every ten minutes. I have often seen an allergic response start, then retreat as the herbs take effect. You *must* remember, though, that allergic reactions can have serious consequences. If you know that someone is allergic to a bite or sting from a particular insect, do *not* depend solely on herbal first-aid—immediate medical attention is required. Wheezing, swelling and hives are all indications of a serious, possibly fatal problem that requires immediate medical attention.

Most bites and stings are likely to occur when you are away from home, perhaps on a hike. At these times you may not have your first-aid kit handy, but you can always turn to wild plants for help. Be certain, however, that you correctly identify them and that the plants are clean and have not been sprayed with herbicides. If you are not familiar with wild herbs, check your local bookstore for a good wild-plant identification book that covers the plants in your area. Better yet, check with local herb experts about herb walks offered in your area; herbalists throughout North America give herb walk classes and will personally introduce you to the healing herbs.

In the meantime, I'll start you off with two easy-to-spot herbs you might already be familiar with: plantain and jewelweed. Both of these herbs not only soothe the pain and itching of a sting or bite, but also reduce swelling and even slow down allergic reactions. Since plantain grows wild through lawns and meadows in many parts of the world,

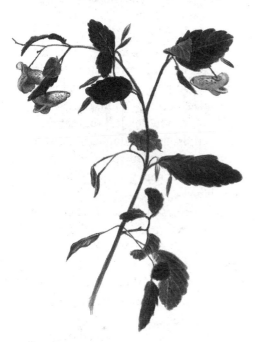

Jewelweed's pretty flowers will liven up any wildflower garden, and the whole plant can be used to produce a yellow dye.

once you're familiar with it you will have a remedy on hand no matter where you travel. Jewelweed is not nearly as common, but it does grow wild in the northeastern part of the United States and in Canada.

For an instant treatment while on the go, chew plantain leaf into a poultice and put it on the injury. Sometimes called "nature's bandage," plantain has the wonderful trait of being able to adhere to the skin without any artificial means. Jewelweed, if handy, is even easier to use than plantain. Simply break a leaf and rub its sticky, soothing juice into your skin.

One of my favorite poultice stories comes from my mechanic, Chris, who decided to investigate the world of herbs by attending one of my herbal first-aid classes with his wife, Darhl. When their dog, Sutter, got an infection between his toes as a result of an embedded foxtail grass, Darhl immediately took action, putting her newfound herbal knowledge to use. Several plantain poultices later, two foxtails had worked their way out and the infection was gone. (This treatment works just as well for stubborn splinters and the infections that can result from them.) Chris was impressed, and when he attended a party at his brother's house and found the family lamenting about yet another $50 veterinary bill for the removal of an embedded foxtail from their dog's paw, Chris offered to treat the dog himself. Not surprisingly, everyone was skeptical, and they were really shocked when he walked into the backyard and began chewing some of the weeds found on the lawn. But Chris knew what he was doing, and the dog's foxtail problem was soon solved. By now, the tale of this herbal feat has been repeated so often that the story—and the cure—is destined to become one of Chris's family traditions.

I can't tell you how many times I've been out collecting herbs in the wild and have brushed up against a patch of nettles. I've also encountered more than my share of red ants. The pain that arises from being "stung" by nettles or bitten by ants is caused by formic acid. Fortunately, this acid can be neutralized by a poultice of yellow dock leaf tincture and baking soda. Yellow dock has long been popular in treating formic acid stings. (The Old English rhyme "Nettle in, dock out, dock rub, nettle out" is a reminder of the effectiveness and tradition of using yellow dock for this purpose.) Of course, there is always a chance you will run into ants or nettles without having any baking soda nearby. If this happens to you, just reach for some yellow dock leaves, crush them between your fingers, and as the rhyme says, rub them on.

Ant Bite/Nettle Remedy
1 teaspoon baking soda
½ teaspoon yellow dock leaf tincture
🌤 Stir the baking soda and tincture together into a thick paste. Apply directly to bite. If remedy dries out, simply add enough yellow dock tincture to turn it back into a paste.

As an herbalist, I spend a lot of time outdoors foraging for medicinal plants, so I've certainly come to appreciate the importance of an effective repellent—a nontoxic, herbal one, of course. Natural,

essential oil–based repellents have become so popular that you can find them not only at natural food stores, but also at most drugstores and sporting goods stores. Or you can make your own, using my recipe.

Insect Repellent
2 ounces vegetable oil or vodka
¼ teaspoon each citronella and
*   eucalyptus essential oils*
⅛ teaspoon each pennyroyal, cedar
*   and rose geranium essential oils*
🌤 Combine ingredients and apply mixture directly to all exposed skin. Keep oil away from eyes and mouth—take care not to rub your eyes right after applying the repellent with your fingers. This repellent will keep for at least a year.

While I can't prove that herbal insect repellents work any better than the standard drugstore variety, they do present some stiff competition. Herbal repellents have a more pleasant fragrance than their drugstore counterparts, and using them is certainly preferable to rubbing toxic chemical repellents into your skin.

I've successfully used this herbal repellent in my own backyard and have sent bottles all over the world: into the insect-filled tropics of Thailand, India, the Caribbean and the Amazon and to the high plains of China and Tibet, not to mention the southeastern United States. Everyone who has used this bug "dope" has given me glowing reports on how well it works.

Because insects have an amazing sense of smell, odor is used as the basic element in most repellents. Mosquitoes, ticks and many other crawling and flying pests hate the smell of herbs like eucalyptus, pennyroyal and citronella; unfortunately, so do quite a few people. Combine these herbs and you end up with a great insect repellent that also fends off your friends. I have found that the pungent smell of eucalyptus and citronella becomes more pleasant with the addition of rose geranium—but only for humans, not for insects. Despite its sweet smell, rose geranium is great for keeping bugs away.

Another herbal method for reducing the insect population hovering around you is to light a citronella candle. These candles release the citronella scent continuously as they burn. They are available from most camping goods and household stores and catalogs. Or you can make your own by taking a votive candle and using a dropper to slowly saturate the wick with about 20 drops of citronella oil, which is available at most drugstores. Allow two hours for the wick to absorb the oil; the candle is then ready to use.

BLEEDING

If the sight of blood makes you woozy, you are not alone. I find, however, that being prepared by knowing what to do in an emergency really makes a difference.

The next time you are confronted with an injury, consider that a small amount of bleeding has its advantages. Bleeding cleans dirt and foreign particles from a wound, and when blood is exposed to air, it forms an important fibrous substance called fibrin. This fiber creates a netting that entangles other blood cells so that they clot into a scab.

I've been in quite a few situations where bleeding was serious and something needed to be done right away. Certain herbs can be applied directly to the wound. If this does not stop the bleeding, place an herbal compress over the injury and apply pressure. A flat object, such as a credit card, inserted into the folds of the compress can help distribute the pressure. While administering herbal remedies, you should also try to slow the flow of blood by raising the injured area higher than the heart. For deep cuts, or if bleeding does not stop within a minute or two, be sure to get medical help.

While preparing dinner you cut yourself with a knife. What do you do? Reach for the spice rack! Powdered cayenne, the same pepper used in chili powder, will quickly staunch bleeding when sprinkled directly on a wound. It will also reduce the time it takes for a scab to form. I realize that putting cayenne on a wound sounds as if it might be more painful than the injury itself, but the pepper not only arrests bleeding but also contains a substance that reduces pain: capsaicin, the same stuff that makes cayenne peppers hot. Researchers have discovered that capsaicin suppresses a chemical that carries the pain messages from nerves in the skin to the brain.

Powdered kelp (a seaweed used as a salt substitute) has been used in England for centuries as a folk remedy to arrest bleeding. During World War II, when medical supplies became scarce, British medics used it extensively in the field.

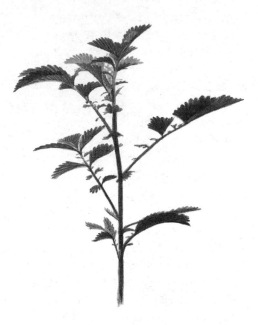

Because of its tall flowering stalks, agrimony is nicknamed "church steeples."

Agrimony, plantain and yarrow are versatile herbs that arrest bleeding and encourage scabbing. You can either sprinkle the dried and powdered leaves of these herbs directly onto a bleeding wound or make a poultice from the fresh plant. I have nicked myself so often on stakes or rosebushes while gardening that it has become second nature when this happens to grab a leaf of plantain, agrimony or yarrow, mash or chew it into a poultice and press it on the bleeding area. I know that a few readers will cringe at the idea of chewing their medicine, but in an emergency, most people out on a stroll or having a picnic would rather staunch a sudden cut with a wild plantain leaf than bleed all the way back to the house. Just be certain that you properly identify your herbs.

Legendary in its ability to arrest bleeding, yarrow is a common wild plant that also decorates herb and flower gardens. Its Latin name, *Achillea,* comes from Achilles, the name of a soldier-doctor who dressed the wounds of Greek troops during the Trojan War. Plantain, like yarrow, has a long history as a treatment for battle wounds. English children still refer to it as "soldier's herb" or "kemp" (from *cempa,* the Anglo-Saxon word for "soldier"). Plantain is a good herb for you to be able to recognize because it seems to grow everywhere—in the United States, you will even find it growing in vacant city lots.

Like many herb gardeners, I grow agrimony and have always been impressed by how quickly it slows bleeding. Various kinds of agrimony grow in many parts of the world, including China, and studies reported in Chinese medical journals, as well as the *American Journal of Chinese Medicine*, found that this herb stops bleeding and doubles the speed of formation of scabs. The same studies cited the discovery that agrimony controlled hemorrhaging after surgery within two minutes. Actually, I knew that agrimony slowed bleeding long before I read these reports. It was mentioned in the English poet Geoffrey Chaucer's fourteenth-century work "The Yeoman's Prologue" and was made into a famous sixteenth-century wound wash called arquebusade water, which is still sold in France.

Keep in mind that treatment with powders and poultices made with these herbs is an emergency tactic only. Although the herbs quickly arrest bleeding, they are not antiseptic enough for long-term healing. Unseen infection can hide beneath a lumpy scab thickened with herb powder. Once bleeding is arrested, the area needs to be cleaned and disinfected with an antiseptic.

Another way to arrest bleeding is to swallow two capsules of cayenne or a tincture of shepherd's purse. Both herbs take only a few minutes to begin working—which is hard to believe until you've seen them in action. They are useful whenever there is substantial bleeding or when direct pressure with a compress isn't possible—for example, if you are treating a wound near your eye. This is exactly what happened to me one day. I had a blood blister on my eyelid that was very bothersome. I kept thinking that it was a bug and trying to flick it off. After one really strong flick, I could hardly stop the bleeding. But I was in my kitchen, and cayenne powder was within arm's reach. I mixed about half a teaspoon into a quarter-cup of water and drank the mixture. The bleeding ceased within a minute. The only disadvantage to this treatment is that on an empty stomach it occasionally creates a slight burning sensation; to avoid this unpleasant feeling, have a light snack or something to drink as soon as the emergency is over.

A few years ago, I went on a camping trip in the mountains with some of my students and their families. One of the teenagers was slicing a watermelon with a deer-skinning knife that was at least three times larger than was required for the job. I was wondering if I should remind him to be careful when the knife slipped and went into his hand. We

were an hour away from the nearest doctor. I ran to get my first-aid kit, and everyone nearby went into action. We coated the wound with cayenne powder, and the boy's father pressed an antiseptic compress soaked in lavender water over it. We also had the boy take two capsules of cayenne with some water. The cloth quickly became blood-soaked, but we were ready with more cayenne and another compress. The bleeding quickly subsided. We also put a cool lavender compress over the boy's eyes, since he was starting to feel faint. (I also had to lay the poor father down and place a lavender compress on his forehead before he fainted.) We followed up with herbal treatments to prevent infection, and the wound quickly healed.

Incidentally, the same herbs that work for bleeding wounds also work well for nosebleeds. You might also hold a compress—the colder, the better—firmly over the bridge of the nose. Then sit down and lean forward, tucking your head between your knees so that the blood doesn't run down your throat and choke you. As an added measure, or if the nosebleed is severe, place another compress (also cold) on the back of your neck and apply pressure directly to your upper lip.

Many things can provoke a nosebleed. Among the most common are a sinus infection, a blow, excessively dry air conditions or weak blood vessels. Frequent nosebleeds may indicate that you have a serious problem, such as anemia or high blood pressure, so see a doctor if you are prone to this condition.

In addition to using a compress, you can also stop a nosebleed by sniffing one of these powdered herbs. I assure you that this sounds much worse than it really is. It takes only a small amount and the results are dramatic.

Herbal Compress to Stop Bleeding

1 teaspoon tincture of yarrow (or other suitable herb)
½ cup water
Soft cloth

🌿 Combine ingredients. Soak the cloth in the liquid, wring it out and apply it with pressure over the wound.

BRUISES

Medical dictionaries define a bruise as "an injury just below the skin where the skin is not broken," although most of us would settle for describing it as an uncomfortable nuisance with unsightly discoloration. Actually, many bruises are so minor that after announcing themselves with a few moments of intense pain, they seem to go away. Be warned, however—if the bruising was caused by a heavy impact, the underlying muscles, bones or organs could be injured, so call a doctor if you're in doubt as to the severity of the injury.

If you bruise easily and seem never to be without a few discolored spots, you should probably look beyond simple first-aid remedies. Easy bruising may be an indication that you have weak blood vessels or a problem with blood clotting. See chapter 4 for suggestions of herbal treatments to strengthen blood vessels. You should also consult a physician, because easy bruising may indicate a serious problem.

For simple, uncomplicated bruising, herbs can be quite helpful. One day I

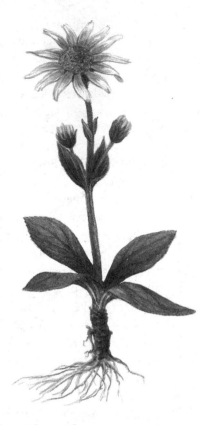

The eighteenth-century writer Johann Wolfgang von Goethe gave arnica credit for saving his life by relieving his angina attacks.

was potting some herbs and went prancing at high speed across my stone-filled driveway, arms full of plants. I tripped and went sailing across the rocks, herbs flying in all directions. I received a deep scrape on my knee, but that was nothing compared to the assortment of bruises inflicted by those rocks. I limped over to pluck a plantain leaf to stop the bleeding. Then I thought to put my misery to some good, so I tried an experiment. I put Saint-John's-wort tincture on half the bruises and arnica tincture on the other half. Like a true scientist, I even left a few small bruises untreated. The result was a tie between the two tinctures: By the next day, the discoloration was fading on both sets of bruises, and in a few days my skin no longer looked like a calico quilt. The untended bruises, however, did not fare so well. Even though they were very minor, they remained visible and painful long after the other bruises disappeared.

The best herbs for treating bruises are those that discourage swelling and promote quick healing, such as arnica, chamomile, lavender, Saint-John's-wort and witch hazel. In Germany, pharmacies sell more than 100 different arnica preparations to reduce inflammation caused by bruises. Arnica is also popular in North America, although many herbalists use Saint-John's-wort instead because it grows much more abundantly. Another classic North American folk remedy for the treatment of bruises is witch hazel tincture, which is conveniently sold at drugstores. The distilled witch hazel that is commonly sold in drugstores does not contain the astringent tannins that reduce bruising, but folks still swear by it. For even better results, purchase a witch hazel tincture at a natural food store.

I was at a picnic once when a young boy fell out of a tree. He received several bad bruises that began to swell almost immediately. My herbal first-aid kit was in my car, a good 20-minute walk away, but growing right near the tree was some Saint-John's-wort. While I collected some leaves, I thought, "How can I best chop this to release its healing properties?" The answer was obvious— I popped the herb into my mouth and

chewed it. And yes, it tasted terrible. A few minutes after the poultice was on the child's bruises, the swelling receded and his crying was reduced to an occasional sob.

Whichever herb you choose, the sooner you dab on the oil or tincture, the better. To further diminish swelling, apply a tincture-soaked compress that has ice slipped inside its folds. Or use herbal ice cubes, which you can make from a strong tea (use two teaspoons of herb per cup instead of the standard one teaspoon) of any of these herbs. (Do not place ice directly on the skin.) Keep your Herbal Ice in the freezer so that it is always handy for an emergency.

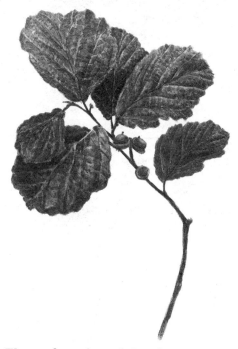

The medicinal witch hazel tree, which grows some 15 feet high and about as wide, is an excellent choice if you're looking for some shade in your garden.

Bruise Compress

1 tablespoon tincture of arnica flowers,
Saint-John's-wort flowering tops,
witch hazel bark or chamomile
flowers
4 drops lavender essential oil
2 tablespoons cold water
Washcloth

Combine ingredients. Soak a washcloth in the herbal water to make a compress. Wring it out and place it directly on the bruised area. To keep the compress extra-cold, insert an ice cube (regular or herbal) inside the folded cloth.

Herbal Ice

1 cup water
1 teaspoon chamomile flowers
1 teaspoon lavender flowers

Pour boiling water over the herbs and let steep in a covered pan for about 15 minutes. Strain out the herbs and freeze the tea in medium-size ice-cube trays. Once the cubes are frozen, pop them out and store them in a plastic bag in the freezer. Herbal Ice can be applied directly to the bruise or wrapped inside the Bruise Compress.

BURNS AND SUNBURN

I confess that I am attracted to hobbies that often lead to burns. I like to make scented candles with hot wax, boil up herbal jellies and candies and use a hot-glue gun on dried herbal wreaths. It's no wonder I learned early to keep an herbal burn remedy nearby! I'm sure you are familiar with the discomfort of a burn, whether it is caused by an herbal hobby like mine, a hot kitchen pan or a long day under the sun. Sunburn, after all, is essentially just another kind of burn,

usually less severe in intensity but dangerous at times because of the large area of skin affected. Although the causes of these burns are not the same—sunburns are the result of prolonged exposure to ultraviolet light, and standard burns are caused by physical heat—the symptoms are the same. The burned skin swells, blisters and sometimes even peels off. Underneath, dilated blood vessels leak toxins into the inflamed area, which causes further skin irritation. For the most part, burns and sunburns respond equally well to the same herbal treatments.

Whenever you are in doubt about a burn's severity, seek help from a professional health care practitioner. Burns from chemical and electric shocks require special treatment, and a superficial burn over a large area can be more serious than a deep, small burn, because extensive nerve damage and dehydration are possible. After a doctor has treated even serious burns, herbal remedies are wonderful elements to incorporate into your follow-up care.

For any minor burn that you can confidently treat yourself, the rule is immediate action. First, cool the burned area by immersing it in cold water or applying ice for about a minute—the cold numbs the pain and prevents further injury. Then reach for the herbs. Whether you treat your burns with an herbal remedy of your own making or with a commercial treatment, you should avoid using oil-based products, such as salves, on all but the most minor burns. Oil retains heat and inhibits air circulation and drainage, all of which combine to slow the healing of a burn.

According to John P. Heggers, M.D., director of research for the Division of Plastic and Reconstructive Surgery at Wayne State University in Detroit, it is the center of a burn that receives the most heat, and it is the skin there that suffers the greatest damage. Surrounding tissue is often injured, but seldom destroyed; it will, however, die in two days if not treated.

I have been impressed by the burn-healing effects of certain herbs since I went to an herb retreat more than 20 years ago. All those who attended spent a lot of time in the sun that weekend—too much time. The staff and some of the students traveled there and back in a school bus; on the way home, everyone compared sunburns. As I worked my way from seat to seat, burn remedy in hand, the bus became an herbal burn clinic on wheels. The "oohs" and "ahs" of my patients communicated their instant relief. After a couple of rounds at my "clinic," bright red skin had dulled to a healthier pink. Everyone asked what herbs were in my magic formula.

Actually, the recipe contained only two primary ingredients: aloe vera and lavender. Both of these are star performers when it comes to burns. They ease pain and swelling, help repair damaged cells, deter infection and help prevent burns from scarring. It's no wonder that many hospitals use aloe and that it is the main ingredient in many burn remedies sold in pharmacies and drugstores. (If you buy your burn remedy already prepared, look for one that is at least 90 percent aloe.) Studies conducted at Wayne State, the University of Chicago Hospital and the University of Miami Medical School show that aloe vera not only reduces burn damage and promotes new skin growth, but also stops cell destruction caused by inflammation.

If you are lucky enough to have your own aloe vera plant, remove an outer leaf from the plant (leaving the younger, inner leaves undisturbed). Peel off the thin, green skin from a small section of the leaf, and rub the gel-like substance from the inside directly onto the burn, as often as needed for relief. Stored in the refrigerator, the unpeeled leaf should keep for at least a week.

Homemade Aloe Gel

¼ cup peeled aloe vera leaves
150 International Units vitamin C
    powder

🍃 Puree aloe leaves in an electric blender, using enough leaves to make ¼ cup of puree. Stir in vitamin C powder as a preservative. Store in the refrigerator—cold helps burns to heal.

Aloe is not the only herb that can be used to heal burns. There are a number of other herbs and essential oils that can help injured skin to regenerate, including calendula, chamomile, comfrey, Saint-John's-wort, plantain and, as mentioned earlier, lavender. The last one is my favorite. Time and again I have seen the almost miraculous burn-healing power of lavender essential oil at work. Like other essential oils, lavender needs to be diluted; I combine it with aloe vera. It was lavender that came to the rescue of the French chemist Dr. René-Maurice Gattefossé when his hand was badly burned in a freak laboratory accident. He was so impressed by how quickly this essential oil healed his hand that he began a study of medicinal essential oils and later became known as the "father of modern aromatherapy."

I heard a similar story from an Oregon woman who runs an essential oil distillery. After badly burning her arm when the distiller's boiler exploded, she plunged it into the essential oil she had just distilled. By the time she got to the hospital, her burn was already healing—the emergency staff was amazed. They could not believe that the accident had occurred less than an hour earlier.

One of the best ways to apply a burn remedy is to spray it on. (The spray can also be gently dabbed on very minor burns.) In this way, you don't have to touch sensitive, burned skin. Also, a spray feels cool on a burn.

Aloe Burn Spray
4 ounces aloe vera juice
½ teaspoon vitamin E oil
  (or 2 400–International Unit capsules)
⅛ teaspoon lavender essential oil
🖎 Combine ingredients. Pour into a spritzer bottle (which can be found at most drugstores). Shake well. Spray on burn as needed. The vitamin E will promote healing. Make sure that you use aloe vera juice, not gel, which will clog the sprayer.

Another good treatment for burns is a cool wash or bath that contains lavender and oatmeal. (This is especially good for a light sunburn that covers a large area.) My friend Terry was badly burned when she tripped and fell into a camp-

fire. Terry knows her herbs well. Her mother and friends spread a concoction that was mostly aloe vera on the burns, and Terry took nutritional supplements and drank an herbal tea to promote healing. As soon as she could bathe, she spent four weeks taking daily baths of skin-healing comfrey, plantain, calendula and lavender. I saw the burns during their various stages of healing and watched as new, unmarked skin gradually replaced the old without leaving a trace—not even one scar—of that unfortunate accident.

Bath for Burns
1 quart boiling water
¼ cup each comfrey leaves, plantain leaves and calendula flowers
3 drops lavender essential oil
1 cup colloidal oatmeal (a finely milled oatmeal available in most drugstores) or regular oatmeal milled in a coffee grinder
🖎 Pour boiling water over herbs. Steep for 20 minutes. Strain. Pour the "tea" into a cool bath. Stir in lavender essential oil and colloidal oatmeal.

CUTS AND SCRAPES
Minor cuts and scrapes will probably cause you to reach for your herbal first-aid kit more often than any other injury. The first step with wounds of this kind is to bring the flow of blood to a halt (see "Bleeding" on page 249). Once you've stopped any bleeding, you must treat the wound to prevent infection and promote speedy healing. I cannot count the number of times that people have shown me a wound that they have treated with

herbs and asked, "Can you believe how fast this is healing?"

My computer's hard drive is filled with file upon file of research studies about the effects of different herbs. Some of these studies show that tea tree, lavender, lemon, thyme, sage, eucalyptus and garlic function as powerful germ fighters. Others show that lavender, lemon, bergamot, thyme, chamomile, pine and sandalwood (in that order) increase the number of white cells, which gobble up infection-causing bacteria. According to world-renowned essential oil expert Ernest Guenther, Ph.D., tea tree essential oil was added to machine oils used in ammunition factories in Australia during World War II. This greatly reduced the number of infections that occurred when workers cut themselves on the metal filings. One very popular antiseptic herb is goldenseal, but I prefer to use barberry or Oregon grape root, since goldenseal is endangered in many parts of the United States. To encourage healing, try plantain, comfrey, aloe vera, lavender, baptisia, calendula, Saint-John's-wort and rose geranium. Although they are not quite as effective, cinnamon, eucalyptus, garlic, lemon, oregano, sage, sandalwood, tea tree and thyme can be used for the same purpose. In clinical studies, aloe vera has been shown to increase blood flow to the injured area, thus accelerating the healing process.

Antiseptic and healing herbs like these can be used in salves, sprays, diluted essential oils or poultices. The type of injury and its location dictate the most appropriate application. Salves, for example, adhere to the skin and form a protective layer to protect minor scrapes and cuts. A salve generally promotes healing and also has some antiseptic properties.

Herbal Healing Salve

2 ounces dried comfrey leaves
1 ounce dried calendula flowers
2 cups olive oil
1 ounce pure beeswax (available at bee
   supply stores and crafts shops, or
   from a beekeeper)
4 drops each tea tree and lavender
   essential oils

Heat herbs in olive oil over low heat for about 5 hours. Do not let the oil boil or bubble. A Crock-Pot or the lowest temperature setting on a range should be suitable for heating this mixture. (If the lowest setting is too hot, turn off the heat once it has warmed the oil—it should keep warm for at least an hour—then repeat the process twice.) After cooking, strain out the herbs while oil is still warm.

Place 1¼ cups of the herb oil in a pan, add beeswax and heat just enough to melt the wax. Add essential oils and stir. Finally, pour the salve into widemouthed jars. Store at room temperature.

Sprays, which can be potent antiseptics, are good for raw wounds or any injuries that you want to avoid touching. When essential oils such as eucalyptus, tea tree and lemon are used as a spray, the germ-killing properties of these herbs are increased by being combined with oxygen.

Lemon and Tea Tree
Antiseptic Spray

⅛ teaspoon each lemon and tea tree
*   essential oils*
½ ounce tincture of goldenseal, Oregon
*   grape root or barberry bark*
1½ ounces aloe vera

~ Combine ingredients in a jar and shake well twice daily for a week to help disperse oils. Keep in an atomizer. Shake before each use. (This formula represents the ideal 2 percent dilution proven in studies to be the most effective.)

Essential oils can also be rubbed directly into the skin to deter or destroy

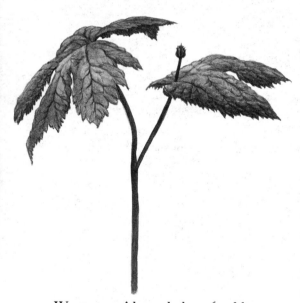

Westerners' knowledge of golden-seal as an antiseptic and healing herb goes back at least as far as 1650, when a French Jesuit in the United States reported that "it closed up all kinds of wounds in a short time."

an underlying infection. Because these oils are diluted in an oil or alcohol base, they should not be applied directly on serious wounds—they should instead be rubbed on the skin surrounding the injury.

Poultices, which can be used to draw out infections, are generally reserved for serious wounds or those that do not heal properly, since they require fresh plants, take time to prepare and can be messy.

The experiences of my friend Ron reveal a successful herbal treatment of a potentially serious infection. One day, when he was cutting weeds, the weed-eater flung a nail into his leg. Ron went to the doctor, but even though the wound looked insignificant and Ron had recently had a tetanus shot, the doctor told him to use an antiseptic and come back the next morning if an infection developed. Within a few hours, the area around the hole had become swollen, red and painful, and the entire leg felt very hot. Ron could not wait until morning to have the wound treated. He decided to try an herbal treatment and allow a few hours for it to take effect before making a trip to the hospital.

Ron needed a strong antiseptic that would penetrate below the skin's surface. Not wanting to take any chances, he decided to use two herbal treatments. He rubbed a diluted antiseptic essential oil around the circumference of the hole. He also crushed garlic into a poultice and put it directly over the wound, binding it in place with a gauze bandage wrapped around his leg. He repeated this treatment every hour.

When Ron removed the first poultice after one hour, there seemed to be little change. If anything, it was slightly worse. However, an hour later, the red color and swelling were noticeably reduced. He continued this treatment for a few hours, then fell asleep. When he awoke the next morning, there was no sign of infection.

Skin-Healing Poultice

1 handful fresh comfrey or plantain
    leaves
½ cup water

Place ingredients in a blender and mix into a thick slurry. Spread on wound, holding the poultice in place. Leave poultice on for 20 to 60 minutes. It will be messy, but it will be effective. To store this poultice for future emergencies, freeze it in ice cube trays, then store the cubes in a plastic bag or freezer container. When you need a poultice, thaw out a cube in a pan.

Infected cuts and scrapes sometimes call for internal as well as external action, especially if an infection is more than skin-deep. Tip-offs include wounds that take longer to heal than seems reasonable and infections that seem to spread, traveling through the bloodstream and reappearing in new areas. When an infection travels from the location of the original wound and takes hold elsewhere, there is usually an accompanying fever. If this happens to you, it means you have

a spreading systemic infection, in which case you must see a doctor immediately.

While Ron applied a poultice to treat the external infection, he also swallowed a tincture of echinacea to encourage quick healing and to build up his immunity from the inside. For recurring or extremely stubborn infections that you are unable to conquer, try the Wound-Healing Tea. (You can also drink this tea periodically as a tonic to help keep you healthy.)

Wound-Healing Tea

1 teaspoon each astragalus root, baptisia
    root (if available) and echinacea root
3 cups water

Combine herbs and water in a saucepan. Simmer for 2 to 3 minutes, then remove from heat and steep for 20 minutes. Strain and serve. Drink 3 to 4 cups throughout the day to fight an active infection. (These herbs can also be taken as tincture: 30 drops, 3 or 4 times a day.)

Researchers have begun to find explanations for some of these age-old herbal treatments. Studies conducted in Germany show that a compound found in echinacea stabilizes hyaluronic acid, a substance found in the body that protects cells and connective tissue from caustic chemicals secreted by germs that can often penetrate cell walls. Researchers have found that drinking aloe vera juice once a day speeds healing, probably because it increases the amount of oxygen carried by blood to cells and strengthens collagen, the fiber that supports cells. You can purchase an aloe juice tonic in some stores, or you can make your own by mixing half a cup of aloe juice with half a cup of fruit juice.

FAINTING AND DIZZINESS

Standing up too quickly or overexerting yourself can cause you to feel faint, and a strong emotional shock or the sight of blood is enough to set some folks' heads swimming. Fainting may be accompanied by a cold and sweaty feeling, or an uncomfortable sensation in the pit of your stomach. All this happens because your brain is not receiving enough blood. If you become dizzy on a regular basis, see your doctor to rule out a deeper physical problem. Probably no one was better prepared for fainting than the Victorians, who revived themselves by sniffing lavender and camphor salts as well as inhaling the aroma of "swooning" pillows filled with lavender flowers. Although fainting is not nearly as common these days as in the Victorian age, almost everyone has a dizzy spell or becomes faint once in a while.

Lavender is still the herb of choice to relieve occasional dizziness and fainting, although any herb with a sharp fragrance, such as rosemary, eucalyptus and tea tree, will do. To take advantage of these herbs' revivifying effects, place a hot compress on the back of the neck and another on the forehead. The fragrance and heat work together to in-crease circulation. Combine this treatment with the conventional helpful hint offered by doctors: Get your blood flowing into your brain by placing your head between your knees or by lying down. When you are able to swallow, take a hot drink.

Lavender Compress
5 drops lavender essential oil
2 cups water
Soft cloth
❧ In a small bowl, combine essential oil and water. Soak cloth in lavender water and wring it out. Fold cloth and apply it to back, neck and forehead.

For your traveling first-aid kit, you can take a hint from the Victorians and carry smelling salts. After I smashed a vial of rosemary in my car door and later found the lid of a bottle of lavender essential oil loose in my purse, I decided that salts are more practical to carry than bottles of essential oils. Although you can no longer buy smelling salts, you can easily make your own.

Lavender Smelling Salts
½ teaspoon rock salt
5 drops lavender essential oil
❧ Place salt in a nonporous container. Add essential oil drop by drop. The salt will readily absorb the oil. Carry your salts in a closed container. Open and sniff as needed.

FROSTBITE

When winter arrives, most people have a tendency to spend more time inside. But for those who work or play outdoors, cold can be a real danger. Fingers, nose, ears, toes and cheeks are most vulnerable to Jack Frost. Normally, blood keeps these extremities warm, but when extreme cold restricts the flow of blood, frostbite can occur. At first, the skin turns red and feels tingly, then it becomes white and numb as cells begin to die from lack of blood. A person suffering from frostbite needs to be quickly warmed both inside and out by drinking warm water (or tea) and by having warm water poured over the chilled area. This brings blood and warmth back into chilled areas and stops further damage. *Warning:* Be sure that the water is warm, not hot, as frostbite makes skin more vulnerable to being burned.

Because frostbite can be serious enough to lead to amputation, seek medical help immediately if sensation and color do not return quickly to the skin. If your toes and fingers get cold easily even when you are bundled up, you may have poor circulation; for herbal ways to improve your circulation, see chapter 4.

You may be surprised to learn that aloe vera works as well for frostbite as it does for burns, and for many of the same reasons: It promotes new skin growth, fights off infection and soothes injured skin. According to studies from the Department of Surgery at the University of Texas Medical School in Galveston, aloe vera also warms a frostbitten area by increasing blood flow. And aloe will help heal blisters that form as a result of frostbite. When treating frostbite, it is also advisable to take herbs that stimulate the circulation.

I live in snow country and love to ski and explore the winter countryside, but I have never personally experienced

frostbite. I use herbs to prevent it. I sprinkle small amounts of powdered cayenne pepper and ginger into my socks and gloves before heading outside. Ski resorts have also discovered the secret of these herbal warmers. On a ski trip to a resort near Lake Tahoe, I saw foil packets of foot- and hand-warming herbs in the ski store—at five times the price the same herbs sell for in the grocery store! One problem with these herbs is that cayenne lightly stains white socks. My solution? Wear colored socks.

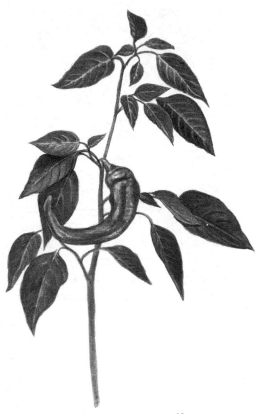

Cayenne certainly is hot stuff—and not just on your tongue. It can also be used to keep your extremities warm and prevent frostbite.

Foot-Warming Powder

1 tablespoon cayenne powder
1 teaspoon ginger powder

👃 Mix the powders together and store. Sprinkle ⅛ teaspoon into each sock to keep your toes warm. And remember, if you touch the powder with your fingers, be sure to wash your hands thoroughly before getting them near your eyes—cayenne burns!

HEAT EXHAUSTION AND SUNSTROKE

Just like your car, your body can get overheated when the air temperature soars or when you overexert yourself. This sometimes results in heat exhaustion or, even more serious, sunstroke.

Heat exhaustion typically begins with a wave of dizziness and is often accompanied by weakness and tingling sensations. The skin becomes pale, cool and clammy, and the pulse weak, but the body's temperature remains normal. These are signs that you have lost too much fluid and too many important minerals. In an attempt to cool down, the body begins to sweat; as a result, you lose even more water and salt. The opposite symptoms—high fever, lack of sweating and a bounding pulse—indicate sunstroke, which should be treated by a health care professional as soon as possible. While waiting for medical help, cool down the victim with ice water, by having him drink it and/or by applying compresses, or by placing him in a cold bath (if possible).

Heat exhaustion can generally be self-treated, but your body needs to cool down quickly to avoid further damage, such as delirium, elevated blood pressure and even coma. A person experiencing heat exhaustion might be confused and in need of your help. Keep this person quiet and comfortable. To replace lost fluid and minerals, give him miso soup, fruit juice or one of the drinks designed to replace electrolytes lost by athletes during a workout. Also, place the cool Lavender Compress suggested for dizziness (see page 260) on the victim's forehead.

Heat stroke can occur in the most unexpected places. I once experienced it in a Native American sweat lodge. I'd just flown across the country and had had far too little water to drink on the way. I recall feeling very dizzy and disoriented once I got into the lodge. Fortunately, I was among herbalists. An herbalist friend named Cascade Anderson looked at me and summed up her diagnosis in one word: electrolytes. Another herbalist friend, Michael Tierra, produced some miso soup, and I swear that soup never tasted so good! Since then, I have carried packets of instant miso soup in my first-aid kit. Of course, now I am more careful to avoid becoming dehydrated, but I have had occasion to share the soup with others.

To prevent overheating, the Chinese drink a tea of mulberry leaves, licorice, ginseng, peony root and peppermint. I often work in my garden under the hot summer sun, and even though I always wear a large straw hat and cool, light-colored clothing, I occasionally become lightheaded. I find that this tasty tea not only prevents heat exhaustion, but also increases stamina. Mulberry leaves and peony root can be ordered through a natural food store or a Chinese herbalist.

(You can also use the leaves from your own mulberry tree, if you happen to have one in your yard.) For this recipe, the mulberry leaves should be dried and cut into small pieces.

Heat Exhaustion Tea

1 teaspoon each mulberry leaves, peony root bark and peppermint leaves
½ teaspoon each licorice root and ginseng root
1 quart water

❧ Combine the herbs and water in a saucepan and bring to a boil. Turn down the heat and simmer for at least 20 minutes. Remove from heat and strain herbs. Drink a cup before venturing out into the sun. (This formula can also be taken as a tincture: 30 drops in hot or cold water makes an instant tea.) This recipe is adapted from the traditional Chinese formula.

POISON IVY, OAK AND SUMAC

Poison ivy, poison oak and poison sumac are famous for the itching and oozing rashes they can cause. Despite their names, these plants are not really poisonous—their danger lies in an allergen called urushiolir. These notorious plants are related; if you are allergic to one, you are probably allergic to all three. The itching, blistering rash usually associated with the "poison plants" appears any time from a few hours to a few days after exposure. Other possible symptoms include nausea, tiredness, mental disorientation and fever. Very bad cases can cause breathing difficulties and kidney damage, requiring medical attention. Some people are very lucky—they don't react at all to these plants.

The best way to protect yourself from poison ivy, oak and sumac is, of course, to stay away from them. Some people have told me how they have built up an immunity to these plants by eating small amounts of them in the spring. While this may be true, I have also heard from individuals who developed poison oak in their throats by trying this.

If you touch one of these plants, wash the oil off with soap and water, or at least cold water, as soon as possible. (In the wild, I use nature's soaps, such as soapwort, soap root or deer brush blossoms.) Even scrubbing with dirt helps remove the offending oils and possibly offers another advantage—the roots of poison ivy and possibly poison oak exude a substance into the surrounding dirt that is an antidote to the plant's sap.

The pain, swelling, itching and blistering caused by poison ivy, oak and sumac can be alleviated by quite a few herbs. In 1980, after observing that fresh plantain poultices immediately reduced swelling and itching in ten of his patients, Serge Duckett, M.D., reported that plantain was a "blessing for those who must have a constant supply of calamine lotion or cortisone." Jewelweed, also effective in fighting reactions to the "poison plants," grows in the eastern and central United States, and was so well-known in the 1950s that several commercial poison ivy products were based on a jewelweed compound. Comfrey and aloe vera also promote healing and soothe skin irritated by reactions to these plants.

Unlikely as it may seem, the essential oil of simple peppermint can give you hours of relief from itching by soothing inflamed nerve endings. Although lingering in a hot bath is not recommended, a short shower in water as hot as possible and washing with a liquid peppermint soap can provide at least temporary relief for many poison ivy, oak or sumac sufferers. You might also try a lukewarm bath with herbs, oatmeal and Epsom salts. For oozing rashes, mix an herbal paste with ground oatmeal to cover the rash. Your resistance to poison ivy, oak and sumac can also be improved with immunity-enhancing herbs such as chamomile, echinacea and licorice, all of which work specifically to quell the allergic response.

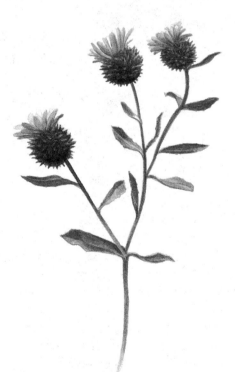

In some areas of the world, children use the "resin" that forms on grindelia's flower heads as a chewing gum.

You may need to experiment a bit to find the remedy that works best for you. My dance teacher, Cathy, seems to come down with at least one really bad case of poison oak each year. Not only is this uncomfortable, it also makes it difficult for her to teach and impossible for her to dance professionally. Just as she begins warming up, the itching increases. In addition to being a dance teacher, Cathy is a registered nurse who studies herbs. She says that she has tried almost every-thing, but being a nurse has made her reluctant to treat her poison oak with powerful steroids like cortisone, which can have long-term side effects. While not all physicians agree that cortisone is a strong medicine when applied exter-nally, most holistic-minded medical doc-tors have another opinion. Andrew Weil, M.D., author of the popular book *Nat-ural Health, Natural Medicine,* calls corti-sone steroids "dangerous drugs" and says that they are "much misunderstood, abused and over prescribed." He goes on to say that they "suppress rather than cure disease, and reduce the chance of healing by natural methods. . . . All of these products are absorbed through the skin to one degree or another, and all of them can suppress activity of the thy-mus, the lymph nodes and the white blood cells." Dr. Weil suggests not using these steroids in any form until you have tried all other forms of treatment. If you must take them, he says, you should limit their use to a few weeks.

Cathy seems to be of a similar mind. Her solution was to use a homemade herbal paste of oatmeal, grindelia, comfrey and peppermint salt. Below are two versions—one liquid, the other paste—of my formula, which uses the same herbs.

Poison Ivy, Oak and Sumac Remedy

2 tablespoons each tinctures of grindelia flowers (or jewelweed leaves) and comfrey leaves
¼ cup vinegar
3 drops peppermint oil
½ teaspoon salt

🍃 Combine ingredients in a jar. Shake well before each use. Apply as needed.

Poison Ivy, Oak and Sumac Paste

⅛ cup Poison Ivy, Oak and Sumac Remedy
⅛ cup distilled water
¼ cup colloidal oatmeal or 1–2 tablespoons bentonite clay

🍃 Stir liquid ingredients into clay or oatmeal to make a paste. (If colloidal oatmeal is not available, you can grind your own by putting whole oatmeal in a coffee mill or blender.) Store in an airtight jar. Reconstitute with distilled water as needed.

Poison Ivy, Oak and Sumac Bath

4 drops each peppermint and lavender essential oils
4 cups colloidal oatmeal
1 cup Epsom salts

🍃 Add ingredients to lukewarm or cool bath water. You can also choose to sponge this formula onto the afflicted area, rather than taking a bath in it.

SHOCK

Treating shock is most certainly a job for health care professionals, but you never know when you might encounter someone in shock. If you do, you can provide interim treatment herbally, but remember that shock must be treated by a medical doctor. A few years ago, my landlady's young grandson ran up to me saying, "Grandma just fell off the roof and wants me to get you." I am afraid I nearly knocked him over in my haste to get to her. Except for a bruised knee, Marion didn't appear to be injured. She kept insisting that she was fine and just needed help getting to her couch, but as I eyed the distance from the roof to the hard ground below, I wasn't so sure. I do not have x-ray vision, so I could not spot internal injury, but it was easy to see that she was in shock. She was chilly, obviously dazed and insisted that she did not feel any pain.

Not to be dissuaded, I encouraged her to stay lying down and placed a lavender compress on her head. What she most appreciated (and remembers to this day) was the Rescue Remedy that I handed her as her son-in-law arrived to take her to the emergency room. This combination of flower essences, which is sold at natural food stores (ask for it by name!), is designed to ease shock and stress. Marion took a few drops every few minutes, and she swears that this is what got her through the ordeal and kept her from falling back into shock. She successfully used it again when she went into the hospital for surgery to repair her knee, which she injured when she fell.

Shock can result from a number of situations, including injury that results in loss of blood, reaction to a drug, poisoning, serious infection, internal bleeding and severe dehydration. Extreme emotions—anger, fear and even joy—

can also cause a person to go into shock. When this happens, the heart's action is reduced—it does not receive or send out enough blood—and the skin pales, lips and fingernails may turn bluish, the pulse weakens and breathing becomes more rapid as the body struggles to get more oxygen.

People in shock may be oblivious to pain or very alert, and they may not realize that they need help. It may be up to you as a bystander to take charge. In assisting a shock victim, have her lie down, and do your best to keep her as warm and comfortable as the situation allows. If possible, elevate the victim's feet so that more blood is sent to the brain. In general, keep a clear head and maintain a reassuring presence. It is often other people's panic that pushes an injured person into shock. Be sure to get professional help, even if the person begins to recover in a few minutes. Shock can also indicate a serious underlying problem, so be concerned if someone goes into shock for no apparent reason.

One day, when a neighbor boy was playing under a car that was supported on a jack, the jack slipped and the car dropped almost to the ground, trapping the child. Fortunately, he was a little tyke, so he wasn't crushed by the vehicle. His sister ran to get me, but by the time we reached the boy, chaos had broken out among panicking neighbors and relatives arriving on the scene. Some family members were not comfortable with the idea of me using herbs to help him. It was too bad. Within minutes, his little teeth were knocking together, his eyes had turned glassy, his pupils dilated and he broke

out into a cold sweat—typical signs of shock. It turned out that he was not hurt a bit, but still had to be treated for shock at the hospital.

To snap a person out of shock, use any strong fragrance, such as lavender, eucalyptus, tea tree, rosemary or peppermint. Gently wave a scented cloth near the victim, put a lavender compress on his forehead, or simply crush a few leaves under his nose. Don't provide anything to drink, even herbal tea, because the victim may not be able to swallow.

SPRAINS AND STRAINS

An active lifestyle generally makes for a more healthy person, but it also has its drawbacks. For one thing, an afternoon of digging up plants, rearranging furniture or participating in your favorite sport makes you more prone to wrenching an ankle or waking up with stiff, painful muscles. Even those who seldom venture from their easy chair find themselves with an occasional sprain or strain, sometimes just from using a muscle in an unaccustomed way.

It's easy to be confused about the difference between a sprain and a strain. Sprains occur at the joints when ligaments, the fibrous tissues that hold together two bones that meet at a joint, are pulled and overstretched. Strains happen when the muscles themselves, or the tendons that hold them in place, are pulled or torn. Either condition can result from exerting the body past the strength of your muscles or joints. Sprains and strains have many things in common, including swelling and pain. The first signs of trouble are rapid swelling, heat, pain and limitation of

YOUR HOME MEDICINE CABINET: QUICK REFERENCE

THE BASICS

Aloe Burn Spray
Arnica Tincture
Bite and Sting Poultice
Herbal Compress to Stop Bleeding
Herbal Healing Salve
Herbal Ice
Herbal Liniment
Homemade Aloe Gel
Insect Bite Oil
Insect Repellent
Lavender Essential Oil

Lavender Smelling Salts
Lemon and Tea Tree Antiseptic Spray
Miso Soup Packet
Poison Ivy, Oak and Sumac
    Remedy/Paste
Roll of Gauze Bandage
Saint-John's Strain and Sprain Oil
Skin-Healing Poultice
Soft Cloth for Compresses
Wound-Healing Tea/Tincture
Yarrow Tincture

OPTIONAL EXTRAS

Ant Bite/Nettle Remedy
Comfrey Leaves
Foot-Warming Powder
Heat Exhaustion Tea

function. A sprain often becomes bruised and discolored as blood from broken blood vessels and fluid from surrounding tissues seep into the damaged area (this sometimes happens with strains as well).

Treat a sprain or strain as soon as possible. There are two options for home treatment: herbs and RICE, which stands for rest, ice, compression and elevation. In other words, raise the injured area, higher than the heart if possible, to drain excess fluid. Keep the injured area from moving. Decrease swelling with ice and a compress of arnica or Saint-John's-

wort, applied with light pressure. (Never apply ice directly to the skin; wrap it in a towel first.) After about 20 minutes, remove the ice for 15 minutes, then apply more ice. Repeat process as often and as long as necessary to reduce the swelling.

Strain and Sprain Compress

1 to 2 teaspoons tincture of arnica flowers
    or Saint-John's-wort flowering tops
2 tablespoons cold water
Soft cloth

Combine the tincture and water in a bowl. Soak a soft cloth in the mixture and apply compress to injured area.

It is important that you take good care of these injuries; if left untreated, they can cause repeated problems. Untended ankle sprains, considered the most common athletic injury, can plague you for years, sometimes for your entire life. A simple strain or sprain seldom needs a physician's care, unless the joint feels loose or unstable, or the injury is extremely swollen or painful. If you're at all unsure about the severity of an injury—it can be difficult, for instance, to know whether or not a bone has been broken—treat it first with herbs, then see a doctor. After a serious sprain, strain or even broken bone has been treated by a doctor, you can enhance long-term healing with the Skin-Healing Poultice suggested for cuts and scrapes (see page 259) applied over a generous layer of Saint John's Strain and Sprain Oil.

Saint-John's Strain and Sprain Oil

2 ounces Saint-John's-wort oil
⅛ teaspoon lavender essential oil
8 drops marjoram essential oil
2 drops chamomile essential oil

Combine ingredients. Apply to skin over injury as needed.

At a recent herb seminar I found myself rooming with another herb teacher named Suzanne, who had become a good friend during the last few years. I was surprised when she said to me, "I suppose you don't remember when I was an herb student and you helped treat my sprained foot, but I want to thank you again."

Years ago, when we were participating in a traditional Native American dance on uneven ground, Suzanne stepped into a gopher hole and badly wrenched her ankle. Someone who knew that I habitually carry first-aid herbs tapped me on the shoulder and I was soon at Suzanne's side, rubbing Saint-John's-wort essential oil onto her ankle. She was in so much pain that she had to be carried back to her cabin. I handed her the bottle and suggested she apply the oil liberally every 20 minutes. The next morning, Suzanne, walking as if almost nothing had happened, returned a half-empty bottle of Saint-John's-wort oil.

Modern fitness specialists advise that one way to avoid injury to your

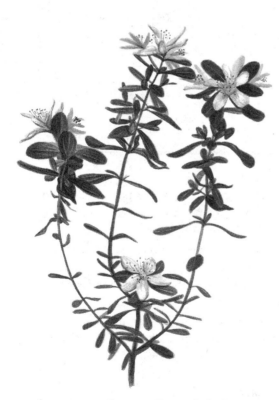

In ancient Greece, Saint-John's-wort was thought to protect against evil.

muscles and ligaments is by doing warm-up exercises that stretch, loosen and warm muscles before you work out or do strenuous labor. Stretching, however, isn't the only way to warm up. Frank G. Shellock, M.D., a research scientist at Cedars-Sinai Medical Center in Los Angeles, found that applying a liniment prior to a workout increases blood flow to the treated area and significantly warms it up. This isn't to suggest that an athlete, or even the occasional jogger, should forgo physical warm-ups in favor of a liniment, but it's not a bad idea to use both.

A liniment also helps after soreness has set in. It has a curious way of relieving pain by tricking the brain. Pain creates a reinforcing loop between the muscle and brain; the muscle cries, "Oh, it really hurts!" and the brain agrees. All this focus on pain makes it hard for the tightened muscle to relax. The heat from a liniment diverts the brain's attention from the muscle to the burning sensation created on the skin, providing the muscle an opportunity to relax. Actually, the peppermint or camphor essential oil in liniment activates both hot and cold nerve impulses in the skin. When the brain receives alternating messages of hot and cold, the contrast between the two makes a liniment seem much hotter than it really is. One way to increase a liniment's heat even more is to rub it into the skin. Experts say that this friction doubles the sensation of heat.

Most liniments also contain other essential oils that provide a sensation of heat, such as cinnamon or cayenne, along with muscle relaxants, such as ginger and rosemary. In fact, many arthritis and sore-muscle liniments from centuries ago have rosemary as their basic ingredient. There is an old story about Elizabeth of Hungary buying a secret beauty formula from a hermit in 1235. The formula turned out to be made up mostly of rosemary vinegar, and rumor had it that the mixture was as much for the old queen's rheumatism as for her complexion. Whatever the case, a young prince fell in love with her, and today you can still find Queen of Hungary's Water along with other herbal liniments at drugstores and natural food stores. Or you can make your own (instead of using rosemary vinegar, as the Queen did, I use rosemary essential oil).

Herbal Liniment

½ cup olive oil
8 drops each eucalyptus, peppermint and rosemary essential oils
4 drops each cinnamon and clove essential oils

Combine ingredients. Rub into sore, cramping muscles as needed. This is hot! Keep it away from your eyes.

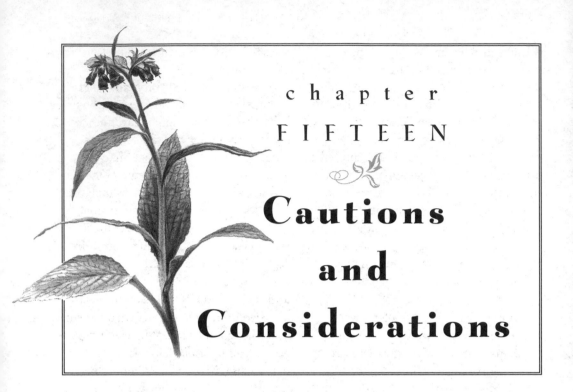

FIFTEEN

Cautions
and
Considerations

One of the great advantages of
using herbs for health and
healing is their relative safety.
Although herbs are generally safer and
carry fewer side effects than pharmaceutical drugs, not all herbs are harmless at
all dosages. Safe and rational use of
herbs requires an understanding not
only of what and how much to use, but
also of what not to use.

Some herbs, including old-time
favorites such as comfrey, are the subjects of hot debate. Some experts believe
that comfrey is completely safe; others
believe that it carries some dangers. In
many of these debates, a lot of contradictory evidence being tossed about. For the
most part, I have played it safe—when
confronted with the choice of whether to
include the most controversial herbs, I

decided to leave them out of this book.
However, since scientific understanding
changes as each new study presents new
data, it is possible that some of these
questionable herbs will once again come
to be regarded as safe.

Potential toxicity is not the only factor to consider when choosing which
herbs to use and which not to use. A few
herbs have become so popular that they
are being overharvested. The use of pesticides and fumigants on herbs are cause
for still more concern.

The subject of which herbs are safe
and which are questionable can be very
confusing, especially since there are so
many unsubstantiated theories floating
around. To help you out, here are some
guidelines and some background information on how some of these debates

got started. This should help as you work your way through the aisles of the natural food store, trying to determine how to improve your health safely.

SAFE IN MODERATION

Herbalists have always known that some herbs need to be used more carefully than others. And some plants are downright poisonous. With a few herbs, however, there is a fine line between toxic and medicinal. That line is often determined by the dose.

Most of the herbs suggested in this book are safe even if you take them in much larger quantities than suggested, but there are a few that must be used in moderation—or side effects may occur. When a certain herb has potential side effects, I have noted it in the text. This possibility should not, however, scare you away from using the herb—since herbal side effects are generally much less significant than pharmaceutical side effects. Even the Food and Drug Administration (or FDA; the government agency that regulates the sale of drugs in the United States) which takes a very conservative stance regarding herbs, has sanctioned the moderate use of many of the herbs mentioned in this book.

One common herb that can have side effects is licorice. We generally think of this herb as being safe—most of us associate it with candy—but taking large quantities can lead to sodium retention and potassium loss, which in turn can cause water retention, high blood pressure, headaches, shortness of breath and

sometimes even heart problems. Experts writing in the *Journal of the American Medical Association* described one licorice lover who ate so much candy (two to four ounces a day for seven years) that he landed in the hospital with weakness and hormonal imbalances.

Just chewing and swallowing licorice-flavored tobacco hospitalized another fellow. As a result, licorice is not recommended in any form if you have high blood pressure or kidney disease or if you are pregnant. If you fit into any of these categories, you should be careful even with drugstore laxatives that contain licorice—most use highly concentrated extracts.

Other herbs that can raise blood pressure when taken in large amounts are ephedra, angelica, black cohosh (which also causes dizziness and irritates the nerves) and ginseng, according to some reports. Ephedra and the caffeine-rich plants coffee, guarana, maté and kola nut stimulate the adrenal glands and can make you nervous, cause your heart to race and make it hard for you to sleep. Chances are that if caffeine were a new drug today, the FDA would approve it for prescription use only. Caffeine and derivatives of ephedra are added to diet and energy formulas that speed up your metabolism in an unhealthy way. These stimulants should be used sparingly or—even better—not at all. Several deaths have been linked to misuse of ephedra, so it's best to use this herb under medical supervision.

Other herbs that affect the adrenal glands include gentian and vervain. Gentian can make your body more sensitive to the adrenal hormone adrenaline.

It is safe for most people to use, but in Germany people with high blood pressure are discouraged from taking it. Vervain has quite the opposite action, slightly depressing the heart rate, at least in animals, and constricting the bronchials. You should avoid it if you have asthma. To be on the safe side, if you have high blood pressure or a heart condition, do not use any of these herbs without professional advice.

There are also a few herbs that can foster digestive problems. Large quantities of hydrangea root or of extremely bitter herbs such as gentian and quassia, for instance, can cause nausea and vomiting. Generally speaking, if you become queasy after taking a particular herb, you are probably taking too much of it. (Remember, if you're sensitive to the herb, what's fine for someone else may be too much for you.)

Other herbs may impair your body's assimilation of vital nutrients. No one is sure, but some herbalists think that long-term use of garlic, goldenseal and, to some degree, barberry and Oregon grape root eventually depletes your intestinal flora and thus reduces the amount of nutrients you assimilate, especially B-complex vitamins. Taking large quantities of horsetail can create a deficiency of vitamin B_1. When it comes to horsetail, you should use only the young plants, since older plants develop a toxic compound.

Long-term use of an irritant-type laxative herb such as cascara sagrada or senna causes potassium loss and electrolyte imbalance, which can irritate an existing bowel problem. (Electrolytes are important minerals such as sodium, magnesium and potassium.) One woman developed hepatitis after a month of taking sennoside B, an active compound isolated from senna, but it turned out that she was taking ten times the recommended maximum dose!

RARE REACTIONS IN SENSITIVE INDIVIDUALS

A few herbs are photosensitive—if you go out in the sun after ingesting them, you might have a skin reaction. There are very few such documented cases, but reactions generally occur within 24 hours and only in individuals who are especially sensitive. Even some very common fruits and vegetables, such as figs and carrots, can cause this reaction. Don quai, the related angelica and yarrow are potential herbal culprits. Lovage causes photosensitivity in animals but apparently not in people (although anyone with weak kidneys should not use it). Applying bergamot essential oil to your skin can also cause this reaction, unless you get a version of the oil from which the reactive compound, bergaptene, has been removed (it will say "bergaptene-free" on the label). Other citrus essential oils, especially lemon, are said to sometimes cause a photosensitive reaction.

A number of fresh plants, such as goldenseal, blue cohosh, mullein, elecampane, motherwort, parsley, hops and dandelion, can cause itching or a skin rash in sensitive individuals. This reaction is rarely more than bothersome, and if you react to one of these plants, this does not necessarily mean that you will react to the others.

Some herbs—cayenne, for instance—can cause a burning sensation on sensitive skin. Researchers at the University of Chicago Hospital dubbed cayenne's painful sting "Hunan hand" because cooks working in Chinese restaurants often experience it. These researchers found that soaking the peppers in vinegar for a few hours neutralizes the reaction. Fat and alcohol can be used to relieve the pain, so next time you accidentally chomp down on a hot pepper camouflaged in a plate of Hunan bean curd, try taking a sip of milk or beer. Garlic and other pungent herbs can irritate and even burn sensitive skin. Large amounts even make some people's eyes more sensitive to light.

It is probably obvious, but if you are a hemophiliac or are scheduled for surgery, you should avoid herbs that have anticlotting properties. These include turmeric, alfalfa and motherwort. Ginseng, feverfew and garlic also thin the blood to some degree.

The immune herb baptisia contains a substance that is known to be toxic to animals in large amounts—it has poisoned animals who have overgrazed on it—but I could find no reports of it producing a toxic reaction in people. Baptisia is commonly used in Sweden, but is classified as a drug there.

THE NEW HERBAL OUTCASTS

Although herbs have been used for centuries, there are some very common herbs whose possible toxic reactions have begun to be noticed only recently. Unfortunately, every time an herb is even remotely connected with toxicity, it makes headlines. At the same time, side effects and deaths from pharmaceutical drugs generally receive less media attention. Actually, toxicity from medicinal herbs pales in comparison with injuries resulting from prescription drugs and even vitamin supplements. For example, according to the Consumer Product Safety Commission in Washington, D.C., six children died in the United States in 1993 and three in 1994 as a result of taking products that contained iron. No deaths have been reported from the low doses in children's chewable vitamins.

I suspect that some undiscovered factors cause certain people to be more susceptible to certain herbs than others. Researcher and herb toxicity specialist Ryan J. Huxtable, Ph.D., who works at the Department of Pharmacology at the University of Arizona, notes that taking anticonvulsant drugs with the herbs comfrey, coltsfoot or senecio increases the toxicity of certain compounds found in the herbs.

Simon Mills of the Centre for Complementary Health Studies at the University of Exeter in England also found evidence of complications when certain pharmaceutical drugs and an herb were taken at the same time. Mills reported on one woman who developed liver toxicity while taking the drug Indapamide in combination with various herbs, including germander. Another woman suffered the same effect with a Lorazaepam/herb combination that may also have included germander. A third case involved a group of Native Americans who were poisoned after eating a species of *Heliotropium;* it was discovered that the two who died were also taking phenobarbital to treat epilepsy.

An existing medical condition may also make you more susceptible to the side effects of certain herbs. An example is a thirteen-year-old boy who developed liver dysfunction after eating comfrey regularly for about three years—he may have been more susceptible because he had an inflammatory bowel disease. There are also cases of people developing liver problems while taking chaparral and senna to correct skin problems, but this connection is less clear—skin problems are often related to existing liver imbalances.

In one laboratory study, when experimental animals were fed a diet that was about one-third comfrey, they developed cancer of the liver. And a few cases of liver damage (although not cancer) were reported in people who had ingested large amounts of comfrey. The offending agent in comfrey has been identified as pyrrolizidine alkaloids. More than 200 types of these compounds are found in various other plants as well, including the medicinal herbs coltsfoot, borage, lungwort, senecio and dusty miller. (Borage seed oil contains such small traces of these compounds that it is considered safe.) When animals were fed large amounts of the pure pyrrolizidine alkaloids derived from coltsfoot, they experienced liver toxicity. In 1987, after a woman who drank tea that included coltsfoot gave birth to an infant with severe liver injury, Germany banned any herb containing these alkaloids.

Most medical researchers assume that comfrey is perfectly safe if used externally—for instance, in poultices and salves—but are wary of using it internally, even though practically no alkaloids are found in the dried leaves. Comfrey's fresh root is especially potent—about ten times stronger than the fresh leaves. Germany and France permit the use of comfrey for external use on unbroken skin. Canada allows the sale of only the species that do not contain the strongest alkaloids, such as *Symphtum officinale.* According to experiments done in Sweden, boiling herbs containing pyrrolizidine alkaloids in water for 20 minutes makes them nontoxic; nevertheless, Sweden classifies both comfrey and coltsfoot as drugs. Until herbs containing these compounds receive a clean bill of health, it is best not to take them for internal use but to rely on other herbs instead.

Another herb in question is chaparral. People take it because it contains NDGA (nordihydroquaiatetic acid), a strong antioxidant and anti-cancer agent. Herb industry surveys show that more than 200 tons were sold in the United States between 1970 and 1990. And during this time, there was not a single complaint of side effects arising from the use of this herb. When two to three cups of chaparral tea or the isolated NDGA were given daily to more than 50 cancer patients, the only side effects were occasional nausea or diarrhea. Very large doses resulted in lowered blood pressure. These and other studies led the National Cancer Institute to state in 1989 that "acute toxicity of NDGA is not great."

With all of these essentially positive reports, FDA chemists, who still have not found any liver toxicity in chaparral, were puzzled when a woman developed hepatitis after taking it for three months to treat breast lumps. It turned out that she was downing a whopping 15 tablets a day—far in excess of the recommended dose. This story did not attract much attention until 1992, when three people who were taking two or three tablets daily developed liver problems that did not go away until they discontinued the herb. As a result of these cases, the FDA issued a public warning that a "casual relationship" exists between chaparral and liver problems.

The herb germander also seems to be problematic. In France, seven people came down with acute cases of hepatitis while taking capsules or a tea of wild germander to lose weight. All seven recovered after discontinuing the herb, but three of them developed signs of liver problems as soon as they resumed taking it—researchers suspect that the problem was the result of an allergic reaction. Because of this situation, French manufacturers voluntarily stopped marketing germander; in 1982 the government banned its use.

The root bark of sassafras contains the compound safrole, which is banned by the FDA for use in food, along with sassafras. This ban was instituted in 1960, after laboratory animals developed cancer when injected with large amounts of safrole. The flavoring used in root beer must be "safrole-free." Smaller amounts of safrole are also found in black pepper, star anise, basil, cinnamon leaf, nutmeg, sage and witch hazel, but

so far these herbs have not come under fire.

The results of some studies suggest that comfrey, coltsfoot and sassafras may have anti-cancer properties—in one study, a comfrey leaf tea was shown to decrease tumor growth. Bruce Ames, Ph.D., Chairman of the Biochemistry Department, University of California, Berkeley, has said that the risk of one cup of root tea is comparable to that of a peanut butter sandwich, a diet soda containing saccharin and one raw button mushroom. Mice given an extract made from the whole comfrey plant had their immune systems stimulated. When people were given small doses of safrole, it did not create any cancer-producing substances. This led researchers to suggest that the toxic reaction in humans is different from that in rats. It seems that we have much more to learn about determining herbal toxicity.

SOME OLD CAUTIONS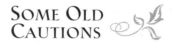

Medicinal herbs with established histories of producing serious side effects are best used only under the supervision of a professional health care practitioner who is knowledgeable about herbs. Lobelia and pokeweed, a strong antiviral agent that stimulates the immune system, are two classic examples. Both irritate the digestive tract, cause vomiting and decrease respiration. The FDA restricts lobelia's general use, but does permit the sale of pills to help stop smoking. Pokeweed leaves are sometimes eaten as a wild vegetable, but in 1981 a group of campers became ill hours after dining on them, even though they had boiled the leaves twice.

USING HERBS AND ESSENTIAL OILS SAFELY

All essential oils need to be used with care because they are so concentrated— generally, one drop equals one to two cups of tea. In many cases, ingesting one ounce of an essential oil can be fatal. Aromatherapists say that unless you are a skilled practitioner, you should use essential oils only on the outside of the body. For internal use, it is far safer to use a tea, tincture or pill. Be sure to keep essential oils away from children.

The essential oils of wormwood and tansy should not be used at all—these plants contain thujone, which can cause seizures. If you want to use the herbs, you must also be careful. The essential oils of wintergreen and thyme can irritate the skin, even when diluted.

Pennyroyal developed a bad reputation in 1978 when one unfortunate 18-year-old woman died after downing an entire ounce (two tablespoons!) of the essential oil while trying to discontinue a pregnancy. After that, the FDA declared that the essential oil and the herb itself must be labeled "for external use only." According to Norman Farnsworth, Ph.D., professor of pharmacology at the University of Illinois, Chicago, an ounce of pennyroyal essential oil equals roughly 75 gallons of the tea!

You should also avoid using any strong herbs or herbal derivatives during pregnancy. This includes goldenseal, barberry and Oregon grape root; laxatives such as senna and cascara sagrada; and coffee, kola nut and guarana, all of which contain caffeine. Also watch out for herbs that produce hormonal actions, don quai, fenugreek and red clover among them, and uterine stimulants such as aloe, fenugreek and rue.

If you are pregnant, you should also avoid large quantities of herbs with aspirin-like actions, such as willow and meadowsweet, because aspirin itself has been linked to birth defects. Chances are that this is not true of aspirin-like herbs, but you might as well play it safe. Black cohosh and blue cohosh are sometimes used during the last few weeks of pregnancy to prepare the uterus for childbirth, but if you are interested in using these herbs, I recommend that you find someone who is experienced in herbs to work with you.

MISTAKEN IDENTITY

When herbs were commonly used as general medicines in the nineteenth and early twentieth centuries, the *U.S. Dispensatory* gave pharmacists detailed directions on how to determine if they had the right plant. Later, as herbalism in North America began to be replaced by medical science, knowledge of herbs became more rare, and herbs offered for sale were often misidentified and mislabeled. Over the years, this has presented numerous problems for the herb industry. Fortunately, herb companies are now beginning to pay more attention to the sources and proper identification of their herbs.

Misidentification is at the heart of the bum rap that some herbs get. As if comfrey does not have enough problems, some toxic side effects ascribed to this plant were actually due to poisonous foxglove leaves that had been mistaken for comfrey. After drinking what they thought was comfrey tea, one elderly couple in Britain developed great thirst and urinary problems. The next day they hallucinated that monkeys, bugs, black clouds and burglars were prancing through their house. After being admitted to a hospital, the man collapsed with a coronary, but then slowly recovered. In 1983, a Mississippi woman who drank comfrey tea to mend a broken hip experienced blurred vision and nausea that were later attributed to foxglove.

Skullcap has also been the subject of mistaken identity. According to an investigation of herbal products in the United Kingdom in 1984, very little real skullcap is sold commercially, since this small plant is not easy to grow or harvest on a large scale. Instead, germander is sold as skullcap. This means that germander was probably responsible for two "skullcap" poisonings reported by the Riks Hospital in Norway in 1991. In Wales, four women who took the stress pills Neurelax and Kalms experienced temporary liver damage. Because the ingredients listed on the label included skullcap and valerian, these herbs were alternately blamed for the adverse side effects; researchers now believe that the culprit in this case was germander. In the 1970s, two women developed hepatitis B after ingesting tablets

allegedly containing skullcap, mistletoe, motherwort and kelp. The doctors who treated the women, apparently not aware that germander often masquerades as skullcap, assumed that mistletoe must have caused the condition.

Researchers studying echinacea at the University of Munich in the 1980s were surprised to find that they were actually working with prairie dock (*Parthenium integrifolium*). The root of the impostor is similar to that of echinacea, but is about five times larger. Testing of commercial products followed, and it turned out that quite a bit of the echinacea on the market was not the real thing. Likewise, Eastern European growers have sometimes supplied British importers with imitation herbs such as German chamomile or, more often, common tansy instead of feverfew.

When the American Herb Association had an independent laboratory conduct chromatographic tests and microscopic analyses of five different products labeled Siberian ginseng, only two proved to be the real thing. The others were probably Chinese silk vine (*Periploca sepium*), which shares with Siberian ginseng the Chinese name *wu-jia-pi* (which translates as "five-leaf, spiny bark").

Siberian ginseng got into even more hot water in 1990, when a baby with hormonal problems was born to a woman who had been drinking a tea labeled "Siberian ginseng." There soon appeared a flurry of negative stories not only about Siberian ginseng, but also about ginseng—many people do not know the difference. It took a while for the dust to settle, but Denis Awang,

Ph.D., then-chairman of Canada's Health Protection Branch of the Department of Health and Welfare, determined that the herbal tea had actually been made with Chinese silk vine. Later, it appeared that the baby's problem had nothing to do with the tea anyway, but rumors continued. Months after, I read in an herbal newsletter yet another warning about Chinese ginseng causing birth defects and hormonal problems.

Although no toxicity has been found in ginkgo leaves, some people have wondered about this herb's safety because of skin reactions sometimes caused by ginkgo's fruit. The fruit contains compounds similar to the rash-producing agents in poison ivy and oak. Likewise, rumors persist that medicinal passionflower, like its relative, the ornamental blue passionflower (*Passiflora caerulea*), contains toxic cyanogenic glycosides. If you plant passionflower in your medicinal herb garden, make sure that it is the medicinal *P. incarnata*.

NOT GUILTY

Today, the FDA considers chamomile a safe herb, but warnings about chamomile can still still be found in many modern herb books. The controversy stems from a *Journal of Allergy and Clinical Immunology* article in which the author said that drinking chamomile tea might produce potentially fatal anaphylactic shock in people who are allergic to the distantly related ragweed. Concerned researchers then reviewed data on chamomile assembled from studies conducted between 1887 and 1982. They found only 50 al-

lergic reactions reported in any chamomile species, and no deaths. Only 5 reactions were from the German chamomile that is commonly used as tea. The researchers concluded that the likelihood of an acute allergy to chamomile is really quite low.

In 1977 Saint-John's-wort was placed on an FDA list of unsafe herbs because animals that ingest it experience a negative reaction to sunlight. In Russia, this common weed is called *zveroboi*, or "beast killer." However, no cases of human poisoning exist in the scientific literature, and many herbalists use Saint-John's-wort extensively—and without complaint from their clients. I have heard a few stories of people—mostly individuals who are HIV-positive—developing a sun sensitivity after taking very large amounts. It is possible that people whose immune systems are compromised are more susceptible to the herb's phototoxic side effects.

In 1989 a controversy developed over psyllium. Fifty-eight people reported allergic reactions from a cereal containing psyllium. It turned out that a few individuals, mostly nurses who had been exposed to psyllium dust in the hospital, had developed a sensitivity to psyllium.

PROTECTING YOURSELF FROM CONTAMINATION

It does not make sense to heal yourself with herbs that are contaminated with chemicals that can harm your liver and kidneys. Organic herbs may cost more, but I strongly recommend them—they are healthier, and health, after all, is the point of using herbs.

Spraying pesticides on herbs in the field is a great concern. In the early 1970s, I was part-owner of an herb company that sold herbal blends. We discovered that it was nearly impossible to find organically grown herbs; we had to grow our own. Today, organically grown herbs are big business.

You should not assume, however, that all herbs and herb products sold in natural food stores have not been sprayed. Even restricted pesticides sometimes sneak into the United States and Canada. When the American Spice Trade Association and McCormick, the world's largest spice company, began monitoring spices imported from India, they found only low levels of pesticide residues. However, the residues they did find included DDT and other chemicals that have long been banned in the United States and Canada. DDT is now restricted by the Indian government, but it is still being used in many other countries.

Pesticides sprayed on growing plants are not the only concern. Chemicals called fumigants are often used to kill pests on dried herbs, sometimes even plants that have been organically grown. Ethylene oxide, ethylene bromohydin and ethylene chlorohydrin are commonly sprayed on herbs to destroy bugs and microbes. The safety of the herbs once they are sprayed is the subject of much debate. Most herb companies argue that the gas residues are long gone before the plants reach the consumer. I certainly hope so—thus far, ethylene oxide has been linked to birth defects and to spon-

taneous abortions in hospital workers who used it to sterilize equipment.

Ethylene oxide is also considered a possible carcinogen. The results of one study conducted in Sweden found that the incidence of leukemia in workers exposed to ethylene oxide was more than ten times higher than that of the general population. In 1990, 800,000 pounds of this chemical were used in California alone—much of this which was released into the air as industrial plant emissions. State officials estimated that this use could result in up to 510 cancers over the next 70 years. In 1990 the Indian government passed legislation requiring that herbs and foods treated with ethylene oxide be clearly marked; U.S. authorities have not even considered setting such restrictions.

Another method of "cleaning" foods is irradiation. This is probably the least of your worries when it comes to herbs, though. This is not because radiation does not pose any risks, but because the process is so expensive that so far it has been restricted mostly to perishable, high-priced items, such as fresh strawberries and a few expensive spices used in prepared foods. Some herb companies make a big deal about not irradiating their herbs. Check to see if they make an equally big fuss about their herbs not being subjected to pesticides or gases.

ENDANGERED HERBS

I am excited about the increasing popularity of herbs. But I am also a bit concerned—that popularity translates into a serious impact on the environment when popular herbs are overharvested. In North America, commercial wild-crafting (picking herbs in the wild) goes back to the days of trappers who sold ginseng along with their furs. Today, it is illegal in many states to wildcraft ginseng without permission, but wild-crafting laws are rarely enforced. Unfortunately, wild ginseng's survival is now threatened.

Traditionally, the backwoods wild-crafters considered different species, and sometimes totally different plants, equally beneficial. As a result, several different herbs may be picked together without regard to the overharvesting of a few threatened species. Some species of echinacea and lady slipper are now so rare that they are on the endangered species list.

Tree barks are often harvested by stripping off all the bark on a particular tree, which kills the tree. I have even heard of oak bark being harvested by bulldozing the trees. There are tech-niques that involve selective stripping (slippery elm is harvested this way), but these methods are more time-consuming and therefore less profitable.

A partial solution to this herb crisis is for you to buy rare herbs only if they have been cultivated instead of wildcrafted. You can also use alternative herbs. For example, I have mentioned Oregon grape root and barberry throughout this book, because in most cases, their similar chemistry makes them an acceptable alternative to goldenseal. I have not even suggested using lady slipper, which has been heavily collected since the nineteenth century and is not cultivated commercially because its actions are so similar to those of the common herb valerian.

If you are truly motivated to use herbs medicinally, the best thing for you to do is to get out your spade and turn a small plot of your yard into an herb garden. This will provide the best assurance that your herbs are of the very highest quality.

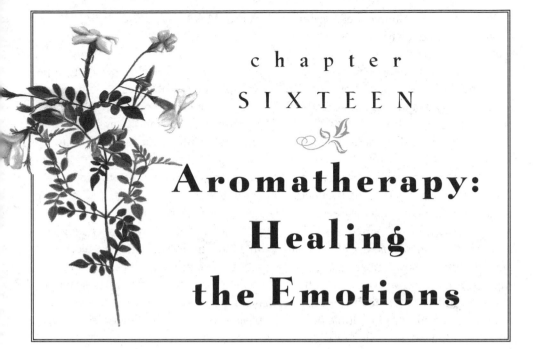

Aromatherapy: Healing the Emotions

Fragrance captures the attention: the sweet smell of a rose, the enticing aroma of a freshly baked cinnamon apple cake, the appealing scent of a cup of warm peppermint tea, the pleasing fragrance of your favorite perfume. Just the word "aromatherapy" conjures up intriguing images, and with good reason. As much as we take our sense of smell for granted, fragrance affects us in a way that is both primal and provocative.

When I first began giving tours through my herb garden in the early 1970s, I couldn't help but notice how each fragrant herb produced its own unique effect. I also observed that each group of visitors responded the same way to particular fragrances. The lavender inevitably produced smiles, and

everyone who sniffed it noticeably relaxed. Chamomile soothed the group even more—so much, in fact, that everyone began speaking much more softly. That is, until they reached the peppermint bed, which sent them chattering a mile a minute!

As a masseuse, I wondered how I could capture such mood-altering properties in a massage oil. I wanted to help send my clients into deeper relaxation and use fragrance to relieve their stress or to perk them up, depending upon what they needed. Lavender has always been one of my favorite scents, so I selected it for my first experiment. It produced such relaxation in the first client I tried it on that he fell asleep—that was all the encouragement I needed! I designed a set of massage oils, each with a different effect: calming or energizing, coping with emotional conflicts and providing mental clarity.

The results from these oils were exciting, but little did I realize how popular aromatherapy would become a decade later. In the 1980s, aromatherapy stepped into the world of modern science and marketing.

The term "aromatherapy" was first coined in the early part of the twentieth century by the French chemist René-Maurice Gattefossé, who used this word to describe the medicinal use of essential oils. In actuality, however, aromatherapy was not a new practice even then; it had always been a part of herbalism. Many traditional remedies had multiple purposes —a single potion often served as cosmetic, perfume and medicine. This is no surprise, since many aromatic herbs that are used as cosmetics are also medicinal.

What makes aromatherapy different from herbalism is that it uses only the herbs that contain essential oils. These herbs are easy to identify because they are all fragrant. When you read an herb book, keep in mind that all the medicinal properties found in an herb are not necessarily contained in its essential oil. Most herbs are filled with other compounds in addition to essential oils. However, the essential oils are often responsible for an herb's antiseptic properties, and many of them perform other medicinal duties as well.

Not all aromatherapy deals with the effects of fragrance on the emotions. For example, fragrant herbs and essential oils are used in massage oils to loosen tight muscles.

AROMATIC RESEARCH

Aromatherapy can help a person to cope with psychological issues, from depression and anxiety to poor memory. That something as noninvasive as natural fragrances can affect our thoughts is quite exciting. Medical researchers hope someday to treat a number of conditions, including Alzheimer's disease and memory disorders, with fragrance. This idea is not as far out as it may seem. When we smell, the information that we receive is sent to specific areas of the brain that influence memory, learning, basic emotions, hormonal balances and even our basic survival mechanisms, such as the "fight or flight" response. Researchers have found that fragrance can even improve interaction and communication among people: Pleasant smells can put people in better moods and even make them more willing to negotiate, cooperate and compromise. Put these same people in an unscented room, and avoidance, competition and conflict are more likely.

Scientific evidence supporting aromatherapy is just beginning to surface. In a 1992 issue of the *British Journal of Occupational Therapy,* aromatherapy is described as a treatment to "promote health and well-being" through massage, inhalation, baths and the application of compresses, creams and lotions. The author of this article suggests that fragrance can reduce stress and depression, sedate or invigorate, stimulate sensory awareness and provide pain relief. Working with International Fragrance and Flavor (IFF), a New York–based fragrance company that has made a multimillion-dollar commitment to research, Gary Schwartz, M.D., a professor of psychology at the University of Arizona, studied how fragrances can be used to alleviate fatigue, migraine headaches, food cravings, depression, schizophrenia, anxiety and irregular heartbeat. Another scientist funded by IFF, Craig Warren, Ph.D., tested more than 2,000 subjects in order to better understand how some fragrances can relieve pain, call up deep-seated memories and generally affect personality and behavior. He is particularly interested in discovering which scents prevent insomnia.

IFF officials believe that companies will eventually market stress-relieving perfumes and that it will someday be commonplace for people to choose everyday items such as shampoo according to their emotional needs as well as their cosmetic requirements. In fact, the mainstreaming of aromatherapy has already begun. The cosmetic firm Redken markets Shinsen shampoo, which features rose, honeysuckle, tuberose and musk scents to "relieve stress and promote peace of mind." (The shampoo's package also provides directions for giving yourself a shiatsu head massage to promote further relaxation.) The Japanese fragrance company Takasago created Avon's popular Tranquil Moments bath line and is investigating aromas that might be used to treat dizziness and nausea. Following Avon's lead, the Estée Lauder cosmetics company formed Origins, an aromatherapy line sold in department stores such as Nordstrom's and New York's Bergdorf Goodman, as well as at a small number of Origins stores

across the United States. Their Green Principles body-care products emphasize botanicals and carry names such as Sleep Time, Stress Buffer, Muscle Easing, Energy Boost and Peace of Mind.

To experience the Esthera aromatherapy and acupressure facial designed by Shiseido, Japan's largest cosmetics company, you would need to visit an exclusive $7,000-a-year health club. But if you do, the effects will certainly be more than skin-deep. Shiseido researchers measuring the brain waves of women while they received the facial found that the waves duplicated those achieved during meditation or deep relaxation! As an added benefit, the facial lowered blood pressure.

Aromatherapy has captured the imagination not only of medical researchers, but also of marketers, who find that fragrance sells. Alan R. Hirsch, M.D., the director of the Smell and Taste Treatment and Research Foundation in Chicago and a psychiatrist and neurologist at the University of Illinois, is studying how different odors change a consumer's reactions. For instance, he analyzes people's responses to television commercials as they smell various odors. According to Dr. Hirsch, "Odors will be the marketing tool of the 1990s." He projects that in less than five years, stores around the world will be counting on fragrances to influence shoppers.

You may not realize it, but you have probably already experienced aromatherapy—maybe when you bought a car or a house, or even laundry detergent. Most of the products we purchase are scented to make them more appealing. Real estate agents know that the smell of freshly baked brownies makes a house more appealing to a buyer. Similarly, used-car salespeople spray a fragrance into cars because customers are more likely to think that the vehicle is in good shape if it smells new. Most detergents are lemon-scented because we tend to associate the smell of citrus with cleanliness.

However, not all aromatherapy-based marketing is successful. Consider the laundry detergent company in England that decided to outsmart competitors by choosing a scent for the product other than the typical lemon. Extensive testing on housewives showed that vanilla was by far the favorite, with musk in close pursuit. Then the company de-

cided to find out why these particular scents rated so high. Imagine the researchers' surprise when they learned that the oils were having an aphrodisiac effect on the women! The company immediately decided to stick with the lemon scent. (I heard that they changed the color of the box instead.)

USING AROMATHERAPY

As mysterious at it might seem, aromatherapy is easy to use. It is also highly individual, built on the concept of finding the fragrances that are appropriate to each person's emotional needs. The simplest way to determine the best healing fragrance for you is to determine which scents you find most appealing. After all, aromatherapy should be enjoyable. The best way to find the scents that are right for you is to try different scents one by one. If you don't like a particular scent, pass it up and go to one that you find more attractive.

Most people prefer familiar fragrances. If a particular odor has a negative or positive association, it may evoke the same emotion the next time you smell it. When students participating in a study at the Olfaction Research Group at the University of Warwick in Coventry, England, were told that they performed poorly after taking a test in a scented room, they became depressed every time they smelled that odor. Students told that they were successful had the opposite reaction: Their self-confidence was boosted whenever they sniffed that aroma.

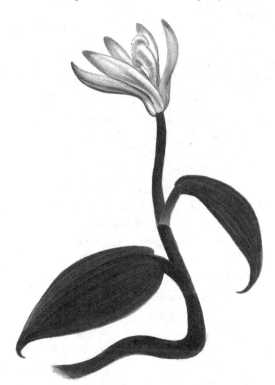

Vanilla is not only great in ice cream—it's also a reputed aphrodisiac.

I know of children who have disliked the smell of strawberries ever since they experienced strawberry-scented masks to help relax them during surgery. Many of us have known people we found romantically attractive, except for something vaguely unsettling. Then you realize that the person's cologne or perfume is the same one that was worn by someone who broke your heart years before.

I once observed a similar phenomenon while giving an aromatherapy lecture. As a sample of lavender was passed around, each student who inhaled its fragrance relaxed and smiled, until it reached one man who immediately stiffened up with the most painful look on his face. When I asked if he had any past association with lavender, he remembered that it was used in his hometown funeral home. Many people he had been close to had died when he was a child, and the scent of lavender produced a flood of painful feelings. I am sure that no matter how much he learns about the positive qualities of lavender, that man will never be able to truly enjoy its fragrance.

Many times I am asked if a person can overcome his or her dislike for a particular fragrance. It is not easy, but you can try to recondition yourself—providing your original negative experience with that scent was not too dramatic. When you are in an enjoyable place and mood, sniff a faint amount of the problematic scent combined with another scent that you do like. After trying this a few times, you may find yourself experiencing the once-disliked fragrance more pleasantly.

AROMATHERAPY TECHNIQUES

In various subtle ways, you probably already use aromatherapy. When you make a tea made from a fragrant herb (such as peppermint or chamomile) or toss such herbs into your bath, you are extracting the herb's essential oils into the water. Likewise, when you make recipes from this book that use fragrant herbs, you are using aromatherapy.

Because essential oils are so concentrated, the safest way to use them is to dilute them in a vegetable oil base and then rub them into the skin as you would a liniment. Essential oils are absorbed into the bloodstream because their tiny molecules pass through the skin. Compounds from lavender essential oil have been detected in the bloodstream only 20 minutes after a lavender massage oil was rubbed on the skin. (You can test this at home by rubbing a piece of cut garlic on the bottom of your foot. Its essential oils will travel through the sole of your foot and within 30 minutes you will taste garlic!)

Essential oils are especially effective when you apply them to the skin over an internal region where they are needed. For instance, a massage oil designed to ease a stomachache can be rubbed over the abdomen. There is a chart near the end of this chapter that details the best proportions to use in creating aromatherapy products.

The most effective way to use aromatherapy is to make the fragrance so subtle that it is barely perceivable. Blend several scents together, as a perfumer does. Use your nose as your guide, and do not be afraid to experiment. I know nurses and other health care professionals who dab scented oil on the backs of their hands before seeing patients.

The most refined way to fill a room with fragrance is by using an electric aromatic diffuser, a glass apparatus that pumps a consistent, light mist of unheated fragrance into the air. (If you decide to purchase one, be sure to get a model with a quiet pump.) A simpler alternative is to dab a few drops of essential oil on a lightbulb or, for a more lasting effect, on one of the special ceramic or metal rings designed to be placed on a lightbulb (these rings are available at stores that sells essential oils). When you turn on the light, the heat causes the scent to fill the room.

A simmering potpourri cooker, heated with either electricity or a candle, will also scent a room for hours. You do not even need the potpourri; you can simply put a little water in the cooker and add a drop or two of essential oil. Or you can heat a pan of water containing a few drops of essential oil on the stove, then turn off the heat and allow the scented steam to fill the air.

Of course, the oldest way to scent a room is with incense (if you do not mind the smoke it produces). Potpourri, sleep pillows and scented bed linens, clothes and stationery offer ways to share aromatherapy with others through fragrant gifts. Aromatherapy can even improve some of your mundane household tasks. Try placing a cotton ball scented with a drop of essential oil in your vacuum cleaner bag.

A fragrant plant often contains less than 1 percent essential oil, but that small amount can be highly aromatic. The oil is extracted from the plant by methods such as distillation or pressing. Once extracted from the plant, these pure essential oils are highly concentrated and must be used with care. Do not use them straight; always dilute essential oils with vegetable oil, alcohol or water before putting them on your skin. The price range of various types of essential oils—from about $4 an ounce to $800 for an ounce of the rarest oils—reflects how difficult it is to extract the particular oil. Bulgarian rose oil, for instance, sells for around $600 an ounce because it takes 600 pounds of rose petals to produce a single ounce of oil.

You can buy the essential oils for aromatherapy at most natural food stores, at some body care stores, at herb shops and through mail order catalogs. In addition to the pure essential oils, many ready-made formulas similar to those provided in this book are available.

AROMATHERAPY FOR THE EMOTIONS

Of all the benefits derived from aromatherapy, the most intriguing are probably its effects on the mind and the emotions. There are many ways to get at the mind-body connection by using aromatherapy techniques.

ANXIETY
Feeling panicked about an approaching job interview or a speech? Then eat an apple, says University of Arizona researcher Gary Schwartz, M.D.—and

be sure to sniff it. Dr. Schwartz, who says he was inspired by the old saying "An apple a day keeps the doctor away," believes that our sense of smell directly affects the part of our brain that controls fear and anxiety. To put his theory to the test, he organized a study in which he asked a group of people questions such as "What kind of person makes you angry?" As expected, everyone tensed up. That is, until they sniffed an apple. When they inhaled that scent, they breathed easier, their blood pressure and heart rates dropped and their muscles even relaxed. They also felt less anxious and embarrassed, and reported that they suddenly felt much happier. When they sniffed a little clove and cinnamon with the apple scent, the results were even better.

In fact, a whole fruit bowl of fragrances may be able to help you overcome fear and anxiety. The researchers at International Fragrance and Flavor found that, for most people, smelling an orange reduces anxiety. They also found that the scent of peaches calms people experiencing panic attacks and combats the sleep disorder narcolepsy.

In the 1970s and 1980s, Paolo Rovesti, M.D., director of the Instituto Derivati Vegetali in Milan, Italy, turned to fragrance to help patients suffering from anxiety. He used scents that perfumers describe as "herbal" or "green," including lavender, rose, marjoram, cypress and violet leaf. To ease migraine headaches caused by anxiety, the twelfth-century Muslim herbalist Al-Samarqandi suggested sniffing violets. Aromatherapists use these same fragrances to help someone who is feeling

lonely or rejected, or undergoing a major life transition. The sixteenth-century herbalist John Gerard also suggested smelling marjoram, "for those given to much sighing," and said that it comforts some specific states of anxiety: grief, loneliness and rejection. In some Greek and Roman texts, it is stated that marjoram "strengthens" the brain and emotions.

A contemporary practitioner who successfully treats anxiety disorders with aromatherapy is J. J. King, M.D., a psychiatrist at the Smallwood Day Hospital in Redditch, Worcestershire, England. He uses pleasant, natural scents combined with relaxation techniques such as deep breathing, positive visualization, soothing music and heat treatments. Once patients learn to associate a particular fragrance with deep relaxation, they relax whenever they are given a sniff. Some of Dr. King's favorite anti-anxiety scents are lavender, rose, bergamot, cedarwood and balsam fir.

One woman I know, Gail, could hardly leave her home for fear of an unsuspected anxiety attack. She felt as if the world were closing in on her. The attacks usually lasted less than an hour, but they were so bad, she said, that she wanted to die. The worst part is that she had no idea when one might occur. A single mom who had to work every day, she found that the condition was making her life unbearable. Gail tried a number of therapies to help her overcome the panic attacks, including psychotherapy and acupuncture, but she also turned to aromatherapy. She was given a combination of orange, marjoram and lavender to carry around. To her amazement, she found that these oils relaxed and calmed her so much that she could begin to control and subdue her attacks. Just the knowledge that she had an instant tool to help increased Gail's confidence in her ability to go out into the world.

Aromatherapy can also help most people overcome episodes of grief and sadness. Most of the research on this subject comes from historical texts. The fragrances used historically correspond to modern ones suggested for anxiety. The ancient Egyptians and Greeks sniffed hyssop, cypress and marjoram to ease grief. Hyssop was said to help clear the mind and help a person think more clearly during trying times. Several ancient cultures, such as Indian and Egyptian, used sandalwood to comfort mourners during funeral ceremonies. Europeans used sage, clary sage and rosemary to help them overcome grief. Rosemary was carried to funerals, then thrown into the grave.

I know several caregivers who work with dying patients, and they have found that fragrances are helpful not only for those who are dying, but also for the family and friends. These fragrances can even be used during an emotional or stressful transition in one's life, such as a job change or while ending a romantic relationship.

Anti-anxiety Fragrance

4 ounces sweet almond oil
10 drops each lavender and orange
*   essential oils*
2 drops each marjoram and cedarwood
*   essential oils*
🌿 Combine ingredients and it's done!

Anti-sorrow Fragrance

4 ounces sweet almond oil
10 drops marjoram essential oil
5 drops each clary sage and cypress or
*   rosemary essential oils*
1 drop hyssop essential oil (expensive,
*   so it's optional)*
1 drop melissa (or lemon) essential oil
🌿 Combine ingredients.

Bath Oil

To make a bath oil from either of these recipes, follow the same formula but use 2 ounces of almond oil instead of 4.

DEPRESSION

Pulling yourself out of the dumps may be as easy as taking a shower—if you use a shampoo containing orange, tangerine and peach that is made by the Japanese cosmetic firm Shinsen and is designed to "lift the spirits." Perhaps someday you will literally be able to wash depression "right out of your hair." Aromatherapy may eventually be accepted by medical doctors as a drugless alternative for depression. According to the latest research by biochemist George H. Dodd, Ph.D., and psychologist Steve van Toller, Ph.D., at the Warwick Olfaction Research Group in England, the effect of fragrance on the brain is similar to that of some antidepressant drugs. This means that certain scents, such as orange, alter brain chemistry that causes depression, anxiety and probably other mood changes.

If Drs. Dodd and van Toller's dream comes true, you will someday be able to get an aromatherapy prescription to treat depression. This is already happening at an experimental convalescent clinic in Baku, Azerbaijan. A prescription from a doctor at this clinic typically recommends spending ten minutes twice a week in a special sunroom sniffing certain live plants. One of the fragrances that they use to overcome general neurosis, headaches and insomnia caused by worry and depression is rose geranium.

Mood swings are a normal part of life, and temporary states of depression are quite normal, but ongoing depression is a complex problem that limits the quality of life for more than 30 million Americans. Statistics show that depression has been steadily increasing in North America since the beginning of the twentieth century. It affects general health by suppressing your immune system and can lead to insomnia and other seemingly unrelated problems by causing changes in the brain's chemistry. Professional psychiatric care is often necessary, but aromatherapy can also play a role (in conjunction with therapy). In fact, many professional therapists are beginning to incorporate aromatherapy into their practices.

When it comes to herbal antidepressants, I find citrus scents to be particularly effective. Orange essential oil, which is produced from orange peel, is easy to find and quite inexpensive. Even smelling an orange as you peel it helps—when you tear the skin, minute amounts of essential oils are propelled into the air to cheer you up. However, this whiff of scent may not be sufficient for someone who is severely depressed. In that case, try the refined scent of the orange blossom, called neroli by aromatherapists, or the less expensive petitgrain, which comes from the stem behind the flower.

Although I did not care for petitgrain when I first sniffed it years ago, I learned to love it after using it in my bath to counter a bout of depression. I figured that money was no object in my pursuit of health, but if a less expensive oil worked, why not use it? It blends nicely with lavender, which is also used as an antidepressant.

Science has not yet investigated the use of aromatherapy to counter compulsive behavior that is associated with depression, including eating disorders. Aromatherapists, experimenting with various oils, have discovered that the fragrance of another citrus, bergamot, along with grapefruit often does the trick. (Do not confuse this with the herb garden plant called bergamot, which is in the mint family.) Children who are depressed usually prefer either grapefruit or tangerine.

Dr. Paolo Rovesti, already mentioned here for his work with anxiety, has helped pull many people out of serious depression using the citrus scents of orange, bergamot, lemon and lemon verbena. He also found that jasmine, sandalwood and ylang-ylang alleviated depression. Here is how Dr. Rovesti described the effect of these aromas: "Patients felt as if transported by the perfume of the essential oil into a different, more agreeable and acceptable world, so that many of their reactive instincts are curbed and they gradually return towards normality."

In sixteenth- and seventeenth-century European herbals, clary sage and lemon balm were suggested to

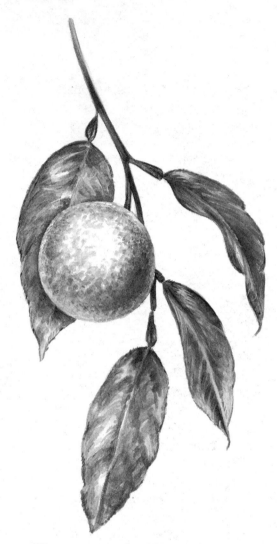

said that sniffing lemon balm, called melissa by aromatherapists, would "gladden the heart" and recommended basil to "taketh away sorrowfullness... and maketh a man merry and glad." Indians traditionally use basil in a similar fashion to prevent agitation and nightmares.

I know of many aromatherapists who have suggested an essential oil for a physical problem, knowing that the fragrance also works as an antidepressant. Only later did their clients confide that they had suffered from terrible depression and were surprised to find their depression lifting with the help of their aromatherapy oil! A good example is Margaret, who was being treated for menstrual disorders with bergamot, clary sage, lemon balm and lavender. The six days of gloom that she always associated with premenstrual syndrome were so dramatically reduced that she was caught by surprise when menstruation occurred without the depression she had come to take for granted.

Antidepressant Fragrance
4 ounces sweet almond oil
10 drops each bergamot and petitgrain
*   essential oils*
3 drops rose geranium essential oil
1 drop neroli essential oil (expensive,
*   so it's optional)*
❧ Combine ingredients. For children, replace petitgrain with grapefruit or tangerine.

Bath Oil
To make a bath oil using this recipe, follow the same formula but use 2 ounces of almond oil instead of 4.

There are two herbs named bergamot—one used medicinally, one in perfumes. The only thing they hold in common is their orangey aroma.

counter depression and to help with paranoia, mental fatigue and nervous disorders associated with depression (though, of course, these disorders were not known then by these names). Modern aroma-therapists concur. Writing in the sixteenth century, John Gerard

Antidepressant Smelling Salts

6 drops Antidepressant Fragrance,
  without almond oil (see page 290)
1 heaping teaspoon rock salt

Drop the essential oil onto the salt. The salt will quickly absorb the oil. Carry smelling salts in a small container with a tight lid.

FATIGUE: PHYSICAL AND EMOTIONAL

Aroma is already assisting people whose jobs and the safety of others depend upon their staying alert, such as long-distance truck drivers. The cosmetics firm Charles of the Ritz markets a fragrance to keep car and truck drivers alert while driving, and there is talk of extending this concept to air-traffic controllers and others who must keep alert while performing monotonous but important tasks. Train conductors in Japan and Russia rely on an "odorphone" developed by Russian professor of biology and odorologist V. Krasnov. Depending on your preference, his little machine spews out hot whiffs of pine, cedar, rose or even seaweed or mushroom.

Air New Zealand and Virgin Atlantic airlines developed kits of floral-scented bath oils to reduce jet lag. These oils, one called Awake and another Asleep, are also sold at Heathrow Airport's International Terminal in London. England's Queen Elizabeth and Princess Diana reportedly used them regularly in their jaunts around the world.

Workers at Tokyo's Kajima and Shimizu architectural and construction companies also benefit from aromatherapy firsthand. Throughout the workday, fragrances are circulated through the air-conditioning system to keep employees attentive. At Kajima, lemon is the morning wake-up call, followed by rose to inspire contented work; after lunch, workers are greeted with an invigorating cypress. Shimizu disperses peppermint into their offices and conference rooms to increase work efficiency, dispel drowsiness and lessen mental fatigue (lavender is also used to help set a positive mood). The company even claims that the scented rooms reduce employees' urges to smoke. Cypress fragrance is sent into the display areas and public relations rooms to promote constructive work. Even the Tokyo Stock Exchange has begun to invigorate the afternoon air with peppermint. Kajima has teamed up with the Shiseido cosmetics company and Shimizu with Toho University to develop environmental fragrancing for businesses.

But aromatherapy does not have to stop at work. During lunch hour, workers in Tokyo can try a peppermint refresher at Club Harry's. Subjects lie on couches in rooms that are filled with aromas. On the way home, they can stop off at one of several atomizer-equipped phone booths to escape from the stress of commuter traffic with a mist of a relaxing scents.

One American paint company is bringing this idea into the American home. City Surplus and Paint in Denver offers more than a wide selection of colors with its West O' Scent Paint. The paint comes in more than a dozen mood-altering scents, including stimulating fragrances such as jasmine, pine and eucalyptus. Sleeping in too late? A Hattori Seiko alarm clock from Japan puffs pine and eucalyptus to rouse you seconds before your alarm goes off.

Some of the first investigation into fragrant stimulants was done in the 1920s by Italian psychiatrists Giovanni Gatti and Renato Cayola. They found that the scents of clove, ylang-ylang, cinnamon, lemon, cardamom, fennel and angelica were stimulating. American studies through IFF also found peppermint and eucalyptus to be stimulating. Later, when brain waves were recorded by researcher Shizuo Torii, Ph.D., of the Toho University School of Medicine in Tokyo, they showed that some of these fragrances and numerous others—clove, basil, ylang-ylang, jasmine, black pepper, cinnamon and, to a lesser degree, rose, patchouli, lemon grass and sage—acted as stimulants.

According to Dr. Torii, these fragrances affect us much differently from the way adrenal stimulants such as caffeine do. They counter the typical adrenal rush caused by caffeine, as well as physiological stress, strain or boredom, reducing drowsiness, irritability and headaches. Dr. Torii has found that stimulating fragrances prevent you from experiencing the sharp drop of sustained attention that typically occurs after 30 minutes of work by arousing the autonomic nervous system, which controls breathing and blood pressure.

To test the effects of such fragrances on alertness, researchers William N. Dember, Ph.D., and Joel S. Warm, Ph.D., gave people at the University of Cincinnati a stressful 40-minute task identifying patterns on a computer. Those working in rooms scented with peppermint had many more correct answers

than people working in unscented rooms. In addition, their performance levels didn't decline as rapidly. In a study conducted by researchers at Rensselaer Polytechnic Institute in Troy, New York, clerical workers set higher goals for themselves and were more efficient when their offices were pleasantly scented. The fragrance worked even when those taking the test did not think that the scent was influencing them.

I travel with a selection of aromatic atomizers to spray into the air or on my face during long drives or airplane flights. Once, while I was flying across the country, a businessman sat down

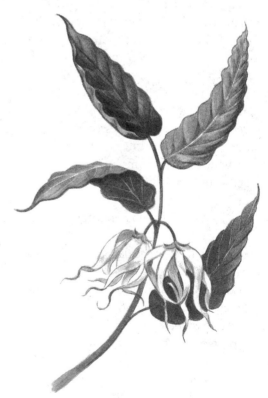

The fragrance of ylang-ylang has been proven to have a stimulating effect, but it also can lull you to sleep.

next to me. He introduced himself as Greg, said he could not stay awake on these long flights and proceeded to fall asleep as soon as the plane left the runway. About every 20 minutes, I reached into my bag and gave my face a gentle rose spray. It was making my trip more enjoyable but I was concerned that I might be bothering Greg. Every time I used the spray, the scent would float across to his seat and he would stir, often waking up to ask if we were there yet. Hours later, we finally arrived in Boston. As the plane landed, he perked right up and told me that it had been the most refreshing and least tiring flight he had taken. He could not imagine why, then looked at me and said, "It must have been you!" (I did not tell him my secret.)

Stimulant for Fatigue
4 ounces sweet almond oil
15 drops lemon essential oil
4 drops eucalyptus essential oil
1 drop each cinnamon, peppermint and benzoin (if available) essential oils
Combine ingredients.

Bath Oil
To make a bath oil using this recipe, follow the same formula but use 2 ounces of almond oil instead of 4.

Some of the fragrances mentioned in this section—including ylang-ylang, rose, patchouli, sandalwood and jasmine—are both relaxants and stimulants. Although it might seem as if these effects would cancel out each other, they actually combine to produce a very enjoyable mood. Indeed, all these scents

also have age-old reputations as aphrodisiac scents.

We know from clinical research, such as the study on vanilla and musk described on page 284, that aphrodisiacs stimulate brain waves. The state of being completely relaxed yet at the same time stimulated offers the perfect combination for an aphrodisiac, since stress and tension are strong deterrents to passion. Other aphrodisiacs include the stimulants cinnamon and coriander (which was used in the famous story *The Arabian Nights*). Aphrodisiacs are especially useful as part of a program to help overcome sexual dysfunctions. For more information, see "Impotence" on page 190.

Aphrodisiac
4 ounces sweet almond oil
10 drops each lavender and sandalwood essential oils
2 drops each ylang-ylang and vanilla essential oils
1 drop each cinnamon and jasmine essential oils
Combine ingredients. Lavender is not an aphrodisiac, but is added to make the fragrance more mellow. It can be a relaxing and emotionally uplifting scent. If you love the fragrance of patchouli, try using it in place of ylang-ylang.

MEMORY
You've probably noticed how a whiff of a certain fragrance that you haven't smelled for years can send you back in time, bringing to mind many images and feelings associated with a particular event. Trygg Engen, Ph.D., a researcher at Brown University and the author of *Perception of Odor*, is interested in

harnessing that power. Dr. Engen has found that memory recall more than doubles if a past event is associated with smell instead of being something we experienced only visually.

Have you ever found yourself trying to grasp a scent as it pulls you back to some past event or long-gone emotion? I know that whenever I smell roses, I am again a little girl sniffing my grandmother's potpourri jar. Lavender recalls the soothing scent of her linens when she tucked me into bed. Psychologists call this experience the Marcel Proust phenomenon, after the famous French writer. One day, when the novelist dipped a biscuit in his tea, the aroma brought back many memories from his childhood; these memories became the basis of his famous multivolume *Remembrance of Things Past*. André Virel, a French psychologist, is a firm believer in the technique—he has clients sniff vanilla to help them recall childhood memories

Rosemary has a long history of increasing memory, concentration and even creativity. Shakespeare, in the last act of *Hamlet,* has the mad Ophelia declare, "There's rosemary, that's for rememberance." In the seventeenth century, herbalist Nicholas Culpeper wrote that rosemary "helps a weak memory, and quickens the senses." Modern research conducted in Japan confirms that rosemary is indeed a brain stimulant. Workers in Tokyo can now visit Club Harry's for a 30-minute morning aroma session of rosemary and lemon designed to improve their concentration.

Other herbal mental stimulants include sage, basil and bay leaf. Bay

JUDGING QUALITY

At first, it may seem difficult to judge the quality of essential oils, but ultimately your nose is the best guide. Essential oils vary widely. Not only are there numerous kinds and qualities of natural oils, but there is also a wide variety of synthetic oils. When I pass around top-quality natural oils in my aromatherapy seminars, I warn the group beforehand that I am about to spoil them for life. Anyone can tell the difference, and once you have smelled the real thing, it is difficult to go back to synthetics or inferior-quality oils.

A number of factors determine essential oil quality—growing conditions, extraction techniques and storage methods all play a role. But the greatest gap by far comes between genuine oils and synthetics. Personally, I don't use synthetic oils, despite their significantly lower cost.

In creating synthetics, usually made with petrochemicals, chemists try to duplicate natural

leaves were used as a brain tonic by both the Romans and Native Americans (who used the North American species). You should know, though, that sniffing too much bay leaf can bring on a headache. During the Renaissance, graduating European students were adorned with bay leaf crowns, and we scents, but in my opinion they never come close. Also, synthetics are potentially harmful since their tiny molecules penetrate the skin and enter the bloodstream directly. Sad to say, synthetic fragrances permeate our lives. Most commercial body care products, even many that are sold in natural food stores, use the less expensive synthetics. Just because a product is labeled an essential oil doesn't mean it is natural.

So how can you distinguish a synthetic oil from the real thing? Labels usually don't say, and you usually can't trust store clerks. Until your nose becomes educated enough to do the job on its own, you can try looking at stores' oil racks for clues. If the display includes carnation and gardenia oils, the entire rack likely contains synthetics—those two essential oils cannot be produced naturally. Next, check for jasmine and rose, two popular and expensive oils. If they are being sold for less than $50 per quarter-ounce, what you are holding is either greatly diluted or a synthetic.

Once you purchase high-quality essential oils, to retain their quality you will need to store them in glass vials with tight lids in a cool place. The glass can be clear or amber, but in either case you must keep essential oils away from direct sunlight. Properly stored, most will keep for years. Citrus oils, such as orange and lemon, are the most vulnerable, but even they will last two years if refrigerated. Some oils actually improve with age. Called fixatives because they are used to keep or "fix" the scent of perfumes and potpourris, these include patchouli, clary sage, benzoin, vetivert and sandalwood. I have a bottle of 25-year-old patchouli that smells so rich that most people don't even recognize the fragrance— even those who usually hate the smell.

There is always a possibility that you might be allergic to an essential oil. I have rarely encountered this, however. When I hear people say that they react adversely to a fragrance such as rose, I am always suspicious. Chances are, they are sensitive only to the cheap synthetic imitation found in most body care products, not to the pure essential oil.

still give graduates a baccalaureate, or "bay laurel," though without a wreath! Of sage, Gerard said it is good for the head and brain and "it quicketh the senses and memory." William Turner wrote in his 1568 *Herbal* that clary sage "helps the memory [and] quickens the senses."

Want to help yourself retain something you are reading? Try sniffing one of these aromas as you read. Next time you need help remembering those facts, sniff the same aroma again and it will trigger your memory. I keep a rosemary plant next to my computer, so that whenever I am at a loss for words I can reach over sleep, or better yet, unwind in a relaxing scented bath. An evening massage will soothe anyone plagued with insomnia that is caused by stress. If you do not have time for that, just sniffing the oil will often work. This method is ideal for cranky children who need to settle down before going to sleep. Sound too good to be true? Not according to research by Susan Schiffman, M.D., professor of medical psychology at North Carolina's Duke University. Dr. Schiffman notes that sedative drugs like Valium and Librium affect a newly

The ancient Romans used the aromatherapy herb clary sage as an eyewash.

and rub a leaf between my fingers. The air immediately fills with a wonderful aroma, and I am able to find the words to continue. In aromatherapy classes, I pass around a vial of rosemary essential oil for everyone to dab on their notebooks to help them remember.

Memory Stimulant
4 ounces sweet almond oil
*10 drops each lavender and lemon
    essential oils*
5 drops rosemary essential oil
1 drop cinnamon essential oil
🌿 Combine ingredients.

STRESS AND INSOMNIA
When stress begins to weigh upon your shoulders, try inhaling an essential oil. Dab it on your bedsheets to promote

---

BASIC ESSENTIAL OIL DILUTIONS

1% dilution: Use 5 drops essential oil per ounce of vegetable oil.

2% dilution: Use 10 drops ($^1/_8$ teaspoon) essential oil per ounce of vegetable oil.

A 2% dilution is most common in body care products. This means the product contains 2% essential oil and 98% vegetable oil. Some products, such as liniments and bath oils, use a 4% dilution to make them stronger.

3% dilution: Use 15 drops essential oil per ounce of vegetable oil.

4% dilution: Use 20 drops essential oil per ounce of vegetable oil.

discovered group of smell receptors in the brain. She reasons that if smell receptors help to sedate us, the fragrance itself should perform similarly.

To test her theory, Dr. Schiffman has even taken aromatherapy to the New York City subway system. She sprayed spicy scents into subway cars to see if that relaxed the passengers enough to improve their dispositions. After comparing the number of pushes, shoves and nasty comments in scented cars to those in unscented cars, she found that certain fragrances appeared to cut aggressive acts almost in half. Scents piped through the heating and air-conditioning systems at Memorial Sloan-Kettering Cancer Center in New York City are already lowering the stress levels of patients, staff and families. Vanilla is used to relax patients who must stay perfectly still while undergoing MRI (magnetic resonance imaging) scans inside a large cylinder, a situation that often makes them nervous. Psychologist Sharon Manne, Ph.D., who initiated the therapy, hopes that aromatherapy will also be used to relax cancer patients during CAT scans and radiation therapy.

Fragrances can also lower your pulse and breathing rate. In the 1920s, the Italian psychiatrists Gatti and Cayola concluded that "the sense of smell has... an enormous influence on the function of the central nervous system." They found that for their patients, the essential oils with the greatest sedating effects were citrus scents such as melissa (lemon balm), neroli (orange blossom) and petitgrain, as well as the fragrances of traditional herbal relaxants —

AROMATHERAPY METHODS

1 drop as perfume
1 drop to scent stationery or handkerchief
2 drops on a cotton cloth in a drawer
2 drops on 1 tablespoon rock salt for smelling salts
2 drops per $\frac{1}{2}$ cup water for compress
2 drops on vacuum cleaner or air filter
3 drops to refresh potpourri
4 drops on a lightbulb (or lightbulb ring)
4 drops in a pan of hot water to inhale
5 drops in bathtub
5 drops per quart of warm water for douche
6 drops ($\frac{1}{16}$ tsp.) stirred in 1 oz. skin cream
6 drops ($\frac{1}{16}$ tsp.) in 1 oz. aloe vera gel for skin care
6 drops ($\frac{1}{16}$ tsp.) in 1 oz. aloe juice for skin moisturizer (suitable for spray bottle)
12 drops ($\frac{1}{8}$ tsp.) in 1 oz. vegetable oil for massage
12 drops ($\frac{1}{8}$ tsp.) stirred in 1 oz. skin salve
24 drops ($\frac{1}{4}$ tsp.) in $\frac{1}{2}$ cup salt for bath salt
24 drops ($\frac{1}{4}$ tsp.) in 1 oz. vegetable oil for bath oil

AROMATHERAPY AT A GLANCE

Here is a brief list of the effective fragrances discussed in this chapter. Many of these scents have been used for centuries to achieve these results. Next time you're feeling a bit off-base, why don't you try one of these?

SCENTS TO RELIEVE ANXIETY

Bergamot	Lavender	Peach
Cedarwood	Marjoram	Rose
Cypress	Opopanax (or Myrrh)	Spiced Apple
Hyssop	Orange	Violet leaf

SCENTS TO ALLEVIATE DEPRESSION

Bergamot	Lemon	Petitgrain
Clary Sage	Lemon Balm	Rose Geranium
Grapefruit	Lemon Verbena	Sandalwood
Jasmine	Neroli	Tangerine
Lavender	Orange	Ylang-ylang

SCENTS TO IMPROVE MEMORY

Bay Laurel	Lavender	Rosemary
Jasmine	Lemon	

chamomile, valerian and opopanax, which is similar to myrrh. IFF researchers have found that neroli measurably lowers stress and blood pressure. In fact, they found a blend of neroli, valerian and nutmeg so effective in helping release tension that IFF has patented it and intends to market a product that will ease stress in the workplace.

One way to understand how fragrance affects us is to measure certain brain waves. W. Grey Walter, Ph.D., and his associates at IFF found that these brain waves slow down when you feel drowsy or take a sedative drug and also when you smell certain fragrances. The scents they tested that proved to have the greatest sedative effect were (in order of effectiveness): lavender, bergamot, marjoram, sandalwood, lemon and chamomile. Scientists at the Japanese fragrance firm Takasago also measured brain waves to determine relaxation produced by lavender. Surgeons found that lavender given to hospital patients after heart surgery proved very effective in reducing stress and worry.

SCENTS TO RELIEVE SORROW

Clary Sage	Fir	Rosemary
Cypress	Marjoram	Sage

SCENTS TO STIMULATE (APHRODISIACS)

Jasmine	Sandalwood	Ylang-ylang
Rose	Vanilla	

SCENTS TO STIMULATE (TO COUNTERACT FATIGUE)

Angelica	Cinnamon	Lemon
Benzoin	Clove Basil	Peppermint
Black Pepper	Cypress	Pine
Camphor	Eucalyptus	Sage
Cardamom	Fennel	Spiced Apple

SCENTS TO TREAT STRESS AND INSOMNIA

Bergamot	Lemon	Petitgrain
Chamomile	Marjoram	Rose
Cinnamon	Melissa	Sandalwood
Cloves	Myrrh	Valerian
Frankincense	Neroli	Vanilla
Hops	Nutmeg	Violet
Lavender	Orange	Ylang-ylang

In nineteenth-century medical books, rose was recommended to reduce nervousness; nineteenth-century psychiatrist W. S. Watson, M.D., reported that it successfully calmed his patients. More recently, at Middlesex Hospital in London, England, fresh roses were used as part of an overall relaxation strategy practiced on patients. After six weeks of treatments, patients found that their muscle tension decreased measurably.

The use of chamomile to relieve stress and promote relaxation goes back at least to medieval European monks who had patients lie on raised beds covered with the low-growing Roman chamomile plant. In his seventeenth-century herbal, Nicholas Culpeper continued the tradition when he recommended sniffing chamomile, which he said "comforts both the head and brain." Aromatherapists know that chamomile is especially useful for calming upset, disturbed or hyperactive children. One woman in an aromatherapy class I was teaching was so enthralled with the idea that chamomile could calm her unruly

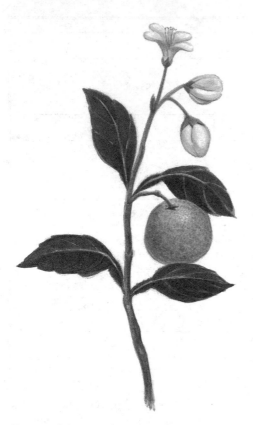

Orange blossom, or neroli, has a comforting, calming scent—this herb is used both to alleviate depression and to send insomniacs off to sleep.

children that she had me make up a spray bottle on the spot. Now, every night around 9:00 P.M. she sprays the television room with chamomile and ylang-ylang! She has found that it not only settles down the kids, but also reduces her irritation as she tries to get them to bed. For an overly active or particularly fussy child, put five drops lavender, one drop chamomile and one drop ylang-ylang in her bath.

Ylang-ylang must be added to the list of sedative essential oils. Although studies show it to be a stimulant,

personal experience has shown that it is also one of the most potent relaxants. Other aromatherapists confirm my observation, and it is a favorite scent when I give aromatherapy lectures at massage schools. The beginning massage students imagine that with ylang-ylang in their massage oil, their clients will be so relaxed that they will not notice the practitioner's inexperience. One student found the scent so calming that he fell asleep while giving a massage!

The aroma given off by pillows filled with hops has been sending people off to sleep for centuries. To encourage sleep, a Japanese firm is designing a device that airs out futons and at the same time makes the bedding smell like flowers. Scents such as neroli and valerian are part of IFF's Sleep for Beauty kit, which comes with a fragrant pillow and 30 vials of essential oils to help customers discover which oils work best for them.

One time when my parents were visiting, my father realized he had run out of sleeping pills. Since he usually had trouble sleeping away from home, he anxiously asked me where we could buy a bottle. Because all the stores close early in my small town, it wasn't possible to make this purchase. I knew he would be reluctant to take an herbal relaxant, so I offered a sleep pillow filled with dill. Of course, he thought it was a joke, but I persuaded him to give it a try anyway. He placed the small pillow under his sleeping pillow and the next morning told me, "I slept like a baby." He was amazed and could not explain what had caused such peaceful sleep, but I knew. If you are interested in making this pillow, see Dilly Pillow on page 238.

CONVERSION CHART

When you are working with recipes that state amounts or dosage in numbers of drops, it's often helpful to be able to know the equivalents of those measurements in more standard form. This chart provides approximate equivalents for commonly used measurements of tinctures, glycerites or other liquid ingredients. Beginning on the left, measures are given in drops (or teaspoons), teaspoons (or tablespoons), ounces, drams (or cups) and milliliters.

8 drops	$\frac{1}{10}$ tsp.	$\frac{1}{60}$ oz.	about $\frac{1}{8}$ dram	about $\frac{1}{2}$ ml.
10 drops	$\frac{1}{8}$ tsp.	$\frac{1}{48}$ oz.	$\frac{1}{6}$ dram	about $\frac{5}{8}$ ml.
20 drops	$\frac{1}{4}$ tsp.	$\frac{1}{24}$ oz.	$\frac{1}{3}$ dram	about $1\frac{1}{4}$ ml.
40 drops	$\frac{1}{2}$ tsp.	$\frac{1}{12}$ oz.	$\frac{2}{3}$ dram	about $2\frac{1}{2}$ ml.
1 tsp.	$\frac{1}{3}$ Tbsp.	$\frac{1}{6}$ oz.	$1\frac{1}{3}$ drams	about 5 ml.
$1\frac{1}{2}$ tsp	$\frac{1}{2}$ Tbsp.	$\frac{1}{4}$ oz.	2 drams	about $7\frac{1}{2}$ ml.
3 tsp.	1 Tbsp.	$\frac{1}{2}$ oz.	4 drams	about 15 ml.
6 tsp.	2 Tbsp.	1 oz.	8 drams	about 30 ml.
24 tsp.	8 Tbsp.	4 oz.	$\frac{1}{2}$ cup	about 120 ml.
48 tsp.	16 Tbsp.	8 oz.	1 cup ($\frac{1}{2}$ pint)	about 240 ml
96 tsp.	32 Tbsp.	16 oz.	2 cups (1 pint)	about 480 ml.

Sedatives for Stress and Insomnia
4 ounces sweet almond oil
2 drops each lavender, sandalwood and bergamot essential oils
6 drops petitgrain essential oil
4 drops each chamomile and ylang-ylang essential oils
❧ Combine ingredients.

Bath Oil
To make a bath oil using this recipe, follow the same recipe but use 2 ounces of almond oil instead of 4.

MEASUREMENTS

Whenever you are using aromatherapy techniques, it is important to create a blend that works well and smells appealing enough to use. The intensity, strength and quality of essential oils varies greatly. If you are intrigued by aromatherapy

and want to learn more about blending therapeutics and formulas, I suggest you read my book *Aromatherapy: The Fragrant Art of Healing* (Crossing Press, 1995), co-authored with aromatherapist Mindy Green.

A note about drops: The standard number of drops in an ounce is 600, which translates to 100 drops per teaspoon. Unfortunately, though, the size of a drop varies according to the oil being used. Some oils are thicker than others and therefore produce larger drops. Drop size also depends upon the size of the dropper you are using. I've provided a conversion chart of measurements to help you convert formulas in this and other books (see page 301). These conversions are also useful when you buy essential oils, which are sold by the milligram, ounce and dram. The conversion from drops to teaspoons is approximate.

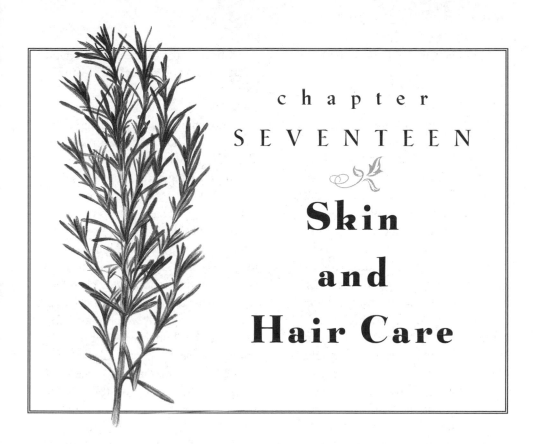

chapter
SEVENTEEN

Skin
and
Hair Care

The beauty products industry can dazzle with packaging and seduce with slick advertising. Perfect skin and hair is its promise, but what it is really selling is hope. The fancy ingredients in most conventional products make them look, feel and smell tremendously appealing—that is, until you read the labels! Chances are you will need a chemical dictionary to decipher them. Chemically altered emulsifiers and synthetic waxes assure that the product will not separate no matter how much heat, cold or shaking that it endures during the long journey from factory to your beauty table. The result is a product that is semi-natural or semi-synthetic, depending on how you look at it. In addition, most cosmetics

are scented with artificial fragrances derived from petroleum products.

In the long run, these cosmetics may be doing your complexion more harm than good. Since your skin does not discriminate when absorbing lotions, creams and the like, potentially harmful chemicals are accepted as readily as the helpful ingredients. Like a growing number of people, you probably are becoming wary about living in a chemical-filled environment. Some cosmetics companies are catching on to this trend toward safer, more natural ingredients and turning to the age-old beauty secrets offered by herbalism. Even so, no matter how natural a product may look, check the label. Some products that claim to be "all natural" contain ingredients that should have stayed in the chemist's lab!

It is no surprise that herbs have caught the attention of the cosmetics industry. Throughout history, herbs have been used to clear complexions, soften hands and make hair lush and silky. Consider some of history's legendary beauties. The Egyptian queen Cleopatra bathed in milk and herbs, anointed herself with costly herbal cosmetics and even owned her own natural cosmetic factory. According to legend, hundreds of years ago, the 80-year-old queen of Hungary bought a secret formula from an herbalist that made her skin so youthful that a young prince fell in love with her. (The main ingredient in this secret formula was rosemary, which is still a popular complexion herb today.) The famous seventeenth-century French beauty Ninon de L'Enclos washed her face daily in chervil water to prevent wrinkles.

BODY CARE THE NATURAL WAY

Herbal body care is important for everyone—while it seems that it is mostly women who concentrate on skin and hair care, men can certainly benefit just as much from these treatments. The best products, whether you are a man or a woman, are those designed for your specific complexion, skin and hair type. Natural skin care products are easy and fun to make in your kitchen and can be prepared with little cost and minimal fuss. Let ground herbs, teas, tinctures and essential oils become your magic ingredients.

Consider the recipes in this chapter a start; when you are feeling creative, experiment with your own recipes. For more inspiration, read chapter 16 to learn how many of the same herbs that are used to make body care products also affect the emotions.

If preparing herbal cosmetics does not appeal to you, look in the cosmetics department of a natural food or department store for their natural body care lines. Since your skin and hair are naturally acid (pH 4.5 to 5.5), the products you put on them should stay close to the same range. You can test a product's pH with nitrazine paper, which is available from your local pharmacy. For directions on how to use this paper, see the label on the box it comes in. You can also increase the effectiveness of store-bought cosmetics by stirring in a few drops of an essential oil that appeals to you.

Warning: There is no such thing as a skin or hair care product—even an all-natural one—that is safe for *everyone*. People can be allergic or sensitive to seemingly harmless substances. Test any new product or ingredient by dabbing a little on the inside of your arm, especially if you tend to have allergies. If you experience a negative reaction such as a rash, swelling, or itching or watering eyes, you should stay clear of the substance.

In one of my classes, we were making cosmetics with glycerin, a natural ingredient sometimes made from coconut oil. Candace, who is allergic to coconut oil, put a drop of glycerin on her tongue. In a few seconds, her mouth swelled up so badly that she could barely speak. Fortunately, her breathing was not affected—a dangerous problem that happens with some allergic reactions. A similar experience happened in another class with a woman who is allergic to olive oil. Rosemary rubbed a salve on the back of her hand, not realizing that it contained olive oil. Her hand broke out in an itchy rash, and to heal it she had to use an herbal remedy for dermatitis—obviously, one that did not contain olive oil!

Beauty is not only skin deep; it also reflects your inner health. Hormonal fluctuations, a poor diet, lack of exercise and stress all adversely affect the health of your skin and hair. So do smoking, alcohol consumption and radical changes in weight. To maintain a radiant complexion and healthy hair, eat a balanced diet and get plenty of rest, relaxation and exercise. A combination of herbs and exercise helps ensure that your skin has a good blood supply that can provide a sufficient amount of nutrients. Scientific studies haven't proven that drinking water improves the health of skin and hair, but aestheticians (professional skin specialists) urge their clients to drink at least eight glasses of water a day to avoid skin dehydration.

BACK TO THE BASICS

Healthy skin begins as clean skin. Cleansing is important to remove dirt, dust, excess facial oil and makeup from your face. But more is not necessarily better—more scrubbing and harsher soaps will not produce finer skin. No matter what your skin type, I recommend using as little soap as possible. Most soaps and liquid skin cleansers are very alkaline (this helps them clean better). For this reason, they have a tendency to alter the skin's natural acidic barrier, which keeps out harmful, infection-causing agents. Ideally, skin should regain its acidity soon after you wash it, but this is not always the case. Diluted vinegar and other toners and even oatmeal make good alternative cleansers.

STEAMING

Steaming is another skin care fundamental. A facial steam or sauna surrounds your face with an herb's essential oils. Steam with fragrant herbs (nonfragrant herbs like comfrey or strawberry leaves contain no essential oils and are therefore useless in a steam) or essential oils. A steam won't remove dirt and grime, but it will soften the skin's surface enough to help cleanse and unclog pores. The heat increases circulation and relaxes facial muscles while the combination of steam and essential oils acts as a moisturizer.

EXFOLIATION

I know exfoliation sounds like a term more suited to reforestation than beauty, but aestheticians consider it one of their most important tools. Exfoliation is the removal of dull, dead surface skin. Carefully scrubbing your face exposes underlying, fresh skin and encourages the growth of the undeveloped skin in the skin's deepest layers. I recommend exfoliation to everyone but those with the most sensitive complexions. It is important that exfoliation be performed properly, using gentle, circular movements. If overdone, too much new skin is exposed before it is ready to face the world. Avoid the chemical exfoliants used by some beauty salons and even natural products containing ground almond shells, which are too harsh for the face. A far better and gentler abrasive can be found in your kitchen—cornmeal. The currently popular vitamin A derivatives used in some cosmetics are also exfoliants, but these are so concentrated that they can produce prolonged skin irritation and are available only by prescription.

TONERS

A toner can be any substance that improves the general appearance and health of the skin. In this chapter, however, the word "toner" is used to describe only lotions and other liquid cosmetics. Facial toners should be misted, dabbed or splashed on after a shower, to cool down on a hot day, after exercising or to freshen your face and attitude on long trips. Instead of rinsing them off, keep toners on your face so that they have a chance to work. For men, toners double as aftershaves.

Aloe vera, with its skin-healing properties and neutral pH, makes an excellent facial toner. Herbs extracted into cosmetic vinegars were the rage for centuries, until they lost their popularity with the arrival of modern cosmetics that do not have vinegar's pungent odor. But do not let the smell deter you from using vinegar—its odor lingers for only a short while, but its beneficial effects last much longer. During the Renaissance, herbs extracted into wine were popular as facial toners. These doubled as edible cordials that women sipped in the privacy of

their dressing rooms! (Marie Antoinette's nightly facial was brandy and milk with lemon.)

Alpha hydroxy acids (AHAs) are also important as facial toners. Both vinegar and wine have the advantage of containing natural AHAs, which restore natural acidity to the skin, improve moisture retention, smooth out fine lines and roughness, lighten dark spots and improve acne. In one study on the AHA lactic acid (the same acid produced by our skin), biochemist Walter Smith, Ph.D., showed that it worked as an excellent moisturizer to improve skin hydration. It made skin almost twice as smooth and one-third firmer than it was before! The regeneration of cells was revved up, and lines and wrinkles were reduced, at least temporarily. To take advantage of the benefits offered by AHAs, use foods that contain these compounds as the base for your masks and incorporate them into your toners. (For examples of foods that contain AHAs, see "Masks" on page 307; for directions for toners and masks, see the recipes in the specific skin type sections in "The Face" on page 308.)

Aromatic hydrosols, by-products of essential-oil distillation, also make excellent toners. They contain water-soluble compounds not found in the essential oils themselves, such as soothing and anti-inflammatory carboxylic acids. Since they are distilled, they will not spoil, as herb tea does. Hydrosols are sold by mail, and at some natural food and cosmetics stores specializing in aromatherapy. You can also buy rose water and orange-blossom water from a liquor store or an Indian grocery. Intended for use in drinks and foods, these waters are

generally less expensive but are also
of lesser quality. Although they do
not have the same moisturizing agents
as hydrosols, floral waters—essential
oils mixed with aloe vera gel or water—
are a viable alternative.

MOISTURIZERS

Moisturizers are also extremely important—healthy skin is at least half water,
which keeps it soft and supple and reduces flakiness, dryness and wrinkles.
Although water is important to your
complexion, by itself it is actually very
drying; it quickly evaporates from the
skin, drawing out moisture in the
process. Oil, on the other hand, makes
cosmetics feel silky, smoothes rough,
scaly skin and forms a protective barrier
that prevents water from evaporating.
But oil cannot moisturize skin all by itself. The perfect skin solution is a moisturizer that combines the best of both
worlds—water to keep skin youthful,
fresh and soft, and oil to stop the water
from evaporating. Typical moisturizers
are creams and lotions held in suspen-
sion by emulsifiers (which prevent sepa-
ration) such as beeswax, glycerin and
lecithin.

MASKS

Our skin care efforts are intended to let
our natural beauty shine through, so we
shouldn't forget the potential of masks—
in private, of course. Roman women
were so fanatical about wearing facial
masks to retain their beautiful complexions that the satirist Juvenal complained
that their husbands could barely recognize them at home. In the words of the
poet Ovid, these masks, which were

made of honey, flour, ground lentils, eggs
and herbs, made the complexion "more
brilliant than a mirror." You might not
care for a face quite that shiny, but a
mask does leave your face with a healthful glow. Masks also pull impurities from
the skin, increase circulation and remove
(exfoliate) dull surface skin.

Clay, which is the most astringent of
the mask bases, is ideal for mixing with
ground herbs, essential oils or both. Use
a cosmetic-grade bentonite, kaolin or
Fuller's earth clay rather than pottery or
building clay, which may contain impurities. Honey, avocado, eggs, fresh fruits,
oats, cream of wheat and nutritional
yeast are a few other possibilities for a
facial mask. So are ginger, papaya,
pineapple and cucumber, which have
skin-softening enzymes. Yogurt, sour
milk, vinegar, apples, citrus fruits and
wine contain AHAs, which are particularly important for a mask because they
loosen the tight bond that holds the old
surface skin (they also restore the skin's
natural acidity). For hundreds of years
(until the beginning of the twentieth century), sour milk was used as a face wash
throughout the Western world; it is still
used today in India. Yogurt is a better
choice since it does not smell as sour, but
either one can be mixed with other mask
ingredients. Acidic fruit such as lemon
and strawberry also help maintain acidity. Feeding your skin with nutritious
foods is not as silly as it may sound. External use of minerals, vitamins and
other ingredients can benefit the complexion just as much as taking them
internally.

If you wish to use a mask, apply it to
your face in an even layer and leave it on

for five to fifteen minutes, as long as it does not become uncomfortable. Then wash the mask off with warm water and gently pat your skin dry. Recipes for masks can be found in this chapter's sections for individual complexion types.

HOW TO CUSTOMIZE YOUR SKIN AND HAIR CARE

Herbs can help all types of skin and hair stay healthy and attractive. But before you can begin any treatment, you need to know what type of skin and hair you have. Facial complexions are divided into eight basic types: normal, dry, oily, combination, problem, couperose (when the capillaries just under the skin are broken, resulting in small red lines on the face), mature and sun-damaged. Basic body skin types include normal, dry, oily, sun-damaged and problem skin. Hair types include normal, dry, oily and problem hair that is limp and lifeless.

Do not expect to find much scientific research on herbs for complexion types in this chapter. Chemists have not yet investigated them, but these herbs have been successfully used for thousands of years and are now used by aestheticians and aromatherapists who specialize in skin care.

If you are blessed with a normal complexion, use the herbs and treatments suggested for either dry or oily complexions. Most complexions, however, fall into more than one category. A combination complexion—oily in the "T-zone" of chin, nose and fore-

head and dry around the eyes, cheeks and mouth—is the most common type. Using the information and recipes for both dry and oily skin, treat your face like two separate faces.

As your skin matures, gradually adjust the way you care for it. Remember that your skin changes with age, menstrual cycle and the seasons. The norm for skin is this: As children we have normal skin, during adolescence it becomes oily, and as we grow older, especially after age 40, our skin becomes increasingly dry.

You probably already have some idea of what type of complexion you have. If you are unsure, you can check how much oil your skin produces with a blotting test. Go to bed without applying any facial products. In the morning, before washing or putting anything on your face, pat a few strips torn from a clean brown paper bag on different areas of your face, especially in the T-zone. Normal skin areas will show a small amount of oil, dry skin won't leave any oil on the paper and oily skin will leave a definite oil stain. Unless you have exceptionally oily skin, your cheeks will not show any oiliness.

THE FACE

The philosopher who said "The eyes are the window to the soul" had it half right. I've long thought that the entire face is the pathway to the heart.

Herbs can be used to lessen the effects of aging, exposure to sunlight and other face-changers—taken properly, they can add a healthy glow, heal facial disorders, prevent premature wrinkling and generally give you a bit more control over the fate of your face.

DRY COMPLEXION

Have you ever considered starting your day with a yogurt, honey and fruit smoothie—not for breakfast, but on your face? If you suffer from dry skin, you've probably considered trying just about anything. This emollient facial mask coaxes water to the surface and does a great job of moisturizing dry skin.

If you have a dry complexion, the skin on your face probably has a fine texture with no visible pores. This type of skin tends to be thin and sensitive, and it may often feel tight and dry, especially after you wash it. It can eventually become sallow and develop a coarse texture. If you have dry skin, chances are it is due to underactive oil glands, probably from a combination of heredity and low hormone production. Skin constantly loses water through sweat and evaporation, but tiny glands secrete an oil to coat skin and stop this loss.

Because women, especially those who are fairskinned, tend to have drier skin than men do, they are more susceptible to premature wrinkling and flaking skin. Escaping summer's damaging heat by jumping into a chlorinated swimming pool or by seeking the cool but dry air of air-conditioning generally increases skin dryness. Dry skin is also vulnerable to winter's wind and chapping cold, which further suppress the oil glands' production. If the air inside your house is particularly dry, consider using a humidifier. You should also consider a humidifier if

you heat your home with a woodburning stove, which has a drying effect on the skin. If you don't have a humidifier, you can achieve the same effect by keeping a pan of water over low heat on the stove.

You can also use herbs to help help bring moisture to your dry skin. Cosmetics experts and aromatherapists suggest the essential oils of palmarosa, rosewood and sandalwood to stimulate oil production in dry skin. According to these authorities, small amounts of peppermint or rosemary increase the skin's oil production and improve circulation. Chamomile, lavender, jasmine, elder flowers, red clover and soothing herbs such as Irish moss, calendula, comfrey, marshmallow root and violets soothe and heal the irritation that so easily develops as outer layers of dry skin flake off. The essential oil of carrot seed soothes extremely raw skin. Elder flowers improve the complexion's tone and texture. In France, dry complexions are treated with an elder-flower water called *eau de sureau*.

If you have a dry complexion, always use as little soap as possible—most soaps dry out your skin. Avoid foaming cleansers, which are far too drying. When you do wash with soap, choose one designed for delicate skin. Otherwise, wash with a water-soluble cleansing cream for dry skin—these are designed not to remove the skin's natural oil—and always pat your face dry very gently. Remove makeup with a face cream instead of soap, and always use makeup that contains moisturizers.

Avoid facial toners that contain alcohol, which will dry your skin. Instead, use a toner with a vinegar base—this will soften your skin, help it maintain its natural acidity and relieve the itchiness and flakiness that often accompany dryness.

The mild astringency of hydrosols is ideal for dry skin because it increases the skin's water content. Hydrosols that contain aloe or glycerin also help skin to retain moisture. Facial creams that are half oil are suitable for dry skin. Heavy, rich creams with even more oil offer greater protection from water evaporation but tend to be greasy; they are usually reserved for the sensitive skin around the eyes where there are no oil glands.

A facial steam can help a dry complexion, but make sure it is not too hot and that it lasts five minutes at the most. Also, don't opt for a facial steam more than once a week because the heat in regular steaming will further dry your skin. Another option is a gentle facial massage with an herbal scrub made with cornmeal and oatmeal. While many people think scrubs are too harsh for a dry complexion, they actually stimulate oil production and remove flaky, dry surface skin. A few minutes per treatment is enough.

Dry skin is sometimes accompanied by inflammations such as blemishes or puffiness around the eyes. Numerous scientific studies on chamomile, lavender, rosemary and Saint-John's-wort show that these herbs reduce these inflammations. In the early 1990s, H.W. Kreysel, M.D., director of the Dermatologic Clinic at the University of Bonn in Germany, conducted three separate clinical studies on chamomile with dozens of men and women. He found that a chamomile cream restored a smooth,

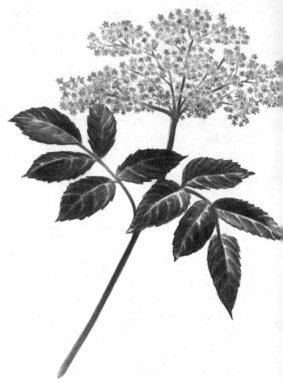

The ancient Egyptians were the first to discover that elder flowers can be used to improve the complexion.

healthy appearance to rough and red skin faster and more thoroughly than other creams did. It also improved "peak and valley" patterns, known more commonly as wrinkles.

Cleanser for Dry Complexion
2 ounces aloe vera gel
1 teaspoon vegetable oil
1 teaspoon glycerin
½ teaspoon grapefruit seed extract
8 drops sandalwood essential oil
4 drops rosemary essential oil
≈ Blend ingredients. Shake well before each use. Apply with cotton balls, then rinse off. I like to substitute grape seed

oil or Saint-John's-wort oil for the vege-table oil. You can also use jojoba oil (re-ally a liquid wax); it is more expensive than vegetable oil but is good for the complexion, and unlike true vegetable oils, it will not spoil.

Toner for Dry Complexion

2 ounces aloe vera gel
2 ounces orange-blossom water
1 teaspoon vinegar
6 drops rose geranium essential oil
4 drops sandalwood essential oil
1 drop each chamomile and jasmine
     (optional) essential oils
800 International Units vitamin E oil

Combine ingredients. Shake before using. For the vinegar, I prefer using elder-flower vinegar, but since it is not sold in stores, you must make it yourself (see Herbal Vinegar Formula on page 18). The jasmine is optional because it is so expensive. You can use liquid vitamin E oil or pop open two 400–International Unit vitamin E capsules. This toner can also be used as a man's aftershave.

Cream for Dry Complexion

3/4 ounce beeswax, shaved
1 cup vegetable oil
1 cup water (or rose water)
24 drops (1/4 teaspoon) rose geranium es-
     sential oil or 6 drops rose essential oil

Heat beeswax and vegetable oil in a pot until beeswax melts. In a separate pot, heat water until it is warm to the touch. Remove the center ring on the lid of your blender (or food processor) and pour the warm water in. With the blender on high speed, slowly add the oil-beeswax mix-ture. (This is just like making mayonnaise. You need to pour the oil steadily at just

the right temperature—you should be able to put your finger in both the oil and the water without discomfort.) The whole concoction should begin to solid-ify when three-quarters of the oil has been added. As this happens, add the essential oils and carefully stir in top edges as they turn solid, staying away from the blender's blades. Keep adding oil until the mixture becomes too stiff to take any more, or when all the water is blended in. Turn off blender. You should have a thick, smooth cream. Using a rub-ber spatula, pour the cream into wide-mouthed jars while it is still warm. (Once it cools, it will be too thick to pour.) Do not try to cut this recipe in half—if you do, there will not be enough liquid to cover the blender blades.

Be sure that you purchase beeswax (sold at craft stores, at natural food and herb stores, and by beekeepers) and not paraffin. Creams, lotions or substances containing water carry a personal invita-tion for bacterial growth, but essential oils, beeswax and vitamin E are natural preservatives and, under most condi-tions, give your creams at least a six-month shelf life. If you store your extra cream in the refrigerator, it should keep three times as long. As an extra precau-tion against spoilage, you might consider using grapefruit seed extract, another powerful antibacterial agent, or vitamin E. Add eight drops grapefruit seed extract or 400 International Units vitamin E per ounce. Be sure that your tools—blender, bowls, measuring cups and containers—are very clean. Even dipping a finger into a cosmetic invites bacteria, so use a small cosmetic spatula or a clean chopstick to scoop cream from the jar.

Facial Steam for Dry Complexion
3 cups water

Method #1: Using Herbs
*1 heaping teaspoon each rose petals, rose-
mary leaves and fennel seeds*
½ teaspoon peppermint leaves
🍂 Simmer water, add herbs, remove
from heat and steep for 5 minutes.

Method #2: Using Essential Oils
*1 drop each rose geranium, rosemary,
fennel and peppermint essential oils*
🍂 Simmer water, turn off heat and add
essential oils.

For either method, set pan in a location where you can comfortably sit next
to it. Cover the back of your head with a
towel and tuck the ends of the towel
around the pan so that steam is captured
inside a "mini-sauna." Hold your head
about 1 foot away from the water. Make
sure that the steam is not so hot that it
feels uncomfortable, and keep your eyes
closed so that the essential oils do not
sting them. Stay in the steam for a few
minutes, then come out to cool your
face. Do this for a few rounds, as long as
it's comfortable.

Scrub for Dry Complexion
2 tablespoons oatmeal
1 tablespoon cornmeal
*1 teaspoon chamomile, lavender or
elder flowers*
6 drops lavender essential oil
🍂 Grind dry ingredients in blender or
electric coffee grinder. (Drugstores sell
colloidal oatmeal, which needs no grind-
ing.) Add essential oil and stir to distribute. Store in closed container. To use,
moisten 1 teaspoon with enough water

to make a paste, dampen your face with
a little water and gently apply scrub.
Rinse with warm water.

Mask for Dry Complexion
1 tablespoon ground oatmeal
1 tablespoon rose water or aloe vera juice
1 teaspoon vegetable oil
1 teaspoon honey
*2 drops rose geranium or palmarosa
essential oil*
🍂 Mix ingredients and apply to face.
Leave on for 5 to 10 minutes, then rinse
off. Castor oil is a good choice for the
vegetable oil because of its emollient
qualities and because it mixes easily with
the other ingredients. Keep any leftover
mask in the refrigerator.

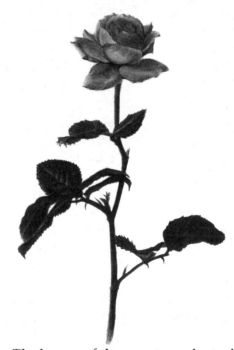

**The beauty of the rose is not limited
to its own appearance—it can also be
used in formulas designed to make us
look better.**

OILY COMPLEXION

People with oily complexions tend to bemoan their genetic fate, at least through their early years. Only later do they start to feel fortunate. There is a positive side to oily skin—it protects and lubricates, so you can expect fewer wrinkles as your skin matures.

An oily complexion tends to be shiny and to have large pores and a thick, coarse texture. It may seem that summer would help an oily complexion, but this is not so. Overexposure to the sun combined with sunburn stimulates already overactive oil glands into even heavier production. Sweating from the heat only increases the skin's oiliness.

In winter, oil buildup is made worse when we bundle up with scarves and hats. All that excess oil attracts dirt, which can breed bacteria, cause infection and clog pores with dead cells.

Nothing you use on your skin should completely stop your skin from producing oil, but some herbs can slow the production. Basil, eucalyptus, cedarwood, cypress, lemon, sage, lemongrass, yarrow, ylang-ylang (sold only as an essential oil) and the fruit and leaves of strawberry help normalize overactive oil glands. I also use lady's mantle, an attractive plant grown by many herb gardeners.

Clean your oily face at least twice a day with a neutral-pH (7.0) soap or cleanser. Wipe away excess oil with cotton pads soaked in witch hazel or a cleanser for oily skin. Steam your face at least once a week—this will unclog pores and eliminate excess oil. Avoid scrubbing; it stimulates oil production. Instead, use a facial mask of oats or clay to draw out and absorb surface skin oils. (Rinse the mask off before your skin begins to feel tight and itchy.) A slight amount of grain alcohol in a toner is okay, but do not use it often. Alcohol is drying, but if you dry out oily skin too much, it will produce even more oil to compensate. Moisturizers that double as toners, such as those with aloe vera or natural ingredients containing AHAs are good—even oily skin needs some moisturizing.

Cleanser for Oily Complexion

2 ounces witch hazel
1 teaspoon vinegar
1 teaspoon glycerin
½ teaspoon grapefruit seed extract
6 drops lemon essential oil
2 drops each cypress and grapefruit (optional) essential oils

🍂 Follow the directions given for Cleanser for Dry Complexion (page 310). If available, you can use an herbal vinegar; I make my own yarrow vinegar.

Facial Steam for Oily Complexion

3 cups water

Method #1: Using Herbs

1 heaping teaspoon each chamomile flowers, lemon grass leaves, lavender flowers and rosemary leaves

🍂 Simmer water, add herbs, remove from heat and steep 5 minutes.

Method #2: Using Essential Oils

1 drop each chamomile, lemongrass, lavender and rosemary essential oils

🍂 Bring water to a simmer, turn off heat and add essential oils.

To steam, follow directions for Facial Steam for Dry Complexion (opposite page).

Mask for Oily Complexion

1 tablespoon witch hazel
1 teaspoon bentonite (or other facial) clay
1 strawberry, mashed (optional)
2 drops each cypress and lemon
    essential oils

Combine ingredients and apply. Leave on for 5 to 10 minutes, then rinse.

Toner for Oily Complexion

2 ounces witch hazel
1 tablespoon aloe vera gel
5 drops cedarwood essential oil
3 drops lemon essential oil
1 drop ylang-ylang essential oil

Combine ingredients. Shake well before using. Without the ylang-ylang, which is too sweet-smelling for most men, this makes an excellent aftershave.

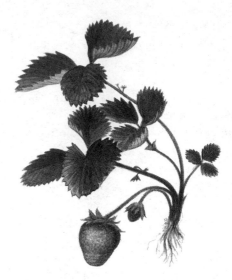

Who doesn't love strawberries? But they're not only yummy; they also help normalize overactive oil glands in the skin.

MATURE COMPLEXION

Your face takes on more character as you mature, but most of us would just as soon keep our immature smooth skin. The legendary French beauty Ninon de L'Enclos, who felt she had no need for lines, once bitterly complained, "If God had to give woman wrinkles, He might at least have put them on the soles of her feet." According to some skin specialists, anyone over 25 has mature skin, but lines typically start to form in your thirties. Your chances of having mature skin and wrinkles when you are young increase if you have a fair complexion or only a thin layer of fat under your skin, if you smoke cigarettes, or if you spend lots of time in the sun.

If you have mature skin, it is likely that it will also be dry, so many of the recommendations for dry skin will apply. In addition, rose geranium, jas-mine, frankincense and myrrh rejuvenate skin by encouraging new cells to develop. So do some unusual essential oils: carrot seed, helichrysum and cistus (better known to gardeners as rock rose). Marshmallow, comfrey and gotu kola heal skin, stimulate skin-cell growth and soothe skin that is irritated from being dry and flaky. For centuries, lavender, neroli, rosemary, rose and fennel have been called anti-aging herbs. These herbs are listed in many old recipes, including one from the diary of the duchess of Alba, whose beauty was recorded in Goya's late nineteenth-century portraits of her. The duchess used rose water and almond oil mixed with egg white to "keep out the wrinkles and preserve the complexion fair" and to promote firmness when "the skin becomes too loosely attached to the muscles."

As you grow older, your body produces fewer of the hormones that keep skin supple and youthful, and supplies less oil, protein and natural moisturizing factors, which attract and hold water in the skin. This process also tends to make the skin drier. As time goes by, collagen and elastin—"elastic" fibers in the skin that are arranged like the meshwork of woven fabric—eventually lose their strength, eliminating the skin's underlying support and causing it to wrinkle and sag. It is these fibers, not muscle, that make your skin strong and keep it toned, firm and unwrinkled.

Like the rest of the fashion world, the cosmetics industry is subject to changing fads and trends. In the 1980s, collagen and elastin derived from animals were acclaimed as cosmetic ingredients to slow the effects of aging on your skin. There doesn't seem to be much point to these treatments—most skin specialists argue that the molecules are too big to penetrate the skin and couldn't mesh with existing fibers even if they did. You can, however, encourage natural collagen production with herbs and foods that contain lots of vitamin C and compounds commonly associated with vitamin C—rutin, flavonoids and hesperidin. For a complete list of these beneficial herbs and foods, see "Couperose Complexion" on page 318. Other herbs, such as gotu kola, echinacea and horsetail, increase skin elasticity and strengthen connective tissue.

So-called antioxidant herbs offer an effective defense against the skin's aging. These herbs encourage cells to regenerate and prevent the formation of free radicals. Free radicals are unstable, quickly multiplying molecules, which are increased by cigarette smoking, inhaling car exhaust and ingesting certain pesticides. They are thought to play a role in the skin losing its elasticity and wrinkling. (In fact, free radicals are thought to play a part in all aspects of aging, including "hardening of the arteries" and the development of cataracts. Due to the effect of these free radicals, a 40-year-old smoker is older, biologically, than a nonsmoker of the same age.) Many natural cosmetics for mature skin include herbs and vitamins that stop free radicals in their tracks. Powerful antioxidants include ginkgo, witch hazel and the essential oils of rosemary, marjoram and lavender.

Antioxidants also are good for treating liver spots, discolorations of the skin that actually have little to do with the liver. A more accurate label for them would be "sun spots" since they appear on the face and hands as a result of sun exposure. There are several natural bleaching agents you can try on these spots and on other types of blotchy skin. Horseradish, vinegar and lemon are favorites, so I suggest using all three.

For a mature complexion, use the cleanser and masks suggested for dry complexions. Drying facial masks, like those made with clay or oatmeal, should not be used often on mature skin and should be completely avoided if your skin is very dry. However, occasional use of astringent masks and toners has one advantage for a mature complexion— the water that they pull to the skin's surface slightly plumps up the skin and makes lines, wrinkles and enlarged pores seem smaller, at least temporarily. Unfortunately, this has a "Cinderella" effect; over the next few hours, the magic wears off as the water is reabsorbed and evaporates. Much like Cinderella's fairy godmother, I offer a warning—be home before the effect wears off. Watch out for commercial toners that plump skin by irritating it and causing inflammation.

Age Spot Remover

1 teaspoon grated horseradish root
½ teaspoon lemon juice
½ teaspoon vinegar
3 drops rosemary essential oil

~ Combine ingredients. If you know how, grating your own horseradish is best, but it is important to add juice and vinegar right away, before the enzymes start to break down. Don't get your fingers near your eyes—horseradish is hot stuff. Simpler, though not as effective, is to buy a bottle of ground horseradish.

Toner for Mature Complexion

2 ounces aloe vera gel
2 ounces orange-blossom water
1 teaspoon vinegar
6 drops rose geranium essential oil
4 drops each frankincense and carrot
   seed essential oils
2 drops jasmine essential oil (optional)
800 International Units vitamin E oil

~ Combine ingredients. Shake before using. I prefer using elder-flower vinegar, but since it is not sold in stores, it must be homemade (see Herbal Vinegar Formula on page 18). It's certainly okay to use plain apple cider vinegar. The jasmine essential oil is optional because it is so expensive. You can use liquid vitamin E oil or pop open 2 400–International Unit vitamin E capsules.

PROBLEM COMPLEXION

A problem complexion is characterized by pimples, cysts, blackheads and whiteheads. If you have this complexion, you know that it can be a constant source of worry and embarrassment. Acne occurs where there are the most oil glands—on the face, back and chest. In severe cases, it scars and pits the skin. Acne usually improves in early summer, as increased sun exposure provides vitamin D and lightly exfoliates the skin, but can worsen if oil glands become stimulated by too much heat and sun.

Oil gets to the skin's surface by traveling up the hair shaft. When your pores become clogged with excess oil and dead cells, the opening narrows; this shuts off oxygen to the pores and encourages bacterial growth, infection and inflammation. Blackheads arise when trapped oil darkens as it oxidizes (this darkening is not from dirt, as many people mistakenly believe). When pores are repeatedly clogged, they enlarge and change the skin's texture.

Most antiseptic herbs, including goldenseal, eucalyptus, sage, rosemary and tea tree, reduce acne. Chamomile, elder flowers, red clover and licorice unclog pores and refine, soften and heal skin. Lavender, neroli and rosemary stimulate new cell growth. In one study of more than 100 people with acne, it was found that a tea tree gel was very effective in combating this problem. Although the gel acted more slowly than an often-prescribed benzyl peroxide lotion, it was better tolerated by everyone's skin. In fact, tea tree produced no adverse reactions at all. You can apply a drop of tea tree essential oil directly a couple of times a day as a spot-application on pimples, as long as you do not rub it on larger areas of your skin and you are not overly sensitive to the oil.

Cleaning your face thoroughly and as often as three times a day is an important step in treating acne. Many people with problem skin like to use foaming cleansers, but if you do, be sure to choose one that is pH balanced. You should also steam once or twice a week, using antiseptic essential oils or herbs.

Scrubbing may seem ideal for an acned complexion, but it actually aggravates the condition. Stick to an astringent mask of clay moistened with a facial toner to promote slight peeling and reduce large pores. Toners with vinegar are antiseptic and maintain the skin's acid balance. You can heal damaged skin with a light lotion that contains mostly aloe vera and little or no oil.

Acne is often caused by hormone imbalances, especially high testosterone levels, which can lead to excess oil production. As a result, problem skin is most common during puberty, when hormones rage; indeed, 80 percent of North American adolescents have skin blemishes. Several studies on vitex berry, an herb that is known to reduce hormone levels and decrease their action, have been reported in various German scientific journals. These studies indicate that vitex helps control acne in young men and women. For women, vitex has been particularly helpful in alleviating premenstrual symptoms, and is especially useful in eliminating acne that flares up right before menstruation. Vitex is available in natural food stores as a tincture, as tea, or in pill form. For more information on the virtues of vitex, see chapter 11.

Unfortunately, acne can also follow you into adulthood, when—if related to hormone imbalances—it generally appears around the chin and jawline. The liver is responsible for keeping hormones like testosterone in balance. Refer to chapter 7 to learn more about herbs that can help fight acne, including milk thistle, burdock, yellow dock, turmeric and sarsaparilla.

Stress may also be partially responsible for causing skin blemishes, especially in women. Not all dermatologists agree that emotions influence the skin, but when researchers at Boston University asked a group of people what triggered their acne, most of them quickly came up with the same answer: stress. The researchers found that, although stress stimulates a rise in adrenal hormones in everyone, women's bodies respond to stress by overproducing testosterone. This finding led psychologists at North Texas State University to teach a group of people with acne stress-countering relaxation methods like deep breathing, biofeedback (in which a person is taught to be aware of unconscious or involuntary bodily processes so that she can learn to control them mentally) and imagery (imagining oneself in a calm, peaceful setting, such as a quiet green meadow). The result was that the complexions of these people improved much more than those in a similar group that did not learn the relaxation methods. If you suffer from acne and believe that stress is a contributing factor, see "Stress" on page 52 for herbs to promote relaxation.

The prevailing opinion of most dermatologists is that diet has little influence on acne. Holistic practitioners, including herbalists, do not share this view and suggest a whole-foods diet with plenty of vegetables and going easy on fatty foods, especially those high on concentrated fat, such as cheese, butter and fried foods. While fatty foods may not directly translate into oil on your skin, they do affect the functioning of your liver and thus your levels of hormones and stress. Fatty foods also reduce the action of important essential fatty acids in the body. Supplements of gamma linoleic acid (GLA), which is found in evening primrose oil, increase these fatty acids and have helped some cases of acne.

Blemish Remover

¼ cup water
1 teaspoon Epsom salts
4 drops lavender essential oil
Small cloth

❧ Bring water to a boil and pour it over Epsom salts. When salts have dissolved, add essential oil. Soak a small absorbent cloth in solution and press this compress on any pimples. In a minute or two, as cloth starts to cool, place it in hot water again and reapply. Do this several times. The lavender is antiseptic and anti-inflammatory.

Intensive Treatment for Acne

½ teaspoon powdered goldenseal root
12 drops tea tree essential oil

❧ Combine ingredients into a paste, adding water if needed. Apply directly on acne spots. Let dry and leave on the skin for at least 20 minutes. Rinse.

Facial Steam for Problem Complexion

3 cups water

Method #1: Using Herbs

1 heaping teaspoon each chamomile flowers, eucalyptus leaves, lavender flowers and rosemary leaves

❧ Bring water to a boil. Remove from heat. Add herbs and steep for 5 minutes.

Method #2: Using Essential Oils

1 drop each chamomile, eucalyptus, lavender and rosemary essential oils

❧ Bring water to a boil, turn off heat and add essential oils.

To steam, follow directions for Facial Steam for Dry Complexion (see page 312).

Mask for Acne

1 teaspoon bentonite (or other facial) clay
1 teaspoon ground strawberry leaves, (optional)
1 drop chamomile, sage or rosemary essential oil
1 drop tea tree essential oil
Water or toner

❧ Mix ingredients into a paste with water or the Toner for Dry Complexion (see page 311) or Toner for Oily Complexion (see page 314), depending on your skin type. Apply to face in a thin layer, avoiding the area around the eyes. Leave on for 10 to 15 minutes, or as long as it is comfortable, then rinse.

COUPEROSE COMPLEXION

If you have a couperose complexion, your skin is filled with broken capillaries (the tiny blood vessels found just under the skin). This makes for redness mostly around the nose or on the cheeks. Any kind of skin can become couperose, but this condition is most common with dry, thin, delicate or mature skin. You increase your chances of having a couperose complexion if you drink, smoke or have fair skin, fair hair or high blood pressure. Exposing your skin to extreme temperatures or rough scrubbing also contributes to the condition and will make the problem worse once you have it.

Though it is often difficult to treat, a couperose complexion can be improved over time, especially if you improve capillary strength with herbs that are high in flavonoids (pigments found in many green and yellow plants). These herbs include hawthorn, ginkgo, Saint-John's-wort, calendula, lemon, peppers, buckwheat and rosehips. Chamomile, lavender, rose and neroli, along with the lesser-known helichrysum, also make weak and broken capillaries stronger and more resilient, soothe delicate skin and reduce puffiness.

A facial also helps combat a couperose complexion, but be sure to take extra care when applying it. Wash your face with lukewarm water and a cleansing cream. Avoid the temperature extremes of a cold water splash or a facial steam because they bring extra blood to the skin's surface. Also, stay away from scrubs and astringent masks, such as those made with clay, which increase surface circulation and encourage capillaries to break in sensitive skin. Instead, use only the gentlest exfoliants and masks, such as yogurt, papaya or honey, and facial toners made of

hydrosols or aloe vera. Look for moisturizers and toners designed for dry complexions.

There is hope. My friend Margaret had one of the worst couperose complexions I have ever seen. She had a good sense of humor, though, and would often laugh while saying she was paying for her old sins. She had lived the "high life" for a long time, and although she no longer drank or smoked, her face betrayed her old ways. She managed to cover most of it with makeup, but was still concerned when she looked in the mirror every morning—her complexion seemed to be getting worse by the day! Margaret's solution was to use the herbal recipes below. While her face still has a few broken capillaries, Margaret is now happy to look in the mirror — her complexion continues to improve.

Facial for Couperose Complexion
1 tablespoon each yogurt and applesauce
2 drops liquid lecithin
2 drops chamomile essential oil
Blend ingredients. Apply to face and leave on for at least 5 minutes. Gently rinse off with lukewarm water.

Toner for Couperose Complexion
2 ounces aloe vera juice
2 ounces rose water
¼ teaspoon glycerin
5 drops lavender essential oil
*2 drops each neroli, chamomile and
    helichrysum (optional) essential oils*
Combine ingredients and shake well before using. Apply with cotton swabs, or spray on using an atomizer. For men with couperose or sensitive skin, this toner can also be used as an aftershave.

THE SIX-STEP FACIAL

One of the best ways to promote a glowing, clear complexion, no matter what your skin type, is by doing an herbal facial. I always bring mirrors to herbal cosmetics classes so everyone can see for themselves how radiant and youthful they look after a facial. Of all the stories from years of conducting these classes, Sharon's is my favorite. She left an evening facial class that was held downtown, and having nowhere else to take her new complexion, went out for a drink with a couple of other women from the class. A handsome young man asked her out, and though she was very flattered, she declined, never telling him that she was almost 20 years his senior! I will not promise you results like this, but you are certain to notice the difference.

If you can afford to have a weekly facial at a salon that uses natural products, by all means indulge! If a salon facial is not in your budget, doing your own facial at home is simple and quick; the entire routine can be completed in only 20 minutes. You will need a washcloth, a facial sponge or soft washcloth, a towel, a pan, a small mixing bowl for mixing a mask or scrub, and all your facial ingredients. If you keep these supplies in a special box or basket, they will be convenient whenever you want a facial. Be sure to wear a shirt or blouse with a wide or low neck, and pull your hair away from your face before you begin your facial.

Step 1: Clean the skin for two minutes.

Step 2: Steam for five to ten minutes (use a quarter-cup herbs or three drops essential oils per three cups water—for specific herbs and steaming directions, see the recipes in the specific skin-type sections in "The Face" on page 308).

Step 3: Exfoliate your skin for two to three minutes —remember to use gentle circular movements.

Step 4: Apply a mask and leave it on for about ten minutes

Step 5: Apply toner.

Step 6: Finish up by applying a moisturizer.

If you do not have time for the full routine, how about a mini-facial? When you are in a hurry or traveling, place two herbal tea bags (chamomile is a good choice) in a cup and pour boiling water over them just as if you are making tea. Hold your face over the cup to steam in the fragrant vapors. Then apply a facial cream or moisturizer. Afterward, you can drink the tea! When your eyes are puffy, strained or bloodshot, make the tea with two tea bags of chamomile or black tea, cool slightly and place one bag on each eye.

THE BODY

The face shows the most obvious signs of sun exposure and aging, but all of your skin suffers equally from these factors. Maybe this is why many people pay close attention to their faces, but forget the rest of their skin. While it is natural to give your face extra care, all of your skin deserves the best treatment. For total body care, treat your entire body with lotions, bathing and saunas.

DRY SKIN

The basic treatments for dry skin are body lotions, scrubs and bath oils. Instead of using soap, which will dry out your skin even more, choose a cleanser or scrub designed for dry skin (some recipes are provided on page 322). If your dry skin itches, add a quarter-cup of vinegar to your bath.

Herbs that encourage oil production in dry skin are the same ones that are used for dry complexions: chamomile, fennel, rose geranium, lavender, palmarosa, sandalwood and small amounts of peppermint and rosemary. Frankincense, jasmine, neroli and rose, which are more expensive, are also beneficial. Putting essential oils of these herbs in your bath is good because they are attracted to your skin and are absorbed more easily in hot water. But be careful; many of them— peppermint, for instance—can sting your skin. If your skin does become irritated, rinse off with cool water and apply vegetable oil to sore areas.

If you have dry skin, try bathing with floating bath oil. If you love soaking for an hour or more in a hot bath, but find that your skin itches and seems to shrivel afterward, your problem will likely disappear. I know several people who were unable to take baths at all because their skin was so dry. That changed when they discovered bath oils. When you emerge, your entire body moves through the water's surface and receives a light coating of oil—just enough to protect the skin from drying out, but not enough to make it feel oily. As an added bonus, the scent of a bath oil will linger for hours as a body perfume.

Dry skin almost always benefits from improved circulation. To improve your circulation, try an herbal steam sauna (a dry sauna is not suggested for dry skin). If the sauna's heating element is designed to have water poured on it, pour a few drops of essential oil or some strong herb tea (lavender, chamomile or rosemary) on the sauna rocks (or whatever element the sauna has). If you cannot pour water on the heating element, place a pan of water containing the herbs or essential oil on it. You should also make sure that no one in the sauna, including you, is sensitive to the oils! Stepping out to rinse with cool water a few times and then returning to the sauna helps increase circulation. (If you have a heart condition or are pregnant, see a doctor before you use a sauna; you will probably be advised against it.)

Sweating may not seem like a beauty treatment, but it does provide some hidden attributes. AHAs, which are produced when we sweat, are so good for the skin that they are now incorporated into the expensive products of many cosmetics companies. Dermatologist Ruey J. Yu,

M.D., of Temple University, who has studied AHAs since the early 1980s, believes that one reason physical exercise contributes to beautiful skin is the AHA lactic acid, which is contained in sweat.

Lotion for Dry Skin
¾ *cup vegetable oil*
1 cup water or aloe vera juice
2 teaspoons liquid lanolin
½ *ounce shaved beeswax*
20 drops lavender essential oil
10 drops sandalwood essential oil
4 drops chamomile essential oil
Follow the directions for making Cream for Dry Complexion (see page 311). Pour lotion into bottles.

Scrub Ball
1 cup Scrub for Dry Complexion (see page 312)
Porous cloth, about 6 inches square
String or cloth tie
Tie the scrub inside the cloth with the string. Throw the ball into your bath water, or hold the ball under hot water in the shower. When you squeeze the ball, a rich and creamy liquid scented with the essential oils will emerge. Wash with this instead of soap, squeezing as you need more liquid. The ball will last for several washes, after which you should toss out the contents, wash the cloth and refill it with new ingredients.

Floating Bath Oil for Dry Skin
2 ounces vegetable oil
12 drops each lavender and rose geranium essential oils
Combine ingredients. Use 1 teaspoon per bath. Contained in a beautiful bottle, this makes a wonderful gift.

Dispersing Bath Oil
½ *teaspoon hydrous lanolin (optional)*
2 ounces castor oil
12 drops lavender essential oil
4 drops petitgrain essential oil
Hydrous lanolin, available at any drugstore, is the easiest form of lanolin to use in any recipe because it contains a small amount of water—just enough to make it easier to mix. Warm lanolin in castor oil just enough to melt it. Add essential oils. Some oils will float on the water's surface and some will blend in the water, making it feel silky. In this oil, I have used petitgrain, made from the twig behind the orange flower, instead of the more expensive flower of the bitter orange, known as neroli.

OILY SKIN
Oily skin, which attracts dirt easily and can take on a greasy appearance, should be treated much like an oily facial complexion—use herbs such as sage, lemongrass, basil, eucalyptus, cedawood, cypress, lemon, yarrow and ylang-ylang to normalize overactive oil glands. Bathing helps oily skin, especially if you use the Aromatic Bath Salts or Aromatic Bath Vinegar (see page 323). A few drops of the essential oils of any of the herbs mentioned above can also be added directly to the bath. If you have oily skin, avoid high heat in saunas; it only encourages your skin to become oilier in an effort to protect the skin from the heat.

Bath salts make the bath water feel silky, remove body oils and perspiration and soften the skin. They are also inexpensive and very easy to make, and the ingredients can be found in any grocery store. You should see the faces in my skin care class when I pull boxes of table salt, baking soda and borax out of my bag, and explain that these are the "mixed salts" used for commercial bath salts! For fancy "mineral" spa salts, ground seaweed or clay is added to increase the mineral content of the salts.

Table salt, borax and baking soda, which are sodium salts, soften hard water and help soap work better by creating more suds. (Epsom salts, which contain magnesium, do not soften water but they do soothe sore muscles.) Sodium salts also eliminate "soap scum"—that dirty, insoluble ring around the bathtub produced when minerals in hard water combine with soap—and the film that hard water and soap leave on skin and hair, making them look dull and feel rough.

Salt can also be used to stimulate oily skin's circulation with a "salt glow," an allover body treatment that you do before washing your body. Before getting into the tub or shower, dampen a handful of regular table salt with a little water or milk (about a tablespoon of liquid to half a cup of salt), then lightly rub the damp salt over your body. After you get out of the shower or tub, you will notice that your body is "glowing."

Aromatic Bath Vinegar

2 ounces vinegar
10 drops each lemon and eucalyptus
 essential oils

🌿 Combine ingredients and let sit for 1 week, shaking the bottle daily. Use 2 tablespoons per bath. Any type of vinegar will do, but for an attractive display in your bathroom, use red wine vinegar stored in a clear bottle.

Aromatic Bath Salts

½ cup table salt
1 tablespoon each baking soda and borax
10 drops each lavender and lemon
 essential oils
5 drops ylang-ylang essential oil

🌿 Mix dry ingredients together, then stir in essential oils. Use ¼ to ½ cup of the salts per bath. Bath salts make wonderful gifts, especially if you package them in elegant bottles.

SUN-DAMAGED SKIN

In the early twentieth century, sunbathing became very popular, at least in North America. It was only in the 1980s and 1990s that people began to realize the dangers of spending long periods of time in the sun to get a tan. Nevertheless, many people still spend too many hours in the sun.

Exposure to the sun can be dangerous because the sun's ultraviolet (UV) rays, which cause the skin to tan and burn, can also cause skin cancer. The long ultraviolet (UVA) rays that are present all day long are particularly destructive. Nicknamed "aging rays," they penetrate into the skin's lower layers, harming collagen, elastin and DNA, which carries a cell's genetic information. UVA rays also make skin more susceptible to the shorter UVB rays, which tan the skin's surface and are strongest at midday. Both of these rays are associated with premature aging and skin cancer, but skin experts believe that very short ultraviolet rays called UVC rays are mostly responsible for the worldwide increase in skin cancer. (One problem with some sunscreens is that they block only the UVB rays.)

With the depletion of the earth's ozone layer, which blocks UV rays, more of these rays are hitting the earth. The National Cancer Institute reports that melanoma, a form of skin cancer associated with sun exposure, increased nearly 90 percent between 1973 and 1990! Skin cancer is now increasing even in dark-skinned people, who used to have few worries about getting it. But you would have a hard time believing any of these facts while spending a day at any beach. North Americans just love to get their sun.

Sun damage can occur at any age, but its long-term effects on the skin, especially premature wrinkling and uneven pigmentation, become apparent only as we grow older. In fact, most skin aging is thought to result from sun exposure. If you doubt this, compare your face and the backs of your hands with areas of your skin that rarely see the sun.

When it come to sun damage, prevention is the key, so do your best to limit your sun exposure, and wear protective clothing or sunscreen when you go outside. Almost 75 percent of sun damage occurs without our even going to the beach or lying out in the sun— as we walk down the street, ride a bike or even drive a car (if the windows are down). Special skin cells spread a dark pigment called melanin through the skin to tan it, protecting sensitive underlying cells from the sun's destructive tendencies. However, this offers only limited protection, and after a few days of repeated sun exposure, the skin also thickens in defense. Margaret Kripke, M.D., of the Anderson Cancer Center in

Houston, Texas, says that sunscreen users may be spending long hours in the sun with a false sense of security. They may not be getting burned, but ultraviolet light also suppresses the immune system, and Dr. Kripke believes that sunscreens do little to prevent this.

No natural ingredient fully protects us from the sun's rays, but some protection can be found in nature's bounty. PABA (part of the B-complex vitamins) and cinoxate (cinnamic acid from cinnamon) are commonly used in sunscreens. However, questions have been raised about the safety of these products, since they can cause allergic reactions and other problems.

According to skin specialists, sesame oil decreases the impact of the sun's burning rays by about 30 percent, while olive, coconut and peanut oils and aloe vera block out about 20 percent of the rays. This is lower than the high rates now achieved with commercial sunscreens, but suitable for less intense exposure. Research shows that a 3 to 6 percent dilution of an extract of helichrysum, sometimes called immortelle, makes an effective sunscreen. And a new sunscreen made from amino acids found in sea algae is currently being tested in Australia.

Ingredients in natural sunscreens are soon likely to include antioxidant herbs, which combat harmful free radicals. Japanese scientists have shown that applying these herbs on the skin not only protects against free radical damage, but also prevents damage caused by UV rays. In one study at the Xienta Institute for Skin Research in Bernville, Pennsylvania, it was found that vitamin E in a 5 percent dilution retards cell damage to underlying skin by decreasing oxidation, and also reduces burning. If, despite all your sensible precautions, you do get sunburned, try using the Aloe Burn Spray on page 256.

Carrot-seed essential oil is especially beneficial to sundamaged skin and is even used to treat precancerous skin conditions. The beta-carotene it contains has been proven to protect against ultraviolet-induced skin cancer. The South American herb pau d'arco is also an antioxidant with a reputation for treating skin cancer.

Warning: If you are planning to go out into the sun, you should avoid bergamot. The essential oil of bergamot contains the phototoxic compound bergaptene, which increases the skin's sensitivity to light and can cause skin discoloration or rashes. I have seen this happen more than once. A bergaptene-free oil is available. If you have very sensitive skin, you should also be careful about using the essential oils of the other members of the citrus family, although they are much less phototoxic.

Natural Sunscreen

2 ounces sesame oil
2 ounces aloe vera gel
1 teaspoon vitamin E oil
24 drops lavender essential oil
Combine ingredients. Shake well before using. Remember, this will not provide total sun protection.

Note: Serious skin disorders such as psoriasis, eczema, dermatitis and skin parasites are discussed in chapter 10.

THE HAIR

Never underestimate the importance of healthy-looking hair. It is nearly impossible to look at people's faces without noticing their hair.

DRY HAIR

If you have dry hair, you probably also have to deal with a dry scalp, split ends and unmanageable hair. You may also have dandruff. Exposure to sun—whether from sailing, skiing or a day at the beach—can also dry out your hair and scalp: Protect them by wearing a hat or scarf. All hair, but especially dry hair, is fragile when wet, so wait to brush it until after it is dry. Hair can stretch to nearly double its length when it is wet, and this can be very damaging.

To understand how best to care for dry hair, it helps to know how hair is constructed. Each hair on your head has an outer layer that holds in moisture and protects the hair shaft. This outer layer is made of transparent, overlapping fibers like shingles on a roof. When these shingles are tight, they give hair a smooth, shiny appearance that reflects light. Chlorine, permanents, hair dye, blow drying, excessive sun exposure and alkaline shampoos all take their toll on dry hair because they strip away the natural oils and lift the shingles, causing a frizzy, flyaway look.

Unfortunately, most shampoos dry out hair and turn it alkaline. If you have dry hair, you should use a mild shampoo containing fatty acids, protein, balsams and moisturizers, and use only as much as needed to get your hair clean. All sorts of protein-rich ingredients, such as milk and egg yolk, have been used to condition dry hair and are still used in modern conditioners. Look for conditioners that contain comfrey—this high-protein herb will help your dry hair. Because hair is made up of dead cells, protein cannot directly feed it, but it can temporarily glue down the outer layer. This not only protects hair, but also helps hair reflect light for a look that is smooth and shiny instead of dull and dry. Hair will also seem thicker, at least until the protein coat wears off.

Herbs that combat dry hair include burdock, calendula, chamomile, rose geranium, lavender, rose, rosemary, cedarwood and sandalwood. These herbs not only encourage healthy hair, but also smell great! But no matter how good your herbal shampoo may smell, it does little for your hair in the brief time it remains in place. To really help your hair, turn to herbal conditioners—and leave them on for a few minutes before rinsing. For dry, wispy ends, put a drop or two of sandalwood or rosemary essential oil on your fingers and gently rub it in.

A hot oil treatment smoothes down the hair shaft to give damaged hair some shine, although it cannot always restore hair's flexibility and bounce. Hot oil also helps treat a dry hair and scalp. The treatment, although simple to prepare, can be a little messy to apply. However, it is usually worth the effort.

Mary's story serves as a good example. Her hair was anything but a crowning glory—it was dry and wispy, and seemed to have a mind of its own when she tried to style it. She took to wearing hats because it was easier than dealing with dry, unmanageable hair. Mary does

look good in hats, but it was not a solution to her problem. It took herbs to provide that.

She began with an herbal conditioner and a weekly hot oil treatment, but then became so involved in her work she had little time to think about her hair. Two weeks later, she finished a major project and decided to go out and celebrate. Just before she put on her hat, she paused to look in the mirror. She was amazed—her hair no longer fell in thin streams exposing her scalp, and it actually had some body. She was so encouraged by how well the herbs had worked that she asked me if I knew of anything else that might help.

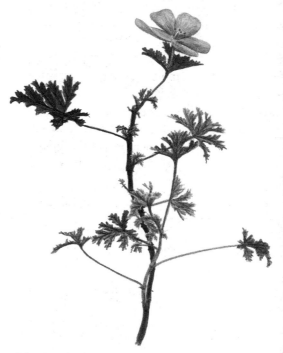

The beautifully scented rose geranium, one of the world's favorite houseplants, was first sent from Africa to England in 1609.

I told Mary that she should also look to her diet to make sure she was getting enough essential fatty acids. If your diet alone is not providing these, one way to supplement it is to take evening primrose oil or some other oil that contains GLA, such as flaxseed oil. Mary thought that her diet was fine, but she tried a GLA supplement anyway. Since diet and supplements affect only new hair at the roots, it took a few months before she noticed that her hair was growing in with more shine and body. Not only that, she was certain that it was growing faster than usual.

Another thing you can do to improve dry hair is to drink a tea made with equal parts oat straw, nettle and horsetail (or take these herbs as a tincture or as pills). These herbs are high in silica and other minerals that are important for hair growth.

Sulfur is also important for producing thick hair. It binds with the protein in the hair, making it stronger and more flexible. You can get sulfur in your diet by incorporating garlic, onions and members of the cabbage family and also by dining on nasturtiums, which you can add to your salad. The French recommend nasturtiums for all sorts of problems that result from having dry hair, and even claim that it prevents premature balding. They also add this flower to hair rinses. As an old country cure for brittle hair, they rub raw onion juice on their hair roots before shampooing!

Dandruff can be a problem with either a dry or an oily scalp, but these dry flakes are most common if you have a dry scalp and dry hair. If dandruff is a prob-lem, use a conditioner that contains burdock and sage. In Asian countries, ginger root is used to stop flakiness and is even said to keep hair from falling out.

Herbal Conditioner for Dry Hair

1 pint boiling water
1 teaspoon each burdock root, calendula flowers, chamomile flowers, lavender flowers and rosemary leaves
1 tablespoon vinegar

Pour boiling water over herbs and steep for about 30 minutes. Strain and add vinegar. Pour over scalp and hair as final rinse after shampooing. Leave on without rinsing out. For dandruff, add 6 drops sage essential oil; shake well before using.

Oil Treatment for Dry Hair

2 ounces aloe vera gel
2 ounces castor oil
6 drops each rose geranium cedar (or sandalwood) and rosemary essential oils
2 drops ginger essential oil (optional)

Combine ingredients. Warm oil slightly. Comb and part hair into different sections, then massage oil into scalp. Cover head with a towel and leave it on for 1 to 2 hours, then shampoo out. Although I use castor oil because it is partially water-soluble and washes out of the hair better, other vegetable oils can also be used—the Italians have long used olive oil for hot oil treatments. In India, hot oil hair treatments are done with sesame oil, the oil of choice in traditional Indian Ayurvedic medicine, and freshly grated ginger. An easy way to add ginger to hot oil is as an essential oil. I like to use Tibetan cedarwood oil for the cedar essential oil.

OILY HAIR

As is true with skin, having too much oil on your hair can be a problem. A little oil makes hair shiny because it smoothes out hair shafts by filling in minute abrasions. But too much oil makes your hair dull and lifeless—because the oil makes the hair heavy and causes it to attract more dirt, which can eventually lead to dandruff. Brushing and scalp massage stimulate circulation and hair growth and help to distribute the oils.

Cedarwood, cypress, lemon, lemongrass, sage and patchouli discourage excess oil production by the scalp. You can add a drop of one of these essential oils into a small amount of shampoo, although you should first make sure that you like the fragrance! A vinegar hair rinse discourages dandruff and rinses excess oil off your hair. It also cuts soap and shampoo residues, leaving hair shiny, smooth and soft. Don't worry about smelling like pickles afterward; vinegar's odor quickly dissipates. A rinse of sage tea also helps to reduce dandruff and excess oil.

If you have oily hair, be sure to use a mild shampoo—the harsh detergents found in many shampoos dry hair too much, encouraging the scalp to manufacture even more oil. A good shampoo cleans your hair without stripping away natural oil or irritating your eyes. Avoid protein and balsam shampoos, which tend to increase oiliness, make hair heavy and attract dirt. Baby shampoos, which are generally made from olive or soy oil, are the mildest and are usually pH balanced. If they are not pH balanced, make them more acidic by adding a teaspoon of vinegar per cup of shampoo.

Many natural cosmetics books give recipes for making shampoos with herb teas and castile soap flakes, but I find castile too alkaline, and it leaves my hair stiff and dull. I prefer using a gentle, nondetergent, unscented shampoo as a base, then adding my favorite herbal ingredients.

Herbal Shampoo

2 ounces unscented shampoo (available at any drugstore)
10 drops lavender essential oil
2 drops chamomile essential oil (optional)
☙ Combine ingredients and shake well before shampooing.

Herbal Rinse for Oily Hair

1 pint boiling water
1 teaspoon each burdock root, calendula flowers, chamomile flowers, lavender flowers, lemongrass and sage leaves
¼ cup vinegar
☙ Pour boiling water over herbs and steep for about 30 minutes. Strain and add vinegar. Pour over scalp and hair as final rinse after shampooing. Leave on without rinsing out.

BEAUTIFYING HAIR

One old-fashioned, natural way to give your hair extra body is to use a setting lotion. Sixteenth- and seventeenth-century herbals boast of rosemary's ability to keep hair curly. Other traditional favorites were lotions made with quince, flaxseed, gelatin, agar, Irish moss or lemon. All of these give thin hair more body and can even be used if you have thick hair like mine.

I do not set my hair very often, but once, inspired by pictures of a local historic beauty, Lola Montez, I decided to go to a fair in her honor, wearing a nineteenth-century dress with my long hair in tight curls—helped by a natural ingredient, of course. I made a solution of agar, a jellylike seaweed thickener used in cooking. I poured this over my hair, which I set in little ringlets all over my head. The next morning, my hair was indeed curled, or rather set. It even shimmered and jiggled when I walked. While this technique proved successful, I find that setting my hair with lemon gives it a much more natural look.

Lola Montez actually wrote her own book, *The Arts and Secrets of Beauty,* in 1853. One of her many interesting recipes is for Honey Water, which she says fashionable ladies all over Europe used as a "celebrated" hair rinse to beautify their tresses. Although the original concoction did indeed contain honey, as well as some other, rather questionable ingredients such as sand, Lola adapted the formula, leaving out the honey but retaining the name. I have turned it into a more modern recipe (see page 330) in case you would like to try beautifying your own hair with a formula that was popular among nineteenth-century beauties.

Another way to perk up hair is by changing the color. Unfortunately, permanent hair dyes, tints and bleaches force open the hair shaft so that they can penetrate inside to alter the color. As a result, your hair may take on the frizzy appearance associated with bleached blondes, particularly if it undergoes repeated dyeing. Commercial natural dyes have become increasingly popular and also more sophisticated, offering a wider range of colors. Because natural hair dyes gradually fade, you do not have to worry about touching up the roots. Be sure to read the list of ingredients carefully, since some companies "cheat" by combining plant dyes with strong chemical dyes.

The color variations offered by natural products are achieved by combining different herbs. Brown and amber colors are usually created by using henna combined with black walnut hull and sometimes iron oxide. For black and dark brown shades, indigo is added; clove, sage and coffee are sometimes used in dark hair dyes. Neutral and blond henna are not really henna at all; most often they are another herbal hair conditioner: *Lyzifus spina-christi.* Chamomile, calendula, turmeric and lemon can be used to increase light highlights. The basic red henna may include safflower or hibiscus to soften the color. If you have light-colored or gray hair, be careful when using pure henna. It may turn your hair carrot-red or a brassy orange. Also, do not mix henna with one of the temporary chemical rinses. This combination can cause Technicolor streaks.

Henna has been used throughout India, Egypt and the Middle East for more than 8,000 years to give hair a red highlight and condition it. It coats dry hair with a vegetable protein that makes it shiny with extra body, and it is drying to oily hair. (Because of this, use henna to treat dry hair no more than once every few months.) Because some people are sensitive to henna, do a patch test on your inner arm before trying this herb on your hair. I have actually seen people get welts on their skin from henna.

Lemon Setting Lotion

2 ounces lemon juice
5 drops rosemary essential oil

That's right, there are only two ingredients to combine in this recipe! Buy unsweetened lemon juice or squeeze and strain your own and use right away since it will not keep. The rest is equally simple—comb it onto your hair before setting. Although using lemon as a setting agent is good because it conditions your hair at the same time, there is also a downside: It often makes your hair feel a little sticky.

Lola's Honey Water

5 ounces white wine
5 ounces distilled water
4 ounces orange-blossom water
8 drops bergamot essential oil
4 drops clove essential oil

Combine ingredients. Rinse through hair after washing.

Henna Protein Pack

1–2 cups warm water
1 egg (optional)
1 teaspoon olive oil
2 tablespoons honey
24 drops lavender essential oil
2–3 ounces henna (for medium-length hair; use more or less, depending on length and thickness of your hair)

Wear a shirt you do not mind staining and keep a cloth handy to wipe the henna paste from your skin (there is always a chance of a stray drip). If you try this inside the house, also protect your floor. Apply salve or cream around your hair line. Put on thin latex gloves to protect your hands from being colored. Mix all wet ingredients and add them to henna, pressing out any lumps. The mixture should be the consistency of cake batter; it should not be too wet or else it will drip. It is better to make more than you need than not to have enough to cover all your hair.

Thoroughly wet your hair, part hair in sections, and apply the henna pack from scalp to hair ends. The mixture will be thick and globby, so expect it to feel a bit strange. Cover your head with a plastic bag or a shower cap, then wrap it with a towel to hold in your natural body heat, which breaks down henna and intensifies the color. You can also use a hair dryer or sit in a sauna or the sun. The longer you leave henna on, the deeper the color will be. One hour is usually sufficient, but up to 2 hours is fine as long as the henna does not dry out. Rinse with lukewarm water. (Do not use hot water—this will cook the egg.) Rinse well—it will probably take a few rinses—and follow with a shampoo and a conditioner. Dry and style as usual.

BODY CARE EXTRAS

Skin and hair aren't the only pieces of your body care puzzle. Healthy and beautiful lips and nails are every bit as important to appearance—left untended, they can become quite irritated.

CHAPPED LIPS

Rough, cracked lips not only feel uncomfortable, but also look unattractive. You can protect your lips from winter's wind and cold and summer's drying heat with a soothing herbal lip balm. The balm I recommend is a good alternative to petroleum oil-based ointment sticks that can dry out your lips more than moisturize them. Indeed, many people complain that lip balm sold in stick form makes their lips even drier, and they find themselves needing more and more of it. Herbal lip balm comes in a tasty selection of flavors, including orange, tangerine, lemon and vanilla. If your lips are very chapped, avoid essential oils that can sting, such as peppermint. Plastic lip-balm containers that snap shut can be purchased in stores that sell backpacking supplies.

Honey Lip Balm for Chapped Lips

¼ cup vegetable oil
¼ ounce shaved beeswax
1 teaspoon honey
10 drops lemon essential oil or 1 teaspoon
*   vanilla extract*

🍂 Heat oil in a pan, adding beeswax until melted. Stir in honey and essential oil or flavoring. (Expect a little residue at the bottom of the pan from the extract and honey.) Pour the balm into lip-balm containers while it is still warm (be sure the mixture is not too hot, or it will melt the plastic containers).

FUNGAL INFECTIONS

Fungal skin and nail infections can be extremely annoying—not only are they unsightly and uncomfortable; they are also difficult to eliminate. Ringworm,

which causes athlete's foot and occurs most often on the feet, scalp, beard, fingernails and toenails, is one of the best-known, but there are many different types of fungal infections. Jewelweed, garlic, yellow dock, pau d'arco, the lichen usnea and the fresh husk of black walnut all contain compounds that deter fungal growth. (The tinctures of jewelweed and usnea are particularly good, but they are also extremely hard to find.) Many herbs high in essential oils are also antifungals, especially tea tree, oregano, lavender, eucalyptus, rose rose geranium and myrrh. Small amounts of peppermint relieve the itching associated with many fungal infections.

An herbal salve can be used on fungal skin infections, but your best bet is an herbal vinegar and/or a bentonite clay dusting powder to dry out the moist environment in which fungus thrives. Although dabbing a gourmet vinegar on your skin may seem odd, oregano and garlic vinegars make excellent remedies. Vinegar itself directly destroys fungal infections, and its effectiveness is increased by adding eight drops of tea tree essential oil per ounce of vinegar.

My friend Dave found great success using herbs to fight fungal problems. He had a terrible case of athlete's foot, which he thought he had picked up at the gym. He tried various pharmaceutical preparations, but they brought only temporary relief. After a few days, these preparations always made his feet burn and feel worse than the athlete's foot itself. Because his feet were so raw and because herbal vinegar stung, he used a salve containing tea tree and lavender essential oils. At first, his feet did not look any better, but they certainly felt better—much better, in fact. It took only a few days for the crusty rings to start subsiding. Dave still needs to use the salve

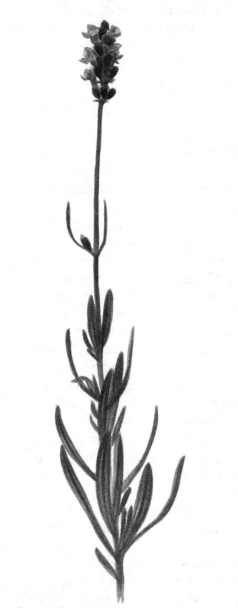

Lavender has been used as a scent for wash water and baths since the time of the ancient Romans.

every once in a while when the athlete's foot flares up again, but he says that the attacks are happening less often. Part of the reason for this may be his discovery that it helps to wear shoes that keep the feet well-ventilated and as dry as possible. He also noticed that the fungal infection becomes worse whenever life becomes stressful.

Antifungal Vinegar
4 ounces vinegar (for extra strength, use oregano vinegar)
2 tablespoons tincture of pau d'arco
¼ teaspoon each tea tree and lavender essential oils
⅛ teaspoon peppermint essential oil
☙ Combine ingredients. Apply a few times daily with cotton balls or swabs or use a compress soaked in vinegar to cover a large area. I use oregano vinegar. You can make this yourself or buy a culinary oregano vinegar.

Antifungal Dusting Powder
¼ cup bentonite clay
⅛ teaspoon each tea tree and lavender and essential oils
☙ Combine clay and essential oils in a plastic bag. Drop in essential oils, tightly close bag and mix well by turning bag over a few times and breaking up any clumps. Let sit three days, then store in an airtight container.

NAIL CARE
Your fingernails are subjected to daily assault. Detergents, fingernail polish, glue for artificial fingernails, formaldehyde-based nail hardeners and household chemicals are just a few of the attackers. You can protect your nails by

wearing gloves while washing dishes or hand-washing clothes, and by avoiding contact with gasoline, paint and other harsh chemicals. Nail polish, lacquers and especially nail polish remover are very drying to nails, often causing them to crack and split. If you use these products, choose formulas without formaldehyde and add half a teaspoon of castor oil to every ounce of an acetone polish remover to moisturize nails and surrounding skin.

Brittle nails that crack easily indicate possible dietary problems. Healthy nails need a sufficient amount of calcium, magnesium, protein and silica. Drinking a tea made of equal parts oat straw, nettle and horsetail or taking capsules or tinctures of these herbs daily can improve your nails from the inside out, since these herbs are high in silica and other minerals important for nail growth. Supplements of GLA in the form of evening primrose, borage or black currant seed oil also help.

How else can you achieve beautiful fingernails? Soaking them in herbal teas or oils of comfrey, oat straw and horsetail strengthens nails and cuticles, the thickened skin at the base of your fingernails. For fungal problems, first soak your nails in the Antifungal Vinegar (see page 332), then follow by rubbing in the Nail Soak Oil.

Nail Soak Oil
2 tablespoons jojoba oil
4 drops each lavender and sandalwood essential oils
Combine ingredients. Soak nails in mixture for 10 minutes. Buff nails to

stimulate circulation and bring out a healthy shine.

PERSPIRATION
Almost all store-bought deodorants are laced with questionable ingredients and loaded with synthetic fragrances. Antiperspirants can also be bad because they actually block sweat glands—this may be asking for trouble since the underarm area is especially sensitive and is susceptible to irritation and rashes. Anyway, once an antiperspirant wears off, underarm sweat glands produce more perspiration to compensate.

There is an alternative. Sweat is odorless until it comes into contact with airborne bacteria. Antibacterial herbs such as chamomile and coriander inhibit growth of underarm bacteria and solve the problem naturally. If you do not perspire much, you may find that a simple aromatic body powder will do. Arrowroot, cornstarch or white clay are good bases for powder.

Natural Deodorant
2 ounces witch hazel
5 drops each sage, coriander and lavender essential oils
Combine ingredients in a spray bottle. Shake well before every application.

Natural Body Powder
1/2 cup cornstarch
5 drops lavender essential oil
2 drops ylang-ylang essential oil
Add essential oils to cornstarch. Put through a sieve and mix well. Let sit a few days to incorporate scents into the powder.

chapter

EIGHTEEN

Cooking

for

Health

Serving medicine for dinner may not seem terribly appetizing, but most cultures traditionally eat much of their medicine. It may not be a coincidence that nature has provided so many of our medicinal needs in herbs that taste good. When you want to take herbs over a long period of time—either to treat a chronic problem or to fend off disease—incorporating medicinal plants into your meals makes a lot of sense.

The next time you add a pinch of this or that, consider that you are doing far more than flavoring your meal. Throughout this book, you have seen many familiar kitchen herbs and spices mentioned as medicines. For example, ginger relieves pain, garlic is "nature's antibiotic" and ginger and turmeric, two of the main ingredients in curry powder, improve liver function.

Almost every cookbook is filled with recipes that rely on herbs for flavor. Once you decide to make herbs part of your diet, you can start by choosing recipes that use the herbs your body needs most—garlic for your heart and ginger to relieve your headache, for instance. In this chapter, I provide many suggestions for herbs you can incorporate into your regular diet. For more ideas, see *Cooking with the Healthful Herbs*, by Jean Rodgers, and my *Herbs: An Illustrated Encyclopedia*.

THE BASICS: SOUP

Herbs of all kinds—including many common kitchen spices—can easily be included in soups and stews. Many of the recipes I've included here use soup stock as a basic ingredient. You can purchase soup stock in cans or you can use bouillon cubes.

One way to use immunity-enhancing mushrooms such as reishi and shiitake is to eat them as part of your regular diet. The mushroom soup recipes provided here are thanks to my friend and fellow herbalist Christopher Hobbs. He says that he has seen soups like these restore vigor and health to adults and children who were weak and ill. It will also benefit your urinary tract, especially if you are prone to bladder infection. Barley is an old European remedy for this problem, garlic treats infection and mushrooms boost the immune system. The Mushroom Barley Soup has been adapted from Hobbs's book *Medicinal Mushrooms*. Here, too, it is a basic soup made using Chinese herbs. You can find many adaptations of this soup designed to treat different conditions in *Between Heaven and Earth: A Guide to Chinese Medicine*, by my friends Harriet Beinfield and Efrem Korngold. I love this soup and cannot imagine a tastier way to good health.

Mushroom Barley Soup

¼ cup barley
¾ cup soup stock
2½ cups water
2 teaspoons tamari (or ¼ teaspoon salt)
½ cup chopped onion
1 or 2 cloves garlic, minced
2 teaspoons olive oil
½ pound fresh medicinal mushrooms
  (such as shiitake)
Black pepper to taste

Cook barley in soup stock until tender. Add water and tamari. In a separate pan, sauté onions and garlic in olive oil. When onions are transparent, add mushrooms. When mushrooms and onions are tender, add them to the barley-tamari mixture. Sprinkle in black pepper, cover and simmer gently for 20 minutes. For variety, add cooked vegetables of your choice, either chopped or grated.

Chinese Soup

2 ounces Chinese herbs (such as astragalus, ginseng, rehmannia, codonopsis, ligustrum, burdock and shizandra berries)
1 tablespoon finely chopped fresh ginger
⅛ cup uncooked rice
4 cups soup stock
1 diced carrot
1 beet or 1 turnip, diced
1 diced yam
¼ cup shiitake mushrooms, slivered

Place the herbs (including ginger) in a muslin bag or tie them together with a string. Simmer the bag and rice in the soup stock for 1 hour. Add the vegetables and mushrooms to the herbal stew, and simmer gently for another 30 minutes. Remove the bag filled with herbs, and serve the soup. If you use burdock in this soup, it can be finely chopped and need not go in a bag.

OILS AND VINEGARS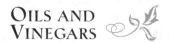

Herbal oils and vinegars give you a quick and easy way to spice up meals. Herbs can turn an ordinary bottle of vinegar or oil into a gourmet delight. Of course, you can use them as salad dressing—standard salad dressing recipes combine two parts oil with one part vinegar. You can always use an herbal recipe in place of commercial vinegars or oils. Thyme, rosemary and bay leaves lend a Mediterranean flavor, and basil, oregano and marjoram give foods an Italian edge. Cilantro and cumin are common in Mexican and Indian meals. Chinese favorites include black pepper and ginger, while tarragon, sage and parsley are much loved by cooks in Northern Europe. You can even use onions and garlic. All of these herbs provide healthful benefits as well as wondrous flavors. I typically make many different types of vinegars and oils so that I have a wide range to choose from.

The tastiest herbal vinegars and oils are made using fresh herbs from the garden or a farmer's market. Most grocery stores sell fresh basil, parsley and cilantro. If you do not have an herb garden, dried herbs will do— the end product just won't be as flavorful. To really show off your herbal vinegar or oil, keep it in a fancy glass bottle. To add flair, add a decorative sprig of dried herb.

Herbal Vinegar

1 cup coarsely chopped herbs (any of those mentioned above will do)
1 pint vinegar (any type; white vinegar produces the best colors)
Fill a widemouthed jar loosely with herbs (do not pack them down).

Pour in enough vinegar to cover herbs. If any herbs do not sink, poke them down with a spoon. Stir to release any trapped air bubbles, and put a lid on the jar. Store at room temperature for 2 weeks; this will extract the herbs' flavor. Strain out herbs. Dilute the final product with plain vinegar; start with half a cup, and adjust according to taste. I store my vinegars undiluted because they take up less storage space in that form.

Herbal Oil

1 cup coarsely chopped herbs (any of those mentioned above will do)
1 pint vegetable oil (any type, though strong-tasting oils, such as virgin olive, will overpower mild herbs)
Fill a widemouthed jar loosely with herbs (do not pack them down). Pour in enough oil to cover herbs. If any herbs do not sink, poke them down with a spoon. Stir to release any trapped air bubbles, and put a lid on the jar. Store in a warm place—one that is slightly above room temperature—for 3 days (an upper kitchen cabinet will do). Strain out herbs, and store your oil in the refrigerator.

Some people like to keep whole, fresh herbs in vegetable oil so as to have a supply throughout the year. If you are interested in preserving whole herbs, such as garlic cloves, you should be careful to refrigerate them and use them within a month, according to the Agricultural Extension Service in Oregon.

SPICE OF LIFE: SEASONING BLENDS

One tasty—and easy—way to use healthful herbs in cooking is with an herbal seasoning blend. Sprinkle powdered herb blends on salads and sandwiches and add them to bread dough, casseroles, pastas, soups and stir-fried vegetables. You can even create Italian, Chinese and Indian meals with a few shakes of an herb blend.

There are several variations on this theme. Here are some of my favorites. For the best herb blend, start with high-quality dried herbs from your garden or buy whole or cut herbs; preground herbs will have lost much of their flavor. It is very easy to grind your own herbs in a coffee grinder, blender, flour mill, mortar and pestle or whatever is convenient. Garlic and onion are exceptions—it is much easier to buy them in powdered form.

Herbal "Salt"

1 tablespoon each basil leaves, coriander
    seeds and thyme leaves
2 teaspoons each cumin seeds, onion
    powder, parsley leaves, whole sesame
    seeds (optional), garlic powder,
    mustard seeds, paprika pods,
    cayenne pods (optional) and kelp
    (optional)

🌿 Grind and combine herbs. Keep a small jar or saltshaker on the table. Store the excess in a jar with a tight lid.

Herbes Fines
(All-Purpose Seasoning)

Equal parts chives leaves, chervil
    leaves, parsley leaves and
    tarragon leaves

🌿 Mince herbs with a sharp knife. Keep in a small jar alongside the rest of your spices. To use, add to food at the last minute. Store extra in the refrigerator in a jar with a tight lid.

Curry Powder

1 tablespoon each cumin seeds, coriander
    seeds and turmeric rhizomes
½ tablespoon each ginger rhizome and
    dried chili peppers
¼ tablespoon each black mustard seeds
    and fennel seeds

🌿 Grind ingredients into a powder and mix well. Store in a container with a tight lid. Add to recipes as needed.

MIDDLE EASTERN CUISINE: GARLIC AND PARSLEY

Garlic is one of nature's most versatile foods. This pungent herb aids poor digestion, reduces high blood pressure, improves circulation and fights high blood pressure, cholesterol, colds, bronchitis and intestinal infections. Heavily used in Middle Eastern cooking, garlic is one of the main ingredients in hummus, a dip made of ground chickpeas and sesame paste and typically served with lettuce and crisp vegetables, sometimes as a sandwich on pita bread (which is also called "pocket bread" because you can open it and fill it). Hummus can also be used as a spread in a sandwich with small patties made from beans or meat.

Hummus

2½ cups cooked chickpeas (about 1 cup dried)
4 cloves garlic, minced
½ cup tahini (sesame seed paste)
¼ cup stock or water
6 tablespoons lemon juice
2 tablespoons olive oil
1 teaspoon coriander leaves, minced
Paprika to taste
🌿 Combine all ingredients except paprika and process in a blender or

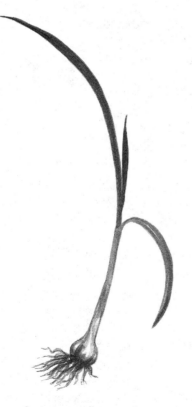

Garlic is known as "nature's antibiotic."

food processor until smooth. Sprinkle with paprika. Makes 2 to 3 cups.

Hummus is often served with the traditional Middle Eastern dish known as tabbouleh. Made from bulgur (cracked wheat) combined with lots of parsley, mint and vegetables, this salad has been a favorite food in the Middle East and Asia since biblical times. Bulgur is made by boiling wheat berries, then drying and cracking them. Because it has been precooked, this nutritious food can be stored longer than other grains. Like rice, it fluffs up when properly cooked. In ancient Greece, parsley was used to treat urinary tract infection and inflammation. Herbalists use mint to soothe nerves, ease stomachaches and fight cold and flu symptoms.

Tabbouleh

1 cup soup stock
1 cup uncooked bulgur
⅓ cup minced scallions
⅓ cup minced mint
⅓ cup minced parsley
2 peeled and chopped tomatoes
¼ cup lemon juice
3 tablespoons olive oil
1 tablespoon tamari
🌿 Bring the soup stock to a boil in a pan and stir in the bulgur. Cover the pan and remove from heat. Let sit until liquid is absorbed, about 20 minutes. Fluff the bulgur with a fork. Mix in scallions, mint, parsley and tomatoes while bulgur is still warm so that it absorbs their flavor. Combine lemon juice, oil and tamari and drizzle over the bulgur mix. Toss to mix. Let sit to marinate at least 1 hour before serving.

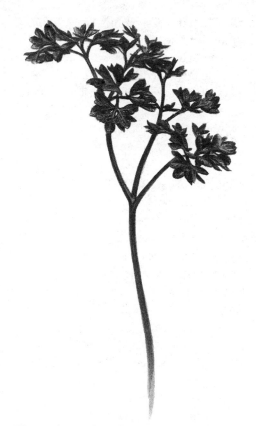

The ancient Greeks used parsley to decorate graves.

Garlic is used in many different ways all over the world—in stuffing, in pasta sauces and even as the main ingredient in various dishes. My favorite ways to use this tasty wonder worker are as a spread and as a dressing.

Garlic Spread
¾ cup olive oil
7 garlic cloves
1 tablespoon onion powder
2 tablespoons chopped parsley
🌿 Blend all ingredients until smooth. Bake in oven set on low heat for 15 minutes. Serve as a side dish or spread on bread.

Garlic-Ginger Dressing
½ cup olive oil
2 tablespoons lemon juice
1 tablespoon each tamari and tahini
   (sesame seed paste)
1 teaspoon grated ginger rhizome
1 clove garlic, minced
🌿 Combine all ingredients in a blender. Use on vegetable or bean salads and vegetable dishes.

PESTOS: BASIL AND SAGE

Pesto is an Italian word that comes from the Latin verb "to pound" or "to crush." Herb pestos are pastes that are used in all sorts of dishes. Pesto with pasta is probably most common, but these pastes also go well with vegetables. You can even use pesto to make a dressing (dilute it with vinegar) or a sauce (dilute it with milk). I like to add a spoonful of pesto to soup. It is also great as a spread—a little pesto turns a plain sandwich into an explosion of flavor!

Basil, the typical main ingredient of pesto, is a gentle sedative, and helps to relieve high blood pressure and the symptoms of peptic ulcers, colitis and asthma. In Japan, India and West Africa, various species of basil are used to treat colds, flus, fevers, joint pain, stomach cramps, nausea and headaches. Other herbs can also be used as the basis for this tasty paste—you might try using parsley, cilantro (the fresh leaves of coriander and one of my personal favorites), sorrel or watercress. Even sharp-flavored herbs that are not as fleshy—thyme and oregano, for instance—can be turned into pesto; just combine them with one of the other herbs or with spinach to provide bulk and soften the flavor.

You might also consider the distinctly different flavors of lemon and cinnamon basil. You will probably have to grow these yourself or go to a farmer's market to buy them, but they are well worth the effort. I have provided two recipes below. If you would like to try others, read Dorothy Rankin's *Pestos! Cooking with Herb Pastes*. The Sage Pesto and the Fresh Shiitake and Sage Pasta Sauce below are both Dorothy's delicious recipes. She serves the Sage Pesto over hot fettuccine and garnishes the meal with sage leaves. For the shiitake recipe, use fresh mushrooms if you can find them; they have a better flavor than the dried fungi and will keep refrigerated in plastic bags for days.

Once you have made your pesto, pack it tightly into a jar, being sure to push out all the air pockets. Cover the pesto with a thin layer of olive oil and put it in the refrigerator. It will keep for a few weeks. For longer storage, freeze it in small quantities that you can thaw out as you need them. If you have lots of fresh herbs on your hands, but do not have the time or all the ingredients to prepare pesto, simply blend the herbs in oil and refrigerate them. When time allows, thaw and prepare.

Basil Pesto

1½ cups fresh basil leaves
2 cloves garlic
¼ cup pine nuts or walnuts
½ cup grated Parmesan cheese
½ cup olive oil

❧ Chop the basil in blender. Add the garlic and nuts and blend into a puree, then add cheese. Slowly add most of the olive oil until the mixture is the consistency of creamed butter. Pack into a container, removing air pockets, and pour the remaining 2 tablespoons of oil on top to keep the pesto from darkening.

Sage Pesto

½ cup fresh sage leaves
1½ cups fresh parsley leaves
2 large garlic cloves
½ cup grated Parmesan cheese
½ cup pine nuts or walnuts
½ cup olive oil
Salt and freshly ground pepper to taste

❧ Combine the sage, parsley, garlic, cheese and nuts in a food processor or blender. Process to mix. With the machine running, slowly add the olive oil. Season to taste with salt and freshly ground pepper, and process to the desired consistency. Let stand for 5 minutes before serving. Makes about 1 cup.

Fresh Shiitake and Sage Pasta Sauce

3 tablespoons melted ghee (clarified butter) or vegetable oil
½ cup thinly sliced shallots
¼ pound julienned shiitake mushrooms
Salt and freshly ground pepper
¼ cup soup stock
1½ cups cream
1 tablespoon Sage Pesto (see above)
¼ to ½ teaspoon lemon juice

❧ In a large skillet, sauté the shallots in ghee or oil very slowly for about 10 minutes. Do not let them brown. Add the shiitakes, salt and pepper and continue sautéing, stirring frequently. Add the soup stock, a little at a time, as you sauté. Pour in cream and simmer very slowly until sauce is reduced by half (about 15 to 20 minutes), stirring frequently. Add Sage Pesto and lemon juice to taste. Serve hot.

GREENS: DANDELION AND NASTURTIUM

Dandelion leaves are nutritious, rich in vitamins and useful for relieving many liver, gallbladder and kidney problems. They also improve digestion. When I was traveling on an herbal tour of Greece, a dish called *horta* was served everywhere. People could be seen out in the fields, collecting baskets full of wild greens such as dandelion and chicory to make horta. I enjoyed horta steamed, fried and raw—the cooked version is the least bitter and the most acceptable to the North American palate. Boiled greens are also common in Greece, though they are less nutritious this way. If you wish to make horta, you can serve it raw or combine the greens with other vegetables. If you pick your own dandelions, go for the fresh, young leaves in the early spring before the plant flowers and turns bitter. Make sure that the plants have not been sprayed with pesticides.

Horta
15 young dandelion leaves
1 small onion
8 black olives
2 tablespoons olive oil
1 tablespoon apple cider vinegar or
    lemon juice
Salt to taste

Steam the dandelion leaves and onion until soft. Add olives and top with the oil and vinegar or juice. Season with salt.

Nasturtiums are flowering plants that are native to South America. When British explorers returned home from the New World carrying these plants, among numerous other goodies, the English eagerly adopted the nasturtium and began growing it for color. They soon found that it also made a tasty food. The Nasturtium Capers recipe comes from *The British Housewife,* written in 1770 by Martha Bradley, who asserted that this snack "will be one of the finest Pickles in the World." She was right! You can also toss small pieces of nasturtium flowers with salad greens to make a colorful blend. For pretty hors d'oeuvres, roll finely chopped herbs and cream cheese into small balls and stick them inside individual nasturtium flowers. The flowers and leaves of nasturtium are more than just tangy—they contain a strong antibiotic that is similar in many ways to the active compounds found in garlic.

Nasturtium Capers
Nasturtium buds to fill a 1-quart jar
1/4 teaspoon nutmeg
1/2 teaspoon whole black pepper
6 cloves
1 quart vinegar
Stir buds in cold water, drain and repeat, then lay on a sieve to dry. Loosely fill a well-washed quart jar with buds, sprinkling in spices as you go. Fill the jar with vinegar and put on lid. Let sit 6 weeks before opening.

HOT STUFF: MUSTARD, HORSERADISH AND PEPPERS

Mustard and horseradish are used to treat many ailments. These herbs improve circulation and aid liver and lung health. They also clear congested sinuses and can even help relieve constipation. Horseradish stimulates digestion, especially of the fatty foods with which it is traditionally eaten.

Mustard can be fun to play with. You can easily give it an international flair just by changing one or two ingredients. To turn mustard French, use red wine vinegar or wine instead of plain vinegar. The true French Dijon mustard uses champagne! Make Chinese mustard with flat beer. A dash (¹/₈ teaspoon) of powdered cloves, dill or both enriches mustard's flavor. For even more variety, add one teaspoon of an herbal spice blend such as the Herbal "Salt" described on page 337. The addition of whole mustard seeds (1 tablespoon) will make mustard slightly crunchy, and black mustard seeds add color. Once made, mustard lasts for months, although its flavor does change as it ages. In fact, this is one condiment you may want to make at the last minute—mustard connoisseurs say that mustards are best when they are not more than a few weeks old.

English Herb Mustard

2 tablespoons ground mustard
2 tablespoons finely ground flour
¹/₂ teaspoon each ground turmeric, ground ginger and grated horseradish (this is quite hot, so it's optional)
¹/₂ cup apple cider vinegar
¹/₄ cup warm water
1 tablespoon honey
Fresh lemon slice

⚘ Mix the mustard, flour and spices together. In a separate bowl, mix the vinegar, water and honey together. Combine dry and wet ingredients in a pan.

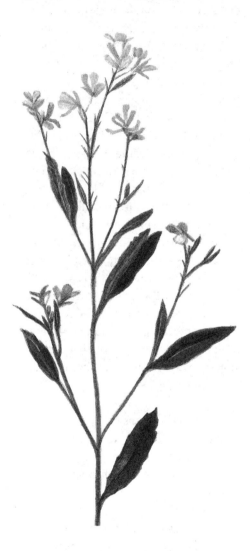

In ancient Rome, black mustard seeds were crushed and mixed with wine to make an early version of our table mustard.

Bring to a boil, turn down heat and simmer for 2 minutes. While the mixture is still warm, pack it into clean jars, pushing out air spaces, and refrigerate. Keep mustard fresh by placing a slice of fresh lemon inside the jar, on top of the mustard. Replace the lemon with a fresh slice every few days. The consistency may be thinned with extra water or thickened with more flour, but watch out: Water makes mustard hotter. For a very hot mustard, switch the amounts of vinegar and water: use ½ cup water and ¼ cup vinegar. If you prefer a mellow version instead, use oil or mayonnaise instead of water.

Mustard can be combined with horseradish to make a dressing for your salad or a sauce for vegetables (see the Dresden Sauce recipe below). Horseradish can also be put in potato salad and cocktail sauces. You should know that this plant turns bitter with age—always buy firm, young roots that have not begun to sprout or turn green, and try to use them fresh. The trick is to grate the fresh root directly into lemon or vinegar so that it gets as little exposure to air as possible. Be careful, though—the fumes can make your eyes burn.

If all this sounds like too much work, you can buy the root already dried as wasabi powder. This is the amazingly hot paste served with some Japanese dishes. (The bright green color is from a dye, but you can get it without dye at a natural food store.) Reconstitute the powder a half hour before serving by soaking 1 tablespoon of powder in 2 tablespoons of water. Keep reconstituted wasabi in the refrigerator.

Dresden Sauce
1 cup sour cream or yogurt
½ teaspoon English Herb Mustard
¼ teaspoon soy sauce
Combine ingredients and serve with main course.

Black pepper has the distinction of being an important spice all over the world. Once literally worth its weight in gold, the humble peppercorn has played an important role over the ages. The trade routes from India to ancient Rome were established mainly because of this spice, and its trade made Venice, Genoa, Amsterdam and Bruges, Belgium, wealthy cities. Today, the United States imports more pepper than any other country. I have heard many people claim that black pepper is not healthy. I am not sure how pepper fell into disfavor, but perhaps it was guilt by association. After all, it does often sit right next to the salt, which is known to cause health problems. But black pepper is not at all risky. In fact, it aids food digestion by increasing digestive juices, including natural stomach acid. In India, practitioners of Ayurvedic medicine still use it medicinally to treat colds, flus and other infections.

Chili peppers are also great herbal foods to incorporate into your cooking— unless your palate does not let you enjoy "hot" food. Chilies contain capsaicin, which, among its other advantages, is a natural painkiller. I found the Berber Spice Mix—named for a group of tribes who live in North Africa—in *The Encyclopedia of Herbs, Spices and Flavorings: A Cook's Compendium*, by Elisabeth Lambert Ortiz. This is hot stuff, since it uses red chilies and cloves (which stimulate digestion by increasing stomach acid levels) as well as pepper, but if you like your food spicy, as I do, you'll enjoy this mix.

Berber Spice Mix

10 dried red chili peppers
½ teaspoon black peppercorns
½ teaspoon ground ginger
5 whole cloves
½ teaspoon coriander seeds
¼ teaspoon ajowan or cumin seeds
(the more traditional ajowan is hard to find)
8 allspice berries
6 cardamom seeds (from green pods if you can find them)
½ teaspoon fenugreek
½ teaspoon cinnamon

🍃 Heat a medium-size skillet. Add the chilies and cook them for 2 to 3 minutes. Add the remaining spices and roast for 3 to 4 minutes longer, stirring constantly and shaking the pan to prevent burning, until the mixture begins to brown. Transfer to a bowl and let cool. Scrape the chili seeds out with a spoon. Grind the mixture to a fine powder and store it in an airtight container for up to 4 months. (If you cannot find ajowan, it can be omitted or replaced with cumin seeds, which have a similar flavor.)

Red chili comes with its own set of health benefits, including improving circulation. Like black pepper, chilies are used all over the world—as an essential ingredient in Indian curry, African peanut sauce, Chinese Szechuan vegetables and Thai food, for instance. And in their Mexican homeland, chili peppers are contained in most of the food. In fact, every time I make a fresh salsa like the one described below, it takes me back to memories of wonderful trips along the coast of Mexico—its warm sunshine, friendly people and relaxed living.

Green Salsa (Salsa Verde)

2 cloves garlic, chopped
¼ cup each chopped fresh cilantro leaves and chopped fresh parsley leaves
1 seeded and chopped chili pepper
1 seeded and chopped medium green bell pepper
Juice of 1 lemon
⅛ cup olive oil
Dash of ground black pepper

🍃 Combine all ingredients. Toss well. Serve with chips (baked, not fried, for your liver's sake), tortillas or bread or on top of a vegetable dish. Of course, salsa is appropriate for serving with almost any Mexican dish.

SAUCY DISHES: CRANBERRY, ELDERBERRY AND TAMARIND

Elderberries and cranberries are extremely high in vitamin C. For centuries, New England sea captains took cranberries with them on long voyages to prevent scurvy. Cranberries are also useful in treating and preventing urinary tract infections. You can buy cranberry juice in the grocery store, but commercial juices are loaded with sugar (to overpower cranberry's sour taste)—

not the best thing to eat when you have any type of infection. You're better off with an unsweetened cranberry sauce. Some find this recipe a bit tart, but I like the taste. For those who find it too sour, I have included some honey in the recipe.

Cranberry Sauce

1 cup cranberries
1 whole orange
¼ cup orange juice
½ cup apple juice
1 tablespoon honey (optional)
1 teaspoon agar powder (if you want to make gelatin)

Grind the fruits in a food processor, then add juices. Add honey if desired. Store in a covered jar in the refrigerator. This dish tastes even better after it sits for a day. You can also make this sauce into a gelatin dessert: Bring the sauce to a boil and stir in the agar. Continue simmering for 5 minutes, stirring occasionally to make sure that agar is dissolved and evenly dispersed. Pour into a bowl or pan. Let cool to thicken.

For centuries, elderberry has been used to cure flus and colds. According to one story, a sailor told a physician in Prague about his sure cure for rheumatic pains—he simply got drunk on port wine. It turned out that it was not the wine that provided the medicine, but the elderberries used to darken and "age" it. In the seventeenth century, Martin Blokwich wrote a book in which he listed more than 70 diseases that could be treated with elderberry. Recently, this plant's age-old reputation sparked new research into its curative powers. It turns out that elderberries, along with other deeply colored berries, contain strong antioxidant compounds that improve circulation, eyesight and connective muscle tissues. Any berry can be used as the basis for a jam or a jelly—not to mention wine—but the easiest recipe by far is a syrup. If you do not have access to elderberries, you can use this recipe to make a syrup out of any similarly colored berry.

Elderberry Syrup

2 cups dried elderberries
1 quart boiling water
¼ cup honey
¼ cup lemon juice

Place berries in an uncovered saucepan and pour boiling water over them. Cover and let soak overnight. The next day, simmer the berries for 30 minutes. Purée the warm berries in a blender, adding remaining ingredients as you blend. Pour the syrup into a clean bottle, and store it in the refrigerator.

The Indian herb tamarind lends its fruity, sweet-and-sour flavor to sauces, chutneys and yogurt dishes. It can also be served by itself as a side dish. The pods of this fruit are a gentle laxative. In Iran, they are combined with rose to mellow the harsh effect and taste of the laxative herb senna. In the 1600s, the Spanish brought tamarind to the West Indies and Mexico, where it has remained a popular part of their cuisine.

This versatile food is not well-known in North America, although it is one of the secret ingredients in

Worcestershire sauce. Unless you enjoy ethnic cooking, you probably have not heard much about it. Look for the sticky, dark paste in Indian and Mexican stores. The easiest form to use has the seeds and fibrous pods already removed. If you want to try tamarind paste in other dishes, use it to replace vinegar. You can also make your own sauce.

Tamarind Sauce

2 ounces tamarind pulp
1¼ cups water
1 tablespoon honey, warmed enough to
    liquefy
¼ teaspoon freshly ground black pepper
½ teaspoon cumin seeds
½ teaspoon chili powder
1 tablespoon chopped mint leaves
❧ Soak the tamarind pulp in water overnight. Mash it into the water and blend. Strain the liquid through a sieve and discard any fibers. Stir in the remaining ingredients, except for the mint, and mix thoroughly. Sprinkle with mint and serve chilled.

DOWN TO THE ROOTS: BURDOCK AND CHICORY

For centuries, burdock and chicory have been considered important remedies to help the liver. They have also been used to help rid the body of uric acid, to treat rheumatism and to eliminate skin conditions. By helping the liver, they also improve hormonal imbalances. The Chinese eat burdock to relieve constipa-

tion. Chicory is an effective digestive tonic, and can be used as a coffee substitute—chicory coffee does not contain caffeine, but it does taste somewhat like coffee. Chicory increases bile production, moderates a rapid heart rate, lowers cholesterol and destroys bacteria.

Burdock and chicory roots are versatile. Burdock can be used much like a carrot—it can be grated, sliced or blended. My favorite introductory-level burdock dish is a gravy. One Thanksgiving, I offered to bring the dressing and you should have seen the looks on the faces of the guests when I told them that it was made from burdock. Of course, I waited until after they had told me how delicious it was! Even after I told them it was burdock, no one refused seconds.

Burdock Gravy

1 cup chopped burdock root
    (1 medium-size root)
½ cup yogurt, sour cream or soy milk
1 tablespoon butter or vegetable oil
3 tablespoons flour
1 teaspoon honey
❧ Blend ingredients until smooth. Heat mixture over low heat, stirring until it thickens, about 4 minutes.

Fresh burdock and chicory roots are not hard to find. Many natural food stores carry them, at least in the fall and into the spring. Japanese groceries sell burdock as *gobo*. Even some regular grocery stores sell these roots, especially in Hawaii. You can also grow your own—look for them in the vegetable seed section of a nursery or seed catalog.

In the North American colonies, in the early days of colonization, coffee was cut with chicory so that supplies of the expensive bean would last longer. Later, chicory coffee became a Louisiana specialty. Roasting gives chicory a bittersweet flavor. To roast chicory, chop fresh roots, place a single layer on a cookie sheet and roast in a 325°F oven for about 30 minutes, stirring every 10 minutes. Roasted chicory roots can easily be made into a tea—just grind them in a coffee grinder and steep.

Coffee Substitute

2 teaspoons dried burdock root, chopped
1 teaspoon each roasted chicory root and
dried dandelion root, chopped
½ ounce licorice root
1 quart water
🍂 Combine herbs and water. Simmer on low heat 20 to 30 minutes. Strain out herbs and serve. Sweetener and/or milk can be added to the tea if desired.

SWEET TREATS: GINGER AND HOREHOUND DROPS

Ginger is a versatile herb, and its utility is not limited to the kitchen—its medicinal properties are seemingly endless. Honeyed Ginger and Ginger Snaps are pleasant ways for you to treat colds and flus, encourage sweating, ease morning sickness and help relieve all sorts of painful conditions, such as headaches and menstrual cramps. Ginger also improves the functioning of the heart and circulatory system, warms cold hands and feet, kills intestinal worms and aids liver function. Since I love the taste of ginger, I always double the amount called for in the Ginger Snap recipe.

Honeyed Ginger

½ cup thinly sliced fresh ginger
About ½ cup honey
½ teaspoon anise extract (optional)
¼ teaspoon peppermint extract (optional)
🍂 Fill a clean jar with ginger. Heat honey to liquefy, then remove from heat. Add extracts to honey and pour over ginger. Stir with a knife or chopstick to eliminate all air bubbles. When done, the honey should cover the ginger. After about 3 weeks, it is ready to eat. Stored in the refrigerator, it will last at least a year.

Ginger Snaps

¼ cup vegetable oil
⅔ cup brown sugar
¼ cup molasses
2 teaspoons vinegar
1 beaten egg
2 cups pastry flour (I use whole wheat)
2 teaspoons finely grated ginger
½ teaspoon cinnamon
¼ teaspoon cloves
🍂 Preheat oven to 325°F. Combine the oil, brown sugar, molasses and vinegar, stir in egg, then add the rest of the ingredients. Form the dough into ¾-inch balls. Bake on a greased cookie sheet for about 12 minutes. As the balls melt down during the baking, the cookies develop the characteristic crinkled surface.

Horehound candy was once very popular. Originally, it was used as a cough drop for sore throats. As late as the 1950s, these drops could be found in any pharmacy. In time, people decided that they liked its bittersweet taste even when they were not sick. Horehound drops eventually found their way into candy stores. Since this is really a candy-making recipe, a candy thermometer will come in handy. It will show you when the mixture has reached the proper temperature to harden. Remember that horehound is very bitter—I like to soften the flavor with peppermint. Once you get the hang of making herb candy, try replacing the horehound with other herbs.

Old-Fashioned Horehound Drops

2 ounces dried horehound leaves
     (or 6 ounces fresh leaves)
3 cups very hot water
3½ pounds brown sugar
2 teaspoons peppermint extract

Pour very hot water over the horehound. Steep 30 minutes, while keeping on low heat. Strain. Add sugar and dissolve. Bring to a boil and continue boiling until mixture reaches 295°F (the temperature for brittle candy). Add peppermint, then drop mixture quickly on a buttered board, half a teaspoon at a time, or pour into a shallow, buttered pan and cut into squares before it completely hardens.

Common and Botanical Names

Aloe vera—*Aloe barbadensis*

Anise—*Pimpinella anisum*

Arnica—*Arnica montana*

Ashwaganda—*Withania somnifera*

Astragulus—*Astaragalus membranaceus*

Basil—*Ocimum basilicum*

Barberry—*Berberis vulgaris*

Barley—*Hordeum vulgare*

Bay—*Laurus nobilis*

Bergamot—*Citrus bergamia*

Bilberry—*Vaccinium myrtillus*

Blackberry—*Rubus villosus*

Black cohosh—*Cimicifuga racemosa*

Black current—*Ribes nigrum*

Black pepper—*Piper nigrum*

Blessed thistle—*Cnicus benedictus*

Blueberry—*Vaccinium angustifolium*

Blue cohosh—*Caulophyllum thalictroides*

Brindal berry—*Garcinia camboga*

Bunge—*Anemarrhea asphodeloides*

Bupleurum—*Bupleurum falcatum*

Burdock—*Actium lappa*

Butcher's broom—*Ruscus aculeatus*

Calendula—*Calendula officinalis*

California poppy—*Eschscolzia californica*

Caraway—*Carum carvi*

Cardamom—*Ellettaria cardamomum*

Carrot—*Daucus carota*

Cascara sagrada—*Rhamnus purshiana*

Catnip—*Nepeta cutaria*

Cayenne—*Capsicum frutescens*

Cedar—*Cedrus* species

Chamomile, German—*Matricaria recutita*

Chamomile, Roman—*Chamaemelum nobile*

*Chaparral—*Larrea divaricata*

Chaste berry—*Vitex agnus caste*

Chickweed—*Stelaria media*

Chicory—*Cichorium intybus*

Cinnamon—*Cinnamomum zeylanicum*

Clary sage—*Salvia sclarea*

Cleavers—*Galium aparine*

Clove—*Eugenia caryophyllata*

Club moss—*Huperzia sesrrata*

*Coffee—*Coffea arabica*

*Coltsfoot—*Tussilago farfara*

*Comfrey—*Symphytum officinalis*

Coriander—*Coriandrum sativum*

Corn silk—*Zea mays*

Cramp bark—*Viburnum opulus*

Cranberry—*Vaccinium macrocarpon*

Cypress—*Cupressus sempervirens*

Damiana—*Turnea diffusa*

Dandelion—*Taraxacum officinalis*
Devil's claw—*Harpagophytum procumbens*
Dill—*Anethum graveolens*
Don quai—*Angelica sinensis*
Echinacea—*Echinacea purpurea*
Elder—*Sambucus nigra*
Elecampane—*Inula helenium*
Eucalyptus—*Eucalyptus globulus*
Evening primrose—*Oenothera biennis*
False unicorn root—*Chamaelirium luteum*
Fennel—*Foeniculum vulgare*
Fenugreek—*Trigonella foenum-graecum*
Feverfew—*Chrysanthemum parthenium*
Fir—*Abies alba*
Fo ti—*Polygonum multiflorum*
Frankincense—*Boswellia carterii*
Galangal—*Alpina officinarum*
Garlic—*Allium sativum*
Gentian—*Gentiana lutea*
Ginger—*Zingiber officinale*
Ginkgo—*Ginkgo biloba*
Ginseng—*Panax ginseng*
Goldenseal—*Hydrasits canadensis*
Gotu kola—*Centella asiatica*
Grapefruit—*Citrus x paradisi*
Grindelia—*Grindelia* species
*Guarana—*Paullinia cupana*
Hawthorn—*Crataegus oxycantha*
Helichrysum—*Helichrysum angustifolium*
Hibiscus—*Hibiscus rosa-sinensis*
Honeysuckle—*Lonicera japonica*
Hops—*Humulus arborescens*
Horehound—*Marrubium vulgare*
Horse chestnut—*Aesculus hippocastanum*
Horseradish—*Armoracia rusticana*
Horsetail—*Equisetum arvense*
Hydrangea—*Hydrangea arborescens*
Hyssop—*Hyssopus officinale*
Irish moss seaweed—*Chondrus crispus*
Jewelweed—*Impatiens capensis*

Joe pye—*Eupatorium purpureum*
Juniper—*Juniperus communis*
Kava kava—*Pipermethysticum*
Kelp—*Fucus vesiculosus*
Kola nut—*Cola acuminata*
Kudzu—*Peuraria thunbergiana*
Lady's mantle—*Alchemilla vulgaris*
Lady's slipper—*Cypripedium calceolus*
Lavender—*Lavendula vera*
Lemon—*Citrus limonum*
Lemon balm—*Melissa officinalis*
Lemon grass—*Cymbopogon citratus*
Lemon verbena—*Aloysia triphylla*
*Licorice—*Glyzerriza glabra*
Ligustrum—*Ligustrum lucidum*
Linden—*Tilis platyphlla*
Magnolia—*Magnolia officinalis*
Ma huang—*Ephedra chinensis*
Marjoram—*Origanum marjorana*
Marshmallow—*Althea officinalis*
Meadowsweet—*Filpendula ulmaria*
Milk thistle—*Silybum marianum*
Mo-er—*Auricularia polytricha*
Motherwort—*Leonorus cardiaca*
Muira-puama—*Liriosma ovata*
Mulberry—*Morus nigra*
Mullein—*Verbascum thapsus*
Myrrh—*Commiphora myrrha*
Myrtle—*Myrica* species
Neroli—*Citirs aurantium*
Nettle—*Urtica dioica*
Niaouli—*Melalucca viridiflora*
Nutmeg—*Myristica fragrans*
Oats—*Avena sativa*
Onion—*Allium cepa*
Orange—*Citrus aurantium*
Oregon grape root—*Berberis aquifolium*
Osha—*Ligusticum porteri*
Palma rosa—*Cymbopogon citratus*
Papaya—*Carica papaya*
Parsley—*Petroselinum crispum*
Passionflower—*Passiflora incarnata*

Patchouly—*Pogustemon cablin*
Pau d'arco—*Tahebuia altissima*
Pennyroyal—*Mentha pulegium*
Peppermint—*Mentha piperita*
Petigrain—*Citirs aurantium*
Pineapple—*Ananas comosus*
Pipsissewa—*Chimaphila umbellata*
Plantain—*Plantago lanceolata*
*Poke—*Phyrolacca americana*
Polporus—*Cordiolis versicolor*
Poria—*Poria cocus*
Prickly ash—*Xanthoxylum americanum*
Psyllium—*Plantago ovata*
Pumpkin—*Cucurbita maxima*
Pygeum—*Pygeum africanum*
Quassia—*Picrasma excelsa*
Raspberry—*Rubus* species
Red clover—*Trifolium pratense*
Red root—*Ceonothus americanus*
Rehmannia—*Rehmannia glutinosa*
Reishi mushroom—*Ganoderma lucidum*
Rose—*Rosa* species
Rose geranium—*Pelargonium odorantissimum*
Rosemary—*Rosmarinus officinalis*
Rue—*Ruta graveolens*
Sage—*Salvia officinalis*
Saint-John's-wort—*Hypericum perforatum*
Sandalwood—*Santalum album*
Sarsaparilla—*Smilax officinalis*
*Sassafrass—*Sassafras albidum*
Saw palmetto—*Serrenoa serrulata*
Self heal—*Prunella vulgaris*
Senna—*Cassia senna*

Shepherd's purse—*Capsella bursa-pastoris*
Shiitake mushroom—*Lentinula edudes*
Shizandra—*Shisandra chinensis*
Siberian ginseng—*Eleutherococcus senticosus*
Skullcap—*Scutellaria laterifolia*
Slippery elm—*Ulmus fulva*
Spearmint—*Mentha spicata*
Spikenard—*Aralia racemosa*
Stevia—*Stevia rebaudiana*
Stone root—*Collinsonia canadensis*
Tea tree—*Melaleuca alternifolia*
Thuja—*Thuja occidentalis*
Thyme—*Thymus vulgaris*
Tumeric—*Curcuma longa*
Uva ursi—*Arctostaphylos uva ursi*
Valerian—*Valerian officinalis*
Vanilla—*Vanilla planifolia*
Vervain—*Verbena offcinalis*
Violet—*Viola odorata*
*Wintergreen—*Gaultheria procumbens*
Wild indigo—*Baptisia tinctoria*
Wild yam—*Dioscoria* species
Willow—*Salix* species
Witch hazel—*Hamamelis virginiana*
Yarrow—*Achillea millefolium*
Yellow dock—*Rumex crispus*
Yerba santa—*Eriodictyon californicum*
Ylang-ylang—*Cananga odorata*
Yucca—*Yucca* species
Zizyphi—*Zizphus spinosa*

* Indicates herbs that carry cautions that are addressed in Chapter 15.

Botanical and Common Names

Abies alba—fir
Achillea millefolium—yarrow
Actium lappa—burdock
Aesculus hippocastanum—horse chestnut
Alchemilla vulgaris—lady's mantle
Allium cepa—onion
Allium sativum—garlic
Aloe barbadensis—aloe vera
Aloysia triphylla—lemon verbena
Alpina officinarum—galangal
Althea officinalis—marshmallow
Ananas comosus—pineapple
Anemarrhea asphodeloides—bunge
Anethum graveolens—dill
Angelica sinensis—don quai
Aralia racemosa—spikenard
Arctostaphylos uva ursi—uva ursi
Armoracia rusticana—horseradish
Arnica montana—arnica
Astaragalus membranaceus—astragalus
Auricularia polytricha—mo-er
Avena sativa—oats
Baptisia tinctoria—wild indigo
Berberis aquifolium—Oregon grape root
Berberis vulgaris—barberry
Boswellia carterii—frankincense
Bupleurum falcatum—bupleurum

Calendula officinalis—calendula
Cananga odorata—ylang-ylang
Capsella bursapastoris—shepherd's purse
Capsicum frutescens—cayenne
Carica papaya—papaya
Carum carvi—caraway
Cassia senna—senna
Caulophyllum thalictroides—blue cohosh
Cedrus species—cedar
Centella asiatica—gotu kola
Ceonothus americanus—red root
Chamaelirium luteum—false unicorn root
Chamaemelum nobile—Roman
   chamomile
Chimaphila umbellata—pipsissewa
Chondrus crispus—Irish moss seaweed
Chrysanthemum parthenium—feverfew
Cichorium intybus—chicory
Cimicifuga racemosa—black cohosh
Cinnamomum zeylanicum—cinnamon
Citirs aurantium—neroli, petitgrain
Citrus aurantium—orange
Citrus bergamia—bergamot
Citrus limonum—lemon
Citrus × paradisi—grapefruit
Cnicus benedictus—blessed thistle
*Coffea arabica—coffee

Cola acuminata—kola nut
Collinsonia canadensis—stone root
Commiphora myrrha—myrrh
Cordiolis versicolor—polporus
Coriandrum sativum—coriander
Crataegus oxycantha—hawthorn
Cucurbita maxima—pumpkin
Cupressus sempervirens—cypress
Curcuma longa—turmeric
Cymbopogon citratus—lemon grass,
    palma rosa
Cypripedium calceolus—lady slipper
Daucus carota—carrot
Dioscoria species—wild yam
Echinacea purpurea—echinacea
Eleutherococcus senticosus—siberian
    ginseng
Ellettaria cardamomum—cardamom
Ephedra chinensis—ma huang
Equisetum arvense—horsetail
Eriodictyon californicum—yerba santa
Eschscolzia californica—california poppy
Eucalyptus globulus—eucalyptus
Eugenia caryophyllata—clove
Eupatorium purpureum—joe-pye weed
Filpendula ulmaria—meadowsweet
Foeniculum vulgare—fennel
Fucus vesiculosus—kelp
Galium aparine—cleavers
Ganoderma lucidum—reishi mushroom
Garcinia camboga—brindal berry
*Gaultheria procumbens—wintergreen
Gentiana lutea—gentian
Ginkgo biloba—ginkgo
*Glyzerriza glabra—licorice
Grindelia species—grindelia
Hamamelis virginiana—witch hazel
Harpagophytum procumbens—devil's claw
Helichrysum angustifolium—helichrysum
Hibiscus rosa-sinensis—hibiscus
Hordeum vulgare—barley
Humulus arborescens—hops

Huperzia sesrrata—club moss
Hydrangea arborescens—hydrangea
Hydrasits canadensis—goldenseal
Hypericum perforatum—saint-John's-
    wort
Hyssopus officinale—hyssop
Impatiens capensis—jewelweed
Inula helenium—elecampane
Juniperus communis—juniper
*Larrea divaricata—chaparral
Laurus nobilis—bay
Lavendula vera—lavender
Lentinula edudes—shiitake mushroom
Leonorus cardiaca—motherwort
Ligusticum porteri—osha
Ligustrum lucidum—ligustrum
Liriosma ovata—muira puama
Lonicera japonica—honeysuckle
Magnolia officinalis—magnolia
Marrubium vulgare—horehound
Matricaria recutita—German chamomile
Melaleuca alternifolia—tea tree
Melalucca viridiflora—niaouli
Melissa officinalis—lemon balm
Mentha piperita—peppermint
Mentha pulegium—pennyroyal
Mentha spicata—spearmint
Morus nigra—mulberry
Myrica species—myrtle
Myristica fragrans—nutmeg
Nepeta cataria—catnip
Ocimum basilicum—basil
Oenothera biennis—evening primrose
Origanum marjorana—marjoram
Panax ginseng—ginseng
Passiflora incarnata—passionflower
*Paullinia cupana—guarana
Pelargonium odorantissimum—rose
    geranium
Petroselinum crispum—parsley
Peuraria thunbergiana—kudzu
*Phyrolacca americana—poke

Picrasma excelsa—quassia
Pimpinella anisum—anise
Pipermethysticum species—kava kava
Piper nigrum—black pepper
Plantago lanceolata—plantain
Plantago ovata—psyllium
Pogustemon cablin—patchouly
Polygonum multiflorum—fo ti
Poria cocus—poria
Prunella vulgaris—self heal
Pygeum africanum—pygeum
Rehmannia glutinosa—rehmannia
Rhamnus purshiana—cascara sagrada
Ribes nigrum—black currant
Rosa species—rose
Rosmarinus officinalis—rosemary
Rubus species—raspberry
Rubus villosus—blackberry
Rumex crispus—yellow dock
Ruscus aculeatus—butcher's broom
Ruta graveolens—rue
Salix species—willow
Salvia officinalis—sage
Salvia sclarea—clary sage
Sambucus nigra—elder
Santalum album—sandalwood
*Sassafras albidum—sassafras
Scutellaria laterifolia—skullcap
Serrenoa serrulata—saw palmetto
Shisandra chinensis—shizandra
Silybum marianum—milk thistle
Smilax officinalis—sarsaparilla
Stelaria media—chickweed

Stevia rebaudiana—stevia
*Symphytum officinalis—comfrey
Tabebuia altissima—pau d'arco
Taraxacum officinalis—dandelion
Thuja occidentalis—thuja
Thymus vulgaris—thyme
Tilis platyphylla—linden
Trifolium pratense—red clover
Trigonella foenum-graecum—fenugreek
Turnea diffusa—damiana
*Tussilago farfara—coltsfoot
Ulmus fulva—slippery elm
Urtica dioica—nettle
Vaccinium angustifolium—blueberry
Vaccinium macrocarpon—cranberry
Vaccinium myrtillus—bilberry
Valerian officinalis—valerian
Vanilla planifolia—vanilla
Verbascum thapsus—mullein
Verbena officinalis—vervain
Viburnum opulus—cramp bark
Viola odorata—violet
Vitex agnus caste—chaste berry
Withania somnifera—ashwaganda
Xanthoxylum americanum—prickly ash
Yucca species—yucca
Zea mays—corn silk
Zingiber officinale—ginger
Zizphus spinosa—zizyphi

* Indicates herbs that carry cautions that are addressed in Chapter 15.

Bibliography

Bailey, Liberty Hyde, and Ethel Zoe Bailey. Rev. L.H. Bailey Staff. *Hortus Third.* New York: Macmillan, 1976.

Bauer, Kurt B., Dorothea G. Garbe and Horst S. Surburg. *Common Fragrance and Flavor Materials.* Stuttgart, Germany: VCH, 1990.

Bensky, Dan B., and Andrew Gamble. *Chinese Herbal Medicine: Materia Medica.* Seattle, Wash.: Eastland Press, 1986.

Berkow, Robert, ed. *The Merck Manual of Diagnosis and Therapy.* 16th ed. Rahway, N.J.: Merck & Co., 1992.

Blackwell, Will H. *Poisonous and Medicinal Plants.* Englewood Cliffs, N.J.: Prentice Hall, 1990.

British Herbal Medicine Association. *British Herbal Compendium.* Bournemouth, Dorset, England: BHMA, 1992.

_____. *British Herbal Pharmacopoeia.* Bournemouth, Dorset, England: BHMA, 1990.

Chan, H., and P. But, eds. *Pharmacology and Applications of Chinese Materia Medica.* Singapore: World Scientific, 1986.

Christopher, John R. *School of Natural Healing.* Provo, Utah: Christopher Publications, 1976.

Cracker, Lyle E., and James E. Simon, eds. *Herbs, Spices and Medicinal Plants.* 4 vols. Arizona: Oryx Press, 1986–1989.

Council of Scientific and Industrial Research. *The Wealth of India.* Vols. I–IX. New Delhi, India: Publications and Information Directorate, 1948–1976.

Culbreth, David. *A Manual of Materia Medica and Pharmacology.* Portland, Oreg.: Eclectic Medicinal Publications, 1987.

Culpeper, Nicholas. *Complete Herbal.* 1649. Reprint, England: W. Foulsham & Co., 1981.

DeFuedis, Francis V. *Ginkgo biloba Extract.* New York: Elsevier, 1991.

DerMarderosian, A., and Lawrence Liberti. *Natural Products Medicine: A Scientific Guide to Foods, Drugs, Cosmetics.* Philadelphia, Pa.: George F. Stickly, 1988.

De Smet, Keller, Hänsel, Chandler, eds. *Adverse Effects of Herbal Drugs.* New York: Springer-Verlag, 1993.

Duke, James A. *Handbook of Medicinal Herbs.* Boca Raton, Fla.: CRC Press, 1986.

_____. *Handbook of Northeastern Indian Medicinal Plants.* Lincoln, Mass.: Quarterman Publications, 1986.

Elingwood, Finley. *American Materia Medica, Therapeutics and Pharmacognosy.* 1898. Reprint, Portland, Oreg.: Eclectic Medicinal Publications, 1985.

Erichsen-Brown, Charlotte. *Medicinal and Other Uses of North American Plants.* New York: Dover, 1979.

Felter, Harvey Wickes, and John Uri Lloyd. *King's American Dispensatory.* 18th ed. 2 vols. 1898. Reprint, Oregon: Eclectic Medicinal Publications, 1983.

Foster, Steven. *Botanical Series.* Austin, Tex.: American Botanical Council, 1991.

_____. *Echinacea.* Rochester, Vt.: The Healing Arts Press, 1991.

Foster, Steven, and James Duke. *Peterson Field Guide: Eastern/Central Medicinal Plants.* Boston: Houghton Mifflin Co., 1990.

Fulder, Stephen, and John Blackwood. *Garlic: Nature's Original Remedy.* Rochester, Vt.: Healing Arts Press, 1991.

Gerard, John. *The Herball.* 1597. Reprint, New York: Dover, 1975.

Green, James. *Herbs & Health Care for the Male.* Freedom, Calif.: The Crossing Press, 1991.

Grieve, Maud. *A Modern Herbal.* New York: Dover, 1971.

Guenther, Ernest. *The Essential Oils.* 4 vols. New York: Robert E. Kriefer Publications, 1972.

Halstead, Bruce W., and Loretta L. Wood. *Eleutherococcus Senticosus: Siberian Ginseng.* Long Beach, Calif.: Oriental Healing Arts Institute, 1984.

Harborne, Jeffrey B., and Herbert Baxter. *Phytochemical Dictionary.* London: Taylor & Francis, 1993.

Hobbs, Christopher. *Echinacea: The Immune Herb.* Soquel, Calif.: Botanica Press, 1990.

_____. *Foundations of Health.* Soquel, Calif.: Botanica Press, 1992.

_____. *Ginkgo: Elixir of Youth.* Soquel, Calif.: Botanica Press, 1990.

_____. *Medicinal Mushrooms.* Soquel, Calif.: Botanica Press, 1995.

_____. *Milk Thistle: The Liver Herb.* Soquel, Calif.: Botanica Press, 1984.

_____. *Valerian: The Relaxing and Sleep Herb.* Soquel, Calif.: Botanica Press, 1993.

_____. *Vitex: The Woman's Herb.* Soquel, Calif.: Botanica Press, 1990.

Hoffmann, David. *The New Holistic Herbal.* Rockport, Mass.: Element Books, 1983.

_____. *Therapeutic Herbalism.* Sebastopol, Calif.: Self-published correspondence course, n.d.

Iwu, Maurice M. *Handbook of African Medicinal Plants.* Boca Raton, Fla.: CRC Press, 1993.

Jain, S.K., and Robert A. DeFillipps. *Medicinal Plants of India.* 2 vols. Algonac, Mich.: Reference Publications, 1991.

Jones, Kenneth. *Shiitake: The Healing Mushroom.* Rochester, Vt.: Healing Arts Press, 1995.

Kapoor, L.D. *Handbook of Ayurvedic Medicinal Plants.* Boca Raton, Fla.: CRC Press, 1990.

Keville, Kathi. *American Country Living: Herbs* (O/P, now in *American Country Living Compendium*). New York: Crescent, 1993.

_____, ed. *American Herb Association Quarterly Newsletter.* 11 vols. 1981–1995.

_____. *Herbs: An Illustrated Encyclopedia .* New York: Friedman/Fairfax, 1994.

Keville, Kathi, and Mindy Green. *Aromatherapy: The Complete Guide to the Healing Art.* Freedom, Calif: The Crossing Press, 1995.

Kinghorn, A. Douglas, and Manuel Balandrin. *Human Medicinal Agents from Plants.* Washington, D.C.: American Chemical Society, 1993.

Lebot, Vincent, Mark Merlin, and Lamont Lindstrom. *Kava, the Pacific Drug.* New Haven, Conn.: Yale University Press, 1992.

Leung, Albert Y. *Encyclopedia of Common Natural Ingredients Used in Food, Drugs and Cosmetics.* New York: Wiley-Interscience, 1983.

Lewis, Walter H., and Memory P. F. Elvin-Lewis. *Medical Botany: Plants Affecting Man's Health.* New York: Wiley Inter-Science, 1977.

Lust, John. *The Herb Book.* New York: Bantam Books, 1974.

Maybe, Richard, ed. *The New Age Herbalist.* New York: Collier Books, 1988.

Merck staff, eds. *The Merck Index.* 11th ed. Rathway, N.J.: Merck & Co., 1992.

Mills, Simon Y., ed. *The Dictionary of Modern Herbalism.* New York: Thorsons Pub. Co., 1985.

Moore, Michael. *Medicinal Plants of the Mountain West.* Santa Fe, N.Mex.: Museum of New Mexico Press, 1979.

Morris, Edwin T. *Fragrance: The Story of Perfume from Cleopatra to Chanel.* New York: Charles Scribner's Sons, 1984.

Morton, Julia F. *Major Medicinal Plants.* Springfield, Ill.: Charles C. Thomas, 1977.

Mowrey, Daniel B. *Herbal Tonic Therapies.* New Canaan, Conn.: Keats, 1993.

Murray, Michael, and Joseph Pizzorno. *Encyclopedia of Natural Medicine.* Rocklin, Calif.: Prima Publishing, 1991.

_____. *A Textbook of Natural Medicine.* Seattle: John Bastyr University, 1985.

Murray, Michael, Joseph Pizzorno, and Melvyn R. Werbach. *Botanical Influences on Illness.* Tarzana, Calif.: Third Line Press, 1994.

Rankin, Dorothy. *Pestos!* Freedom, Calif.: The Crossing Press, 1985.

Rodgers, Jean. *Cooking with the Healthful Herbs.* Emmaus, Pa.: Rodale Press, 1983.

Al-Samarqandi. *The Medical Formulary.* 13th century. Reprint, London: Oxford University Press, 1967.

Schumacher, Mildred M., ed. *Physician's Desk Reference.* 49th edition. Montvale, N.J.: Medical Economics Data, 1995.

Scott, Julian. *Natural Medicine for Children.* New York: Avon Books, 1990.

Thomas, Clayton L., ed. *Taber's Cyclopedic Medical Dictionary.* Philadelphia, Pa.: F A Davis Co., 1986.

Tierra, Michael. *Planetary Herbology.* Santa Fe, N.Mex.: Lotus Press, 1988.

Tyler, Varro E. *Herbs of Choice.* New York: Haworth Press, 1994.

Tyler, Varro E., Lynn R. Brady, and James E. Robbers. *Pharmacognosy.* Malvern, Pa.: Lea & Febiger, 1981.

Van Toller, Steve, and George H. Dodd, eds. *Perfumery: The Psychology and Biology of Fragrance.* New York: Chapman & Hall, 1988.

Wagner, H., Hiroshi Hikino, and Norman R. Farnsworth, eds. *Economic and Medicinal Plant Research.* 5 vols. New York: Academic Press, 1985–1991.

Weiss, Rudolf Fritz. *Herbal Medicine.* Translated from German. Beaconsfield, England: Beaconsfield Pub. Ltd., 1988.

Willard, Terry. *Reishi Mushroom.* Issaquah, Wash.: Sylvan Press, 1990.

Wren, R.C. *Potter's New Cyclopedia of Botanical Drugs and Preparations.* (Revised by Williamson, Elizabeth M., and Fred J. Evans.) Essex, England: C.W. Daniel Co., 1988.

Resources

AROMATHERAPY

You will find aromatherapy mentioned often in this book. For more information, contact:

> National Association for Holistic
> Aromatherapy
> 219 Carl Street
> San Francisco, CA 94117

To subscribe to an aromatherapy newsletter, write to:

> *The International Journal of*
> *Aromatherapy*
> P.O. Box 750428
> Petaluma, CA 94975-0428

I have also written an entire book on the subject with aromatherapist Mindy Green. Published in 1995, *Aromatherapy: A Complete Guide to the Healing Art,* is available from The Crossing Press, P.O. Box 1048, Freedom, CA 95019.

EDUCATION

The American Herb Association also offers the *AHA Directory of Herbal Education,* which lists more than 40 herb schools in North America and herbal correspondence courses that you can take at home. The directory is updated every other year and can be purchased for $3.50. To order this publication, write to the American Herb Association.

HERBAL GARDENING

A good network for small herb growers and businesses is the International Herb Association (previously the International Herb Growers and Marketers), 1202 Allanson Road, Mundelein, IL 60060.

There are also many good books on cultivating your own medicinal herbs— something I encourage anyone to try! Here are some of my favorites.

Herbal Emissaries: Bringing Chinese Herbs to the West, by Steven Foster and Yue Chongxi (Healing Arts Press, 1992).

Herbal Renaissance, by Steven Foster (Gibbs-Smith, 1993).

The Herb Garden, by Sarah Garland (Penguin, 1984).

Herb Gardening at Its Best, by Sal Gilbertie (SMI, 1984).

Herbs, by Claire Kowalchik and William H. Hylton (Rodale Press, 1987).

Herbs: An Illustrated Encyclopedia, by
Kathi Keville (Friedman/Fairfax,
1994).

HERBAL PRODUCTS

I recommend herbalist-owned and oper-
ated companies that offer organically
grown tinctures and glycerites and aro-
matherapy-quality essential oils. Oak
Valley Herb Farm and Simpler's Botanicals offer these and other products, as
well as classes on herbalism, at reasonable prices. Catalogs from these companies can be obtained for $1.00 by
writing to:

Blessed Herbs
109 Barre Plains Road
Oakham, MA 01068

Mountain Rose Herbs
P.O. Box 2000
Redway, CA 95560

Oak Valley Herb Farm
P.O. Box 2482
Nevada City, CA 95959

Simpler's Botanicals
P.O. Box 39
Forestville, CA 95436

Glycerites can also be obtained from:

Herbs for Kids
P.O. Box 837
Bozeman, MT 59711

Chinese herbs and tinctures (as well as
out-of-print herb books) can be obtained
from:

Herbalists and Alchemists
P.O. Box 553
Broadway, NJ 08808

If you would like a current list of more
than 75 mail-order sources for dried
and fresh herbs, live plants, herb seeds,
books, essential oils, tinctures, glycerites
and containers, you can purchase the
*AHA Directory of Mail-Order Herb Prod-
ucts* from the American Herb Association for $4. See page 362 for the
address.

If you prefer to buy your herb prod-
ucts in a store, quality organically grown
herbs, tinctures, glycerites and pills from
the following companies are available
in many stores that specialize in alterna-
tive health products and natural foods,
and even in some pharmacies: Eclectic
Institute, Frontier Cooperative Herbs,
Gaia Herbs, Herb Pharm, Herbs Etc.,
Herbs for Kids, Nature's Way, Planetary
Formulas, Starwest Botanicals, Trinity
Herb Co., Trout Lake Farm, Turtle
Island Herbs, WiseWays Herbals and
Yerba Prima.

HERB BOOKS

Many books have been written about the
healing power of plants and the history
of herbalism. Most bookstores can order
almost any book that is still in print. The
library is another wonderful resource. If
you are using the library, research the
card catalog for books that may be helpful. In addition to the obvious category—
herbs—you can try aromatherapy,
botany, cooking (herbs), ethnobotany,
flora, gardening, medicine (botanical),
medicine (history), pharmacology, pharmacy, plants (edible) and wildflowers. If
your library does not have the book
you're looking for, ask them if they can
get it for you on inter-library loan. If
you're looking for historic herbals, try

your local university library; if you're trying to find old botanicals and herbal pharmacy books, check the bookstores in your area that sell used and out-of-print books. Many of these stores will do book searches for you (for a small fee, of course) if they don't have a copy of the book you want.

HERB-RELATED COMPUTER SOFTWARE

Owning herbal software is like having an extensive herbal library at your fingertips. It is particularly good in helping you choose the most appropriate herbs for your needs. The best products that I know of are:

The Herbal Prescriber, by Christopher Hobbs, 1995. Botanica Press, 10226 Empire Grade Road, Santa Cruz, CA 95060. 4 floppy disks, MS Windows–compatible. This mini-library explains and cross-references 250 herbs and 400 conditions, and is illustrated throughout with old botanical prints. The information is drawn from several dozen legendary and contemporary herbalists.

The Herbalist CD-ROM, by David Hoffmann. Hopkins Technology, 421 Hazel Lane, Hopkins, MN 55343-7116. This Windows/Macintosh CD-ROM, which is illustrated throughout with color photographs, describes the actions and strengths of 150 herbs and how they relate to the systems of the body.

IDENTIFICATION OF HERBS

Never use herbs from the wild, or even from your garden, unless you are absolutely sure what they are. If you need to have plants identified, most university libraries and the U.S. forest service have botanists on staff that will help you. Just bring in a sample that is in good shape, with flowers, if possible. There are also many excellent regional plant identification books, some of which focus on medicinal plants. Here are some of the best:

Edible and Medicinal Plants of the Rocky Mountains and Neighboring Territories, by Terry Willard (Wild Rose College, 1992).

Medicinal Plants of the Desert and Canyon West and Medicinal Plants of the Mountain West, by Michael Moore (Museum of New Mexico Press, 1979).

Medicinal Wild Plants of the Prairie, by Kelly Kindscher (University Press of Kansas, 1992).

Peterson Field Guide: Eastern/Central Medicinal Plants, by Steven Foster and James A. Duke (Houghton Mifflin, 1990).

A Practical Guide to Edible and Useful Plants (of Texas), by Delena Tull (Texas Monthly Press, 1987).

LEGAL STATUS

The American Herbalist Guild, Box 1683, Soquel, CA 95073, is a group of professional herbalists who are interested in improving the legal status of herbs and herbalists in the United States. Their dues are $50/year, payable upon acceptance.

NEWS

If you want to keep up on the latest news, current affairs, scientific studies, books, videos, Internet listings, environmental projects and legal issues, join the American Herb Association and receive the *AHA Quarterly Newsletter* ($20/year). Write to:

American Herb Association
P.O. Box 1673R
Nevada City, CA 95959

PRACTITIONERS

Naturopathic doctors, most acupuncturists and many chiropractors use herbs in their practice and can legally prescribe herbs. These practitioners rarely use drugs.

Ayurvedic practitioners always use herbs, but cannot legally prescribe them in the United States unless they are also medical doctors or are otherwise degreed.

Physicians who practice holistic or preventive medicine and nurse-midwives are often familiar with herbs and sometimes use them in their practices, usually along with drugs.

For information on practitioners in your area, contact the following groups.

American Association of Acupuncture and Oriental Medicine
433 Front Street
Catasauqua, PA 18032-2506

American Association of Naturopathic Physicians
2366 Eastlake Avenue E, Suite 322
Seattle, WA 98102
Send $5 for a directory of their members in the United States.

American College of Nurse-Midwives
818 Connecticut Avenue NW, Suite 900
Washington, DC 20006

American Holistic Medical Association
4101 Lake Boone Trail, Suite 201
Raleigh, NC 27607
Send $5 for a directory of holistic doctors.

American Preventive Medical Association
459 Walker Road
Great Falls, VA 22066
This organization can help you locate a doctor offering preventive health care.

Ayurvedic Institute
11311 Menaul NE, Suite A
Albuquerque, NM 87112

Canadian Holistic Medical Association
409-491 Eglinton Avenue W
Toronto, ON M5N 1A8

Holistic Dental Association
P.O. Box 5007
Durango, CO 81301
For a listing of holistic-oriented dentists, send a self-addressed, stamped envelope.

International Chiropractors Association
1110 North Glebe Road, Suite 1000
Arlington, VA 22201
Write for a list of chiropractors in your area.

National Women's Health Network
514 10th A Street NW, Suite 400
Washington, DC 20004
*This organization will supply you with
a list of women's health clinics in
your area. They will also send a
list of information packets on 70
different women's health topics—
at a cost of $8 per packet.*

Ontario Herbalists Association
11 Winthrop Place
Stoney Creek, ON L8G 3M3

RESEARCH

The Herb Research Foundation, 1007
Pearl Street, Suite 200, Boulder, CO
80302, will send you a packet of information from books and clippings on many
different herbal subjects. The $35 mem-
bership includes a subscription to the
magazine *HerbalGram.*

SCIENTIFIC STUDIES

Much of the information in this book
came directly from scientific studies. You
can access these on a computer through
on-line services such as Med-Line or you
can search for scientific or medical journals in the library of a medical university.
To learn more about how to do herb-re-
lated computer and library searches, see
*The Information Sourcebook of Herbal Med-
icine,* by David Hoffmann (The Crossing
Press, 1994).

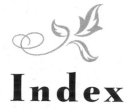

Index

Note: Italicized page references indicate boxed text and illustrations.